Praise for Dr. Jodie A. Dashore

"Dr. Dashore brings an expanded world view of chronic inflammatory response syndrome (CIRS) to clinicians and patients alike. Her book makes for compelling reading for those inside and outside the world of chronically ill patients who never seem to get better. Dr. Dashore works within an academic framework of disciplined science yet liberally uses her knowledge of anti-inflammatory effects of foods, herbs and approaches that are not yet found in American medical schools. Her excellent, safely acquired results show us we all have much to learn from her. When we do, we will have new dimensions of new approaches to treatment to share with our patients."

— RITCHIE C. SHOEMAKER, MD; Pioneer of Biotoxin Illness;
Author of *Surviving Mold* and *Mold Warriors*; Pocomoke, MD

"*The BioNexus Approach to Biotoxin Illness* is a comprehensive overview and treatment guideline that should be in every physician's and patient's bookcase! It has the rare quality of crossing the barriers of traditional and "natural" medicine, simplifying, and clarifying complex issues that few specialists or physicians have mastered. Coming from traditional specialization as a neurologist, Dr. Dashore blends high-level science into the worldwide art of "natural" medicine that is unique. For those seeking answers to their complex health issues, many will find wisdom in these pages and relief from difficult to treat illnesses."

— EUGENE R. SHIPPEN, MD; Endocrinologist;
Author of *The Testosterone Syndrome*; Reading, PA

"I have worked with Dr. Jodie Dashore over many years with many mutual patients. Dr. Dashore's empathy and capacity to think outside the box has helped many patients with complex, chronic diseases to regain their health and pursue productivity. She has helped many who have been frustrated by the rigid dogmatism seen in some medical approaches today. It is encouraging to see that she is willing to share her wisdom with others by writing this book."

— ROBERT BRANSFIELD, MD, DLFAPA; Past President of the
International Lyme and Associated Diseases Society; Red Bank, NJ

"Since I first met Jodie years ago, I've considered her a fresh mind and important thought leader. I look forward to years ahead and what's to come, but most of all, I look to collaborate with her."

— JOSEPH G. JEMSEK, MD, FACP;
Board Certified Internal Medicine, Infectious Disease; Washington D.C.

"I was immediately overwhelmed with the depth of Jodie's knowledge and skill; she clearly has very unique gifts that derive from the wealth of different modalities that she combines against the backdrop of her medical training. Her empathy and compassion as a therapist are also palpable and unparalleled. I have become familiar with Jodie's pioneering and proprietary herbal line that she has created for the treatment of biotoxin illness and inflammation. We are working together to bring her formulas to the UK and Europe."

— GILIAN CROWTHER, ND/NT Dip, mBANT, mNNA, CNHC Reg; Senior Associate of the Royal Society of Medicine Director Research, Academy of Nutritional Medicine (AONM); London, United Kingdom

"Dr. Dashore demonstrated many skills during her studies at Quantum University, including a deep understanding of Herbology, Homeopathy, and Naturopathy, as well as the ability to integrate her knowledge in implementing protocols for many acute and chronic health conditions. Her depth of knowledge and understanding in these fields has allowed her to create her own herbal formulas to address current conditions."

— PAUL DROUIN, MD; Dean and Founder of Quantum University; Author of *Creative Integrative Medicine*; Honolulu, HI

"Dr. Jodie A. Dashore is a dynamic and talented naturopathic scientist, enriched with the great knowledge of plant-based therapy and gut symbiotic principles. She has not only read books but has absorbed a great knowledge of human calmness, health, and well-being from Mother Nature. She is a living story of recovering her son from autism to a normal healthy man by her natural food therapy, mainly herbal medicine, recipes, and camel milk. I have know her for so many years and am honored to work with her as a co-founder of the International Forum for Camel Advocacy and Medicine (IFCAM), Dr. Dashore was the main stimulus of the forum. To me, her book is a practical guide to herbal and natural medicine for complex multisystem medical conditions and to living a calm and healthy life. Jodie, my best wishes for success now and in life ahead."

— ABDUL RAZIQ KAKAR, PhD, DVM; Chief, International Camelid Research and Development, Al Ain Camel Dairy Project; Dubai, United Arab Emirates

"We applaud Dr. Dashore for her time and dedication, assembling her latest publication. For the first time, you can find practical answers too complicated health challenges, never before described in a comprehensive collection. Dr. Dashore's eclectic approach is original, informative, and refreshing."

— ROBBY BESNER; Co-founder and Chief Science Officer, Therasage; Co-author of *Living a Better LifeStyle*; Boca Raton, FL

"Dr. Dashore has been an asset to my family, myself and those dealing with Lyme/ mold and toxin issues. She is passionate, knowledgeable and caring to those who are desperate for answers and care for diseases that are often misunderstood by the medical community. Any physician can be an expert in a field, but I feel Dr. Jodie's greatest gift is her ability to link difficult, often overlapping conditions with holistic herbal treatment and modalities."

— ALBERT WACHA, DPM;
Diplomat, American Board of Podiatric Surgery; Caldwell, NJ

"Biotoxin (mold) illness is the scourge of the 21st century leading to chronic inflammatory response syndrome (CIRS). This serious condition presents in a myriad of ways. CIRS is often mistaken for other disorders, and hence, treatment is often unsuccessful. Dr. Jodie A. Dashore PhD, OTD, BCIP, HHP, CCH, RH (AHG) has written a book about the natural, plant-based approach to CIRS, Mold, and Biotoxin Illness. Dr. Jodie is a recognized expert in plant-based herbal medicine, a sought-after international speaker to both allopathic and complementary health care providers, and treats complex, multifactorial conditions worldwide. She is an eclectic, caring, and compassionate health care provider. Her book, *The BioNexus Approach to Biotoxin Illness* is a 'quantum leap' in the diagnosis and treatment of CIRS. I heartily recommend it to both physician and lay-person alike!"

— JESS P. ARMINE, DC, RN;
Author of *Leaky Gut, Leaky Cells, Leaky Brain*; Upper Darby, PA

"I came to know Dr. Jodie Dashore through her treatment of my wife and daughter, who both have chronic Lyme disease and mold and biotoxin illness. They have had many false starts over many years with so many practitioners. Finally, they discovered Jodie, who has taken them on a healing journey over the past two years. I have been involved as a family member and at the same time, a doctor, who can assess the effectiveness of therapies. What has stood out most for me is the vast body of knowledge that Dr. Dashore has around so many aspects of their illness. She has managed to balance her profound expertise in natural herbal medicine protocols with allopathic treatments to offer a truly holistic treatment of this difficult medical challenge."

— FARREL HELLIG; Interventional Cardiologist Cathlab;
Director, Sunninghill Hospital; Johannesburg, South Africa

"It has been a genuine privilege and always a pleasure to observe and communicate with Jodie Dashore. Opportunities to sit in the audience and learn from one of the finest clinicians in the world is not to be missed. Jodie Dashore is without a doubt one of the finest practising naturopaths and educators, and her clinical expertise and experience make her especially qualified to deal with the complex issues like CIRS/ biotoxin illness and mould, that so many are now facing in an ever-challenging world as is demonstrated by her success rate. Furthermore, she has been able to use her knowledge, clinical experience, and her caring personality to produce a most excellent range of natural herbal formulas and products designed to assist the complex and challenged patient to re-achieve health and well-being."

— JONATHAN COHEN, MSc mBANT, Dip FMU;
Clinic Director, The Centre for Applied Nutrition; London, United Kingdom

"In *The BioNexus Approach to Biotoxin Illness*, Dr. Dashore offers hope, guidance, and a stepwise process for those suffering from chronic inflammatory conditions due to environmentally-related exposures. In doing so, she turns a compartmentalized, conventional medical model on its head.

As a practitioner working with the smallest of patients in pediatrics, I am acutely aware of the need to have Dr. Dashore's book available for the masses. It masterfully empowers with education, a process, and clinically-tested herbal formulas that can be individualized for the most sensitive of patients. Focusing on "plant-smarts," she circumvents the perils of resistance found in single entity pharmaceutics. Recommending BioNexus Herbals for our patients has been a game-changer in our practice and has allowed many children to completely shed prior diagnoses, such as tics, allergies, fatigue, migraines, cyclical fevers, and more. This book will undoubtedly serve as a guide for many people to reclaim the symphony of health."

— DEBORAH M. ALLEN, RPh; Board Certified Pharmacist;
Pediatric Integrative Practitioner, Infinite Health; Charlotte, NC

"Jodie's thirst for knowledge and her extensive training and bold initiatives has been inspiring to me. When I was struggling with my own health challenges, it was Jodie who I turned to for guidance. I continue to refer my most complex cases to her. It has been a blessing to have her expertise and compassion as a resource."

— SHAWN TEPPER-LEVINE, DO; Board Certified in
Neuromusculoskeletal Medicine and Osteopathic Manipulative Medicine;
Kingston, NJ

"I've found that Dr. Dashore's plant-based protocols help even the most difficult cases regain health. Dr. Dashore has thousands of hours of basic and advanced herbology training and is highly regarded as a clinical herbalist. She has created a unique and pioneering line of formulas for her plant-based protocols for chronic inflammation and biotoxin illness. She is invited worldwide to lecture, teach and conduct web-based and/or live practitioner training workshops in plant-based medicine treatment options for today's chronic conditions."

— ERIK HUMS, PT, DPT, CSCS, FAAOMPT; Fellow, American Academy of
Orthopaedic Manual Physical Therapists; Old Bridge, NJ

"Dr. Dashore is an esteemed and cherished colleague of the integrative health care alliance. Decades of learned research and devoted practice makes her a prized resource to the medical community at large, as a skilled naturopath successfully treating inflammatory conditions in the difficult paradigm of vital natural healing. I truly feel privileged to align with her in efforts of finding functional healing for our patients."

— JULIANE EVEREST, PA-C; Lyme Literate Integrative and
Functional Medicine Provider; Middletown, NJ

"As a functional medicine practitioner, I have witnessed firsthand the exponential rise in tick-borne infections, mold-related illness, and autoimmune disorders. I have been disheartened with the lack of available, effective treatment modalities. It has recently struck home, with several family members diagnosed with related disorders. I am beyond grateful to have discovered the gift that is Dr. Jodie Dashore. With her vast knowledge of herbal and integrative medicine, neurology as well as personal experience, she is the real deal when it comes to effectively conquering these frustrating diagnoses. Dr. Dashore is at the top of her field yet can dissect the complexities and convert the science into viable treatment protocols, personalized for each of her patients. I am truly grateful to have her as a mentor and have referred her numerous clients with successful outcomes."

— ADRIA ROTHFELD, DC, MS, CNS; Director, Nutritional Wellness
Centers of NY and NJ; Colts Neck, NJ

"I have known Jodie for many years, and we have collaborated on mutual patients. Her skills and knowledge as an herbalist are outstanding. I know she takes the time to spend with each of her patients and provides individualized treatment plans. I highly respect Jodie's treatment of mold illness and chronic Lyme, which, unfortunately, has not been recognized in the traditional medical community."

— NANCY LENTINE, DO; Medical Director, Integrative Family Medicine;
Little Falls, NJ

"Dr. Dashore helped my family more in six months than traditional medicine had in three years. I tried the "regular" approach for my health issues and was on antibiotics and antifungals for tick-borne infections, and conventional mold binders almost nonstop for over two years. Within two weeks of stopping, all my symptoms would return. My general practitioner finally realized these weren't working and referred me to Dr. Dashore, and life is getting so much better after feeling hopeless for a few years! As a physician myself, I referred several complicated patients to BioNexus Health. The all-natural and herbal approach used by Dr. Dashore is exactly what is needed for people who are resistant to or very sensitive to conventional treatments."

— AARON PAZIK, DC; EPN, ART Corporate Solutions;
Winter Garden, FL

JODIE A. DASHORE
The BioNexus Approach to Biotoxin Illness

Jodie A. Dashore, PhD, OTD, BCIP, HHP, CCH, RH (AHG), is an internationally recognized practitioner, author, researcher, and a pioneering clinical herbalist who is widely known for her plant-based approach to autism, Lyme disease, biotoxin illness and chronic inflammatory response syndrome (CIRS), and camel milk therapeutic protocols. Dr. Dashore earned a PhD in integrative medicine, and is a CIRS Certified Practitioner, Board Certified in Integrative Pediatrics, Board Certified and licensed Doctor of Occupational Therapy (Neurology), Board Certified Holistic Health Practitioner, and has over 20 years of clinical experience. A member of the International Lyme and Associated Diseases Society (ILADS) and Lyme Literate clinician for over a decade, Dr. Dashore also sits on the Scientific Advisory Board of Bio-Regulatory Medicine Institute (BRMI), Global Lyme Diagnostics Lab (GDL), and International Forum for Camel Advocacy and Medicine (IFCAM). She completed eight years of intensive herbal studies under the guidance of renowned master herbalists and is a Registered Herbalist with the American Herbalist Guild. Dr. Dashore brings her love of Ayurveda and bio-regionally abundant western herbs to her work as a clinical herbalist. She created a proprietary line of herbal medicinal formulas used exclusively with patients at the BioNexus Health Clinic in Marlboro, New Jersey, where she is the founder and director. The clinic specializes in scientifically formulated plant-based treatment options; herbal compounded apothecary formulations along with therapeutic camel milk protocols for patients of all ages. Dr. Dashore comes from a multicultural background, is well-traveled, and seamlessly works with families in over 50 countries utilizing local resources, dietary nuances, and honoring cultural traditions.

BioNexusHealth.com

The BioNexus Approach to Biotoxin Illness

A step-by-step guide to sustainable, plant-based treatment options

Jodie A. Dashore, PhD
Director, BioNexus Health Clinic

MASAVITRI PUBLISHING
PARLIN, NEW JERSEY

MASAVITRI PUBLISHING, NOVEMBER 2020

For information about this title, bulk orders, practitioner training, or other book requests, contact BioNexus Health: https://bionexushealth.com/book-request/

The BioNexus Approach(TM), caduceus with vertical cascading chakra or grayscale coloring surrounded by a heptagon with seven numbered circles on the outside connected with six lines, is the trademark of the BioNexus Health Clinic, LLC and Jodie A. Dashore.

Library of Congress Control Number: 2020920265

Trade Hardcover ISBN: 978-1-7346973-0-8
eBook ISBN: 978-1-7346973-1-5
Trade Paperback ISBN: 978-1-7346973-3-9

Printed in the United States of America

Book design by Prosper Suite
Flowers in a row of test tubes photo by rawpixels.com
This cover has been designed using resources from Freepik.com
Illustrations by Prosper Suite
Brain Illustrations adapted from Limbic Systems from Anatomy & Physiology,
Connexions (http://cnx.org/content/col11496/1.6/, Jun 19, 2013) licensed under
Creative Commons Attribution 3.0 Unported License, and Servier Medical Art by
Servier licensed under a Creative Commons Attribution 3.0 Unported License
General Practitioner Guidance icon includes Doctor by Delwar Hossain from the
Noun Project
Macro Leaf by https://unsplash.com/@gildardorh8

Publisher's Cataloging-in-Publication Data
Names: Dashore, Jodie A., author.
Title: The BioNexus Approach to Biotoxin Illness: A step-by-step guide to sustainable, plant-based treatment options / Jodie A. Dashore, PhD, director of BioNexus Health Clinic.
Description: First edition. | Parlin, New Jersey: Masavitri Publishing 2020.
Identifiers: LCCN 2020920265 | Trade Hardcover ISBN: 978-1-7346973-0-8 | eBook ISBN: 978-1-7346973-1-5 } Trade Paperback ISBN: 978-1-7346973-2-2
Subjects: LCSH: Alternative medicine–Information resources. | Environmentally induced diseases–Nutritional aspects. | Diseases–Chronic Diseases. | Environmentally induced diseases–Sick building syndrome. | BISAC: MEDICAL / Holistic Medicine. | BISAC: MEDICAL / Environmental Health. | BISAC: MEDICAL / Diseases.

For Brian Dashore–

For all your sacrifices, courage, and your sweet-loving heart despite all the immense adversity life put upon you. You lost your entire childhood to tick-borne diseases and chronic inflammatory response syndrome but you never once gave up. From the tender age of six, you've been poked, prodded, scanned, misdiagnosed, put through experimental treatments, and were in a wheelchair for several years. You never once lost faith in your family. Thank you for your confidence and belief, and for allowing me the honor of treating you and bringing you out of the dark cloud that enveloped you for so long.

We both firmly believed that the light at the end of the tunnel would be very bright, and indeed it was! You've emerged triumphant from the dense fog of chronic illness to the brilliant, kind-hearted, amazing young man you are and I'm so proud of you. You are my pride and joy, and I love you so very much. Thank you for being my inspiration. Experiencing the multitude of paradigm shifts with you was a profoundly humbling learning adventure. Every puzzle piece we pursued, elevated my ability to heal you and that knowledge allowed me to help other children and adults in over 50 countries around the world!

"The person who takes medicine must recover twice, once from the disease and once from the medicine."
— William Osler, created the first medical residency program; co-founding professor of Johns Hopkins Hospital

Dr. Ritchie Shoemaker's groundbreaking body of work has paved a path for millions around the world suffering from environmental illness. The Shoemaker protocol is undoubtedly efficacious. It is backed by years of clinical data, several published papers and is thoroughly evidence-based for CIRS-WDB and CIRS-Lyme.

From diagnosis to testing and even treatment options, Lyme disease has been a very controversial subject. Lyme Literate medical practitioners often use high dose antibiotics, both oral and intravenous, as part of the treatment protocol for chronic Lyme disease. These treatments can be lifesaving, but a large subset of patients experience debilitating side effects with little improvement (Marzec et al., 2017, p. 607). Almost every child with autism also diagnosed with Lyme disease is unable to tolerate antibiotics, and parents often choose a more natural route. Plant-based treatment options can be far gentler, slower-paced, and customizable to individual constitutions without the fear of developing resistance to treatment or harsh side effects when partaken under the care of a knowledgeable practitioner.

Plant-based treatment options have been shown to be effective, evidence-based and are now the treatment of choice of many patients and practitioners worldwide. The BioNexus Approach can be a viable option for those who are unable to or are unwilling to use pharmaceuticals for various reasons, from a leaky gut and Autism to those who have chosen to adhere to a plant-based lifestyle. The clinical results have been very promising and often a "game-changer," according to the growing number of practitioners globally that use the BioNexus methodology.

CONTENTS

Clinical Notes

Biotoxin Illness Charts

Figures

Recipes

FOREWORD
Scott W. McMahon, MD

Imagine your only child is literally dying, slowly wasting away in front of you. His incredible innate intelligence is being sapped, listlessly dripping like a Vermont maple tree in February. His once strong legs no longer support his thin, short frame, and he uses a wheelchair to ambulate. He's not growing, manifests involuntary movements and suffers from sporadic and widespread pains racking his tiny body. The Orthopedic surgeon just told your family you need to see the oncologist. You are a medical professional – what would you do?

Dr. Jodie A. Dashore, PhD, OTD, BCIP, HHP, CCH, RH (AHG), was in that very predicament just over ten years ago. She was already trained and experienced in neurology in her native India and the United Kingdom. She searched far and wide, found masters and world leaders of various healing disciplines, and discovered the answers her brilliant son needed. In the process, she studied with some of the best of the best for years until she became a master herself at numerous disciplines.

Alternatively, and more personally, tens of millions of you suffer from illness in numerous areas of your bodies and brains. Your medical personnel often do not know what the root cause of your disease is or how to treat you. They have no tests that definitively prove what you suffer from and often "just treat your symptoms," typically with little relief. Where will you look for your answers?

I met Jodie in Phoenix many years ago when we were both presenting at an international CIRS meeting. She spoke considerably about PANDAS (pediatric autoimmune neuropsychiatric disorder associated with Streptococcal infections). Afterward, I approached her and asked if she had ever seen a PANDAS patient who did not also suffer from CIRS. Indeed, neither of us had then nor since. Thus started our warm and productive friendship spanning the years and extending to our children.

Dr. Dashore completed the neurology program at the University of Bombay associated School of Medicine and post-doctoral work focusing on neurology, stroke and traumatic brain injury and sensory integration; and studied alternative and complementary medicine, Ayurveda, herbal and homeopathic healing with emphases in yoga, meditation, bioenergetics and spiritual aspects of medicine. She spent seven additional years mentoring under clinical herbalist Julie McIntyre with additional guidance from master herbalist Stephen Buhner. With compassion and patience, they both helped her to heal herself and her son using herbal medicine to study herbs in greater depth and to spark a deep interest in western herbalism. She worked with such world-renowned mentors as Dr. Joseph Jemsek and Dr. Charles Ray Jones (tick-borne illnesses), Dr. Eugene Shippen (endocrinology as it relates to CIRS and Lyme disease), and Dr. Ritchie Shoemaker and me regarding CIRS (chronic inflammatory response syndrome - a dysregulation of the innate immune system caused by chronic exposure to the interior of water-damaged buildings, the amplified microbial products found in them and by other biologically produced toxins and inflammagens). Dr. Dashore recently completed a second doctorate in integrative naturopathic medicine with a special interest in medical herbalism and quantum physics and is certified in the diagnosis and treatment of CIRS. Jodie is a clinical herbalist and a registered herbalist with the American Herbalist Guild.

Dr. Dashore amassed a varied and tremendous amount of knowledge studying these diverse fields. She presents and regularly teaches about autism, tick-borne illnesses and chronic inflammatory response syndrome (CIRS) worldwide; and created the BioNexus Approach and her own line of herbal formulas to help patients from over 50 countries.

The BioNexus Approach to Biotoxin Illness is an outgrowth of her passion for health and is an amalgamation of the tremendous knowledge she accumulated along her medical and healing arts journey with some of the world's most progressive and creative healing thinkers. Carefully and thoughtfully laid out, you can expect your brain to be opened, your thoughts stretched wide, and your mind blown! Your life as a medical practitioner will never be the same. Your life as a patient suffering multisystem illness and who regularly confounds the medical scholars will now be charmed with treatable answers. Do not put this book down!

In *The BioNexus Approach to Biotoxin Illness*, Jodie takes us on a wild ride surveying the innate immune system, effects of various immune deficiencies, exotic microbial colonizers, standard hormonal patterns, and commonly ignored brain structures until she hones in on what I call "the most common disease of which many doctors have never heard." Yes, it is CIRS, the illness underpinning so many medically unexplained symptoms as well as outright medical enigmas. CIRS, the completely avoidable epidemic that no one wants to talk about and the underlying ego-busting etiology of so many complaints. Kudos to you Jodie for tackling this subject, filleting open for all to see, discussing the vast work of Dr. Shoemaker, the discoverer of CIRS, and then applying the BioNexus Approach for an all-natural treatment plan. This book is a must-read for anyone who sees patients and treats with herbs. CIRS will rock your world, and Jodie's herbal approach will give you options. Got (camel) milk?

Jodie found the answers to her son's health dilemma by searching through diverse healing strategies to synthesize a winning approach. Some solutions came from the wisdom of mentors and other world leaders in health, some through research, and some through her own invention. Today, her son is at the precipice of university and is looking not only at colleges but at combined college/medical school programs. He is exceptionally intelligent, walks without assistance, does research, manages a nationwide teen support group which he founded, and speaks at national medical meetings. Not bad for a 17-year-old! He still endures some challenges, but has overcome the biggest and "baddest" struggles with a host of medical and healing advice and the incredible assistance of his passionate and caring mother and father. *The BioNexus Approach to Biotoxin Illness* takes you to the culmination of Dr. Dashore's medical expedition to date and opens a world of illness which surround us all yet is invisible to many. Once you see what Dr. Shoemaker first saw and what Jodie sees every day, you will not be able to unsee CIRS.

Join my friend Jodie on her journey through medicine, healing, and CIRS as she documents the power of herbal remedies!

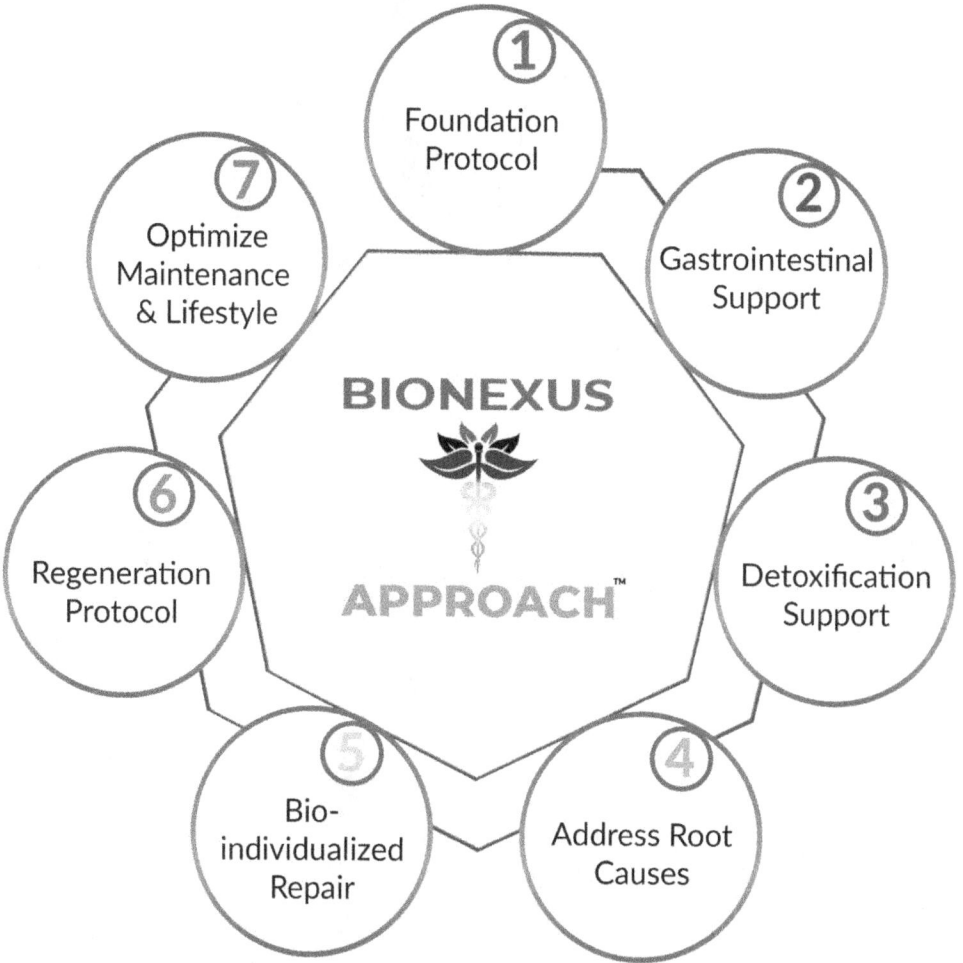

BIONEXUS

APPROACH™

1. Foundation Protocol
2. Gastrointestinal Support
3. Detoxification Support
4. Address Root Causes
5. Bio-individualized Repair
6. Regeneration Protocol
7. Optimize Maintenance & Lifestyle

ACKNOWLEDGMENTS

What a monumental journey this has been! Life has thrown me curveballs almost at every turn. Here I am today, fully healed, and so is my precious child. This book is the culmination of over a decade of intensive study, research, self-experimentation, and clinical experience.

My deepest thanks to my teachers and my mentors for being the voice of truth and right action. I've had the immense good fortune of meeting and learning from the brightest minds in the world – medical doctors, clinical herbalists, healers, and lightworkers. Not only are they trailblazers, but they are also the most wonderful, kindhearted, and down-to-earth human beings. To Ritchie Shoemaker, MD; Scott McMahon, MD; Rosario Trifiletti, MD, PhD; Miloslav Kovacevic, MD; Charles Ray Jones, MD; Joseph G Jemsek, MD, PhD; Eugene R. Shippen, MD; Dietrich Klinghardt, MD, PhD; Stephen Harrod Buhner; Julie McIntyre; Marg Bower; Mary Gint; Dave Gray; and the one and only HH Gurudev Sri Sri Ravi Shankar. My heart is filled with humility and gratitude.

I thank the Universe and all my teachers above for appearing just at the right time. For taking time out from their intense schedules, for opening their hearts to me, and lovingly mentoring me from my humble beginnings towards becoming the practitioner I am today. For instilling faith, resilience, hope, and courage. For sharing their knowledge and allowing me to grow at my own pace. For believing in me, giving me strength when I felt weak and discouraged, and lifting me up when I thought I couldn't go any further.

We have broken bread together; shared laughter and prayers, and you shall all have my deepest gratitude forever. Thank you for allowing me to continue to learn from you. Your diverse wisdom is so appreciated. I am truly blessed.

To Dr. Scott McMahon, thank you for believing in me, being there for my family, your patience, your sheer brilliance, and your open-minded and practical attitude to alternative medical therapies. Thank you for sharing your knowledge so generously and allowing me to shine.

To Guru Babaji, a heartfelt thank you for always being open to helping people, for sharing so many precious pearls of ancient herbal science wisdom, a perfect amalgamation of eastern spirituality and western pragmatism, and for allowing your students to share our own knowledge.

To my divine mentor, cosmic catalyst, the bright light that ignited a transformational spark within me to make all this possible. Thank you for your guidance in awakening my true authentic self that I could not see and for nurturing my inner spirit during times of extreme adversity. From a heart full of humility, you have my utmost respect and eternal gratitude.

My sincere thanks to my behind-the-scenes creative Elle McT, for hours and hours of help to refine this book. For being a true and constant friend.

Last, but not least, the courage and faith embodied by my patients. I've been genuinely inspired by the resolute spirit of those so severely afflicted, where hope infused with a renewed trust has replaced overwhelming doubt and despair. You've given me wings yet humbled me enough to stay grounded day in and day out as we work together towards healing your mind, body, and spirit.

Namaste,
Dr. Jodie A. Dashore

A NOTE TO THE READER

The Food and Drug Administration has not evaluated these statements. Any and all products mentioned herein are not intended to diagnose, treat, cure, or prevent any disease.

Before using any or all products, methods, or information, consult with your physician for approval. In no way should the BioNexus Approach ("BNA"), or recommended and preferred products, methods, and/or information be considered medical advice. The content herein is presented as the opinion of the author based on personal and clinical experience, might be general and/or taken from scientific studies, and is provided for informational purposes only. Never disregard medical advice or delay in seeking it because of something you read herein or on any and all websites, promotional materials, and/or any other materials relating to this book, the BioNexus Approach; BioNexus Health Clinic, LLC ("BNH"); Jodie A. Dashore ("JAD"); and/or any other related website on the internet.

BNH, JAD, and/or the publisher assumes no responsibility for the improper use of, self-diagnosis, and/or treatment using any or all of the methods and/or products described herein. This information should not be confused with prescription medicine or the advice of your physician. The information should not be used as a substitute for medically supervised therapy. If you suspect you suffer from clinical deficiencies, consult a licensed, qualified medical doctor.

You must understand why no claims can be made about the information herein, BNH and JAD cannot suggest the use of any or all products, methods, and/or information that will effect a cure or affect a symptom/ailment. Before starting any supplement, herb, or medicine of any kind, it's always wise to check with a medical doctor. It is especially important for people who are: pregnant or breastfeeding, chronically ill, elderly, under 18, or taking prescriptions or over-the-counter medicines. Certain supplements and herbs can interact with drugs to dangerous levels. None of the products, methods, or information herein are intended to be a treatment protocol for any disease state, but rather are offered to provide information and choices regarding health concerns. None of the information contained herein is intended to be an enticement to purchase and may not be construed as medical advice or instruction.

No action should be taken solely on the content herein, regardless of the perceived scientific merit. Instead, readers should consult health care professionals on any matter related to their health. The information obtained from referenced materials is believed to be accurate, as presented by their respective authors. Still BNA, BNH, JAD, and/or its publisher assume no liability for any personal interpretation. Readers, previous and future customers who fail to consult their physicians before implementing any or all products, methods, or information contained herein and any subsequent use of any product, method, or information, assume the risk of any adverse effects.

The use of any nutritional supplement or herb for any reason, other than to increase dietary intake levels of specific nutrients, is neither implied nor advocated by BNA, BNH, JAD, and/or its publisher.

For any suspected or known illness, or health concern, always consult with your physician or health care provider before to the purchase or use of any nutritional product. BNA, BNH, JAD and/or its publisher have attempted to present information from the author's personal and clinical experiences, literature, books, and other references as well as information about products as accurately as possible. Still, you should be aware that the Food and Drug Administration may not approve of products or information contained herein. Any literature reference or provided link is for your information or convenience. It may not be construed as an enticement to implement, believe, and/or purchase and further, is not intended nor implied to be used in the mitigation, diagnoses, treatment, cure, or prevention of any disease.

Legal Disclaimer

Information contained herein is provided for informational purposes only and is not meant to substitute for the advice provided by your own physician or other medical professionals. The results reported may not necessarily occur in all individuals. The BioNexus Approach ("BNA"); BioNexus Health Clinic, LLC ("BNH"); Jodie A. Dashore ("JAD"); and/or its publisher is providing this book and its contents on an "as is" basis and makes no representations or warranties of any kind concerning the publication and/or its contents. BNA, BNH, JAD, its publisher, and any of their respective directors, employees, contributors, or other representatives will be liable for damages arising out of or in connection with the use of this book. This is a comprehensive limitation of liability that applies to all damages of any kind, including (without limitation) compensatory, direct, indirect or consequential damages, income or profit, loss of or damage to self and/or property, and claims of third parties.

The Food and Drug Administration has not evaluated these statements. Any and all products mentioned herein are not intended to diagnose, treat, cure, or prevent any disease.

The information provided in this book is provided for educational and informational purposes only and is not intended to be a substitute for a health care provider's consultation. Please consult your own physician or appropriate health care provider about the applicability of any opinions or recommendations concerning your own symptoms or medical conditions as diseases commonly present with variable signs and symptoms. Check with a physician if you suspect you are ill or believe you may have one of the problems discussed in this book, as many problems and disease states may be serious and even life-threatening.

Note the publication date of this book because medical information changes rapidly. Therefore, some information may be out of date or even possibly inaccurate and erroneous. The information provided herein should not be considered complete, nor should it be relied on to suggest a course of treatment for a particular individual. It should not be used in place of a visit, call, consultation, or the advice of your physician or other qualified health care providers. Information obtained in this book is not exhaustive and does not cover all diseases, ailments, physical conditions, or their treatment. Should you have any health-care-related questions, please call or see your physician or other qualified health care providers promptly. Always consult with your physician or other qualified health care providers before embarking on a new treatment, diet, or fitness program. You should never disregard medical advice or delay in seeking it because of something you have read in this book. BNA, BNH, JAD, and/or its publisher does not assume any liability for the contents of any material provided.

Reliance on any information provided by BNA, BNH, JAD, and/or its publisher, health experts, commentators, and/or contributors is solely at your own risk. BNA, BNH, JAD, and/or its publisher assumes no liability or responsibility for damage or injury to persons or property arising from any use of any product, method, information, idea, or instruction contained in the materials provided herein. BNA, BNH, JAD, and/or its publisher reserves the right to change or discontinue at any time any aspect or feature within this book. You access this material at your own risk. BNA, BNH, JAD, and/or its publisher, their respective successors, assigns, and/or suppliers have no control over and accept no responsibility whatsoever for such materials.

These statements have not been evaluated by the Food and Drug Administration. This book is not intended to diagnose, treat, cure, or prevent any disease. Please Note: The material herein is provided for informational purposes only and is not medical advice. Always consult your physician before beginning any diet, treatment, or exercise program.

Readers are hereby informed that any and all information contained herein is for educational purposes only.

No Professional Relationship

Your use of this book and any of its associated products or materials - including, but not limited to implementing any recommendations, recipes, websites, or treatments and/or use of any of the resources available in this book - does not create a professional-client relationship between you and BioNexus Health Clinic ("BNH"), LLC; Jodie A. Dashore, or any of their recommendations, partners, affiliates, or assigns. A professional-client relationship requires an initial consultation scheduled through the BNH office, and its associated payments, assessments, and requirements. Thus, you recognize and agree that any information acquired from this book, either by you or others, has not created a professional-client relationship.

Recipes Disclaimer

Please be aware of dietary sensitivities before trying any of the recipes suggested in this book. Various dietary sensitivities like gluten, dairy, histamine, salicylate, oxalate, and sulfur have been noted in people with CIRS. Modifying recipes to a person's dietary restrictions is the responsibility of the reader, physician, practitioner, cook, preparer, or maker.

All recipes, recommendations, and preferences infer the use of naturally grown products, preferably without human interference but at a minimum whole and organic with limited, or no added fillers, colors, and flavors.

Preferences

BioNexus Health Clinic, LLC ("BNH"), and Jodie A. Dashore ("JAD") have not received physical products, incentives, or cash in exchange for mentions in this book. There are no additional disclosures for endorsement or conflict of interest, except those explicitly mentioned in the paragraphs below. All companies and brands mentioned in this book are fully-owned by their rightful copyright, trademark, patent, or registered owners.

JAD and BNH own the proprietary herbal formulas and blends collectively referred to as BioNexus Herbals. The BioNexus Herbals are low-cost, all-natural options developed for BNH patients and practitioners mentored by JAD. A full list of the herbal line may be found in the BioNexus Herbals section within Part 4: Prepping the Approach.

JAD is a Certified Practitioner in Dr. Ritchie Shoemaker's Biotoxin Illness/CIRS protocol. Dr. Shoemaker mentors JAD and has for several years. JAD also discloses that several practitioners and medical doctors mentioned in this book mentored her as a part of her journey to the BioNexus Approach. Mentions of Brian Dashore's practitioners and JAD's mentors, including their medical practices or networks, is a disclosure of their established professional and personal relationships. None of these established relationships exchanged any arrangement or agreement for mentions within the book.

JAD sits on the board of several organizations. These include but are not limited to Bioregulatory Medicine Institute, Global Lyme Diagnostics Lab, and International Forum for Camel Advocacy and Medicine. For a full list of her affiliations, please see the about page on the BNH website (BioNexusHealth.com).

Dr. Ritchie Shoemaker recommends Microbiology DX for MARCoNS testing. Microbiology DX tested and reported results on BioNexus Herbals Formula 1 NSB. The report is available in Part 4: Prepping the Approach.

Reproductions

This book is copyrighted. No part of this publication may be reproduced, copied, or distributed in any form or by any means electronic, mechanical, stored in a database or retrieval system, or posted on social media without the prior written permission from the publisher.

Names

Some names have been changed to protect their privacy.

THE
BIONEXUS APPROACH
TO BIOTOXIN ILLNESS

"The period of greatest gain in knowledge and experience is often the most difficult period in one's life."

—Dalai Lama

Introduction

My journey into the world of all-natural, integrative, and holistic medicinal approaches began only after trying to navigate and balance the plethora of medications and treatments my son required for his multisystem chronic illnesses.

From early childhood, the brain and medical sciences intrigued me. When I met my husband, Alex, during university, we had bright futures and brilliant plans. I turned down offers from London hospitals for us to pursue a new life in America. We settled just outside New York City, where we quickly integrated with our community and enjoyed the luxuries that came with living the American dream. My husband worked for a great firm in the World Trade Center, and I was pregnant with our first child.

A few minutes before Christmas, Brian arrived and was, by all accounts, a healthy newborn. His life-long struggle with multiple illnesses would not begin until he was diagnosed with Pervasive

Developmental Disorder – Not Otherwise Specified (PDD-NOS) at eighteen-months-old. It was during these early years that I prepared myself with an advanced clinical doctorate in OT (neurology) from Rocky Mountain University of Health Professions and a post-doctoral specialization in neurosensory integrative medicine from the University of Southern California.

Raising any child is not easy. Raising one with autism brought its own challenges. Alex and I had moved into acceptance and were incredibly proud of our karate and baseball-loving son. But our world was upended again when Brian was six-years-old and inexplicably lost the use of his left leg. After specialists could not find a reason for his pain or provide an explanation for his symptoms, he ended up in a wheelchair. Then, one morning, he woke up with violent motor tics, eye blinking, head nodding, and vocalizations. The rapid onset of the symptoms gave us enough clues for a colleague to suggest that we see Dr. Trifiletti, a Pediatric Neurologist and CEO of The PANDAS/PANS Institute.

At seven-years-old, Brian received a PANDAS (pediatric autoimmune neuropsychiatric disorders associated with Streptococcal infections) diagnosis. Dr. Trifiletti gave us the first diagnosis that would set us on the correct path to wellness. Soon thereafter, Dr. Charles Ray Jones added Lyme disease and eleven co-infections diagnoses as the root cause of several of Brian's health issues. After each treatment for his various diagnoses, Brian had incredible gains. But, when he was nine-years-old, he rapidly regressed. He lost a pound a day, had intense headaches, and his motor tics returned.

One of his doctors thought it could be cancer, so we went to an infectious disease specialist and a hematologist-oncologist. Both of whom ruled out cancer. When the other tests came back negative, the incredibly well-respected infectious disease specialist brought me into his office. He asked me every conceivable question about Brian's history for any clue to the cause of these returning symptoms. We got to the point where the doctor needed to rule out the possibility that Brian might be doing this for attention simply because there seemed to be no other answer.

What I knew was that my fourth-grader weighed fifty-two pounds soaking wet! The average kid his age weighs seventy-eight pounds. Twenty-five pounds underweight with sufficient nutrition meant it had to be a symptom of something. Whatever

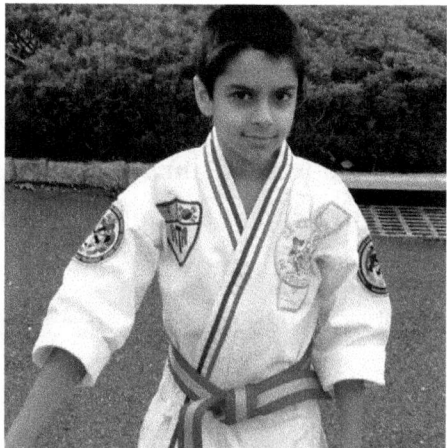

Brian Dashore, age 6, before losing the use of his left leg

New Jersey, 2007

was causing the weight loss was not cancer or anything else these doctors tested. My frustration at this doctor's lack of out-of-the-box thinking made me a fierce advocate for my child. I was determined to prove him wrong.

I went back and combed through Brian's medical records to figure out what we missed. His "cough variant" asthma diagnosis caught my eye. Brian had developed a continuous cough when he was seven-years-old. It became a significant issue in his daily life and became so disruptive that even his teacher complained it constantly interrupted the class. We had taken him to an allergist, immunologist, and even a gastroenterologist because one specialist suggested that it could be acid reflux. Ultimately, he was put on a nebulized steroid treatment three times per day for his cough variant asthma.

In the very early days of Brian's illnesses, I stayed in my lane as a past neurologist and trusted the modern medical process and his specialists. I was shocked to see that none of these doctors tested him for mycotoxins or anything mold-related. The Institute of Medicine connected mold to asthma in 2004 and reported indoor mold as a possible cause of upper respiratory tract symptoms that included coughing. I could not fathom how these specialists failed to ask about mold exposure four years after the report. Several years removed from those appointments, the cough was still a nagging symptom. Brian's mysterious cough was a piece of a more significant underlying issue.

I had seen Dr. Ritchie C. Shoemaker's papers about mold,

biotoxins, and chronic inflammatory response syndrome (CIRS) during Brian's PANDAS treatment. I had even made an appointment. But, while we were in Germany, a bio-energetic test involving muscle testing showed a weak response to mold. So, I canceled the appointment.

Four fateful years later, when we finally got back to mold as a possible underlying cause, I made another appointment with Dr. Shoemaker. The initial consultation included examining potential mold exposures. Fortunately, or unfortunately, Brian's labs hit all the markers for chronic inflammatory response syndrome. He was in the advanced stages of biotoxin illness. As we followed the biotoxin illness treatment protocol, his mysterious symptoms began disappearing, including his cough variant asthma.

Brian improved by leaps and bounds following Dr. Shoemaker's protocol. I could finally see a world where he could excel. After all of his early childhood struggles, perhaps, just perhaps, he could lead a relatively healthy and normal adult life.

Finding Brian's path to wellness did not end there. Six months into his CIRS treatment, we needed to address the damage in his gastrointestinal tract and several other imbalances caused allopathic medicine. A significant pitfall of pharmaceutical drugs is the damage they can cause when used on chronically-ill patients. Biotoxin illness is a life-long, chronic disease with acute capabilities. Brian and other complex patients like him require a strict protocol to prevent relapses and maintain health.

To protect and repair my son's health, I needed to figure out all-natural, organic, plant-based alternatives to the biotoxin illness protocol. Growing up in India, Ayurvedic medicine was a part of my first understanding of medicine. This holistic approach to medicine was developed in India over 3,000 years ago and is still very much a part of the culture, but as my career evolved, I lost that connection to my roots. I had become a product of modern western medicine and believed the philosophies drilled into me during my medical school training.

Reuniting with my Ayurvedic roots alongside my evidence-based medical training helped me realize that I already possessed the resources needed to pursue all-natural solutions. Every practitioner and guide I had sought since Brian's PANDAS diagnosis were kind and generous enough to share their specialty with me. Stephen Harrod Buhner and Julie McIntyre guided my introduction to modern herbalism and plant intelligence, which in turn shined a light on the potentiality of quantum medicine. Learning from the brilliant work of the inimitable Vaidya and medical herbalist, David Crow, added to the therapeutic fabric that blended harmoniously with my background in Ayurveda, homeopathy, and homotoxicology. Dr. Shoemaker provided access to his biotoxin research and his continued developments for diagnosis. Dr. Scott McMahon, the first physician certified in the Shoemaker protocol, elevated my understanding of pediatric biotoxin illness and provided immense support after witnessing my holistic approach at our Art of Living Retreat Center workshop. My retreats garnered interest from the renowned spiritual leader Sri Sri Ravi Shankar, who invited me to discuss my work with the medical board at his Ayurvedic Hospital in India. While there, I was able to learn from the Art of Living's successful permaculture farmers, which propelled the concept of BioNexus Herbals. I feel honored and grateful that our family's struggle allowed me to bring hope to families around the world by embarking upon the creation of safe and effective plant-based CIRS treatment options.

Brian lost his childhood to tick-borne infections and chronic inflammatory response syndrome. His doctors poked, prodded, scanned, and misdiagnosed him, but Brian never lost hope that there would be a silver lining. As he finishes his final year at a top medical magnet high school, Brian is fully recovered from his autism and CIRS diagnoses.

Biotoxin illness is a life-long disease that can spiral into CIRS when symptoms are ignored or left untreated. To prevent relapses, patients must alter their lifestyle, home, diets, and daily

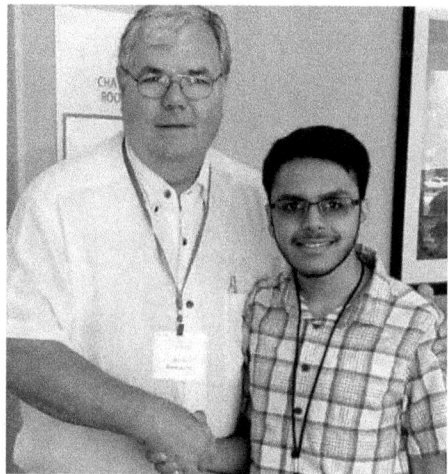

Brian Dashore with
Dr. Ritchie Shoemaker

Mold Conference
New Mexico, 2019

routines to live symptom-free. Some patients choose to custom-build their homes in remote areas while others learn to adapt and lead a normal-adjacent lifestyle by navigating their lives around toxin exposure.

For Brian, university selection involves more than the typical statistics for prospective students. He needs to account for potential exposure to water-damaged buildings (WDBs), organic product accessibility, and other potential sources of toxins. A biotoxin illness patient's new lifestyle includes repair and maintenance protocols that regulate, protect, and train their bodies to function normally to maintain health. Brian's routine requires vigilant awareness of his environment and bio-individualized herbal maintenance to stave off Lyme disease and CIRS relapses. Otherwise, he is a typical teenager who excels in the sciences. Brian received the Presidential Scholarship to an accelerated medical program and is excited about the next chapter of his life and becoming a physician.

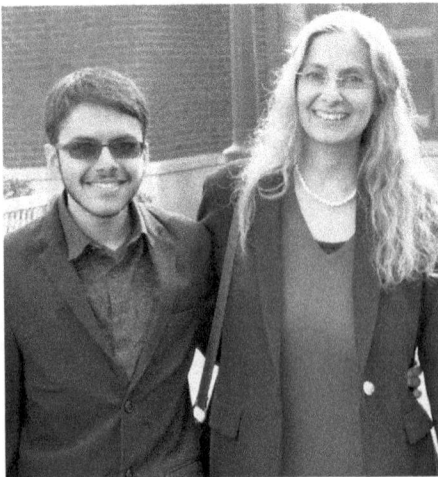

Brian Dashore with
Dr. Jodie A. Dashore

Congressman Chris Smith
Lyme Press Conference
New Jersey, 2019

A Step Back

It took nearly a decade for me to unwind myself from modern medical treatments. The shift coincided with an undercurrent of therapeutic change in America. As I focused on my son, the medical headlines continued to worry me, and friends messaged me with the latest alternative craze. During the early 2000s, any parent of a chronically ill child could have easily been swept up by the mayhem.

Instead of following the latest trend, I decided to track the history of allopathic medicine and dig into my old course books. I needed to understand where the trajectory of modern medicine changed, so I could focus on attaining the training and resources to take my son's health off the roller coaster ride. There needed to be a silver lining to breathe hope into my mindset. I craved to feel strong, capable, and empowered. Most of all, I desired more days where I worried about basic parenting issues and fewer days that felt impossible.

Since the days of Mesopotamia, science has always had a splash of rationalism and a hint of magic. Science is figuring out the things we do not understand and allowing ourselves to seek possible solutions from all of the resources provided. Before the development of Newtonian physics in the 18th century, medicine took a little bit of each of the sciences to propel itself. The introduction of classical Newtonian physics drove a pragmatic approach to science that depends on five assumptions:

materialism, strong objectivity, causal determinism, locality, and epiphenomenalism.

For three centuries, these assumptions were highly regarded and drove the sciences that developed antibiotics, antifungals, and herbicides. In many ways, these discoveries changed the trajectory of humankind — some good and some extremely detrimental to human health.

In acute illness, allopathic medicine has saved millions of lives and improved outcomes for the masses. However, in chronically ill patients, allopathic medicine can cause more health issues, typically treated with more pharmaceutical medications. The World Health Organization (WHO) projected in 1998 that the future posed continuing challenges in the war against chronic diseases. By 2020, chronic illness would account for nearly three-quarters of all deaths worldwide. While several factors contributed to the rapid global spread of chronic disease, the WHO pointed to misjudgment in the effectiveness of drug intervention therapies, commercial pressures, inadequate resources, and institutional inertia as dangerous aspects that needed to be addressed and changed.

As discovered and continually debated for over a century, modern medicine is inherently flawed. Newtonian physics laws fail on high energy (photons) and smaller than matter (subatomic particles) substances. Modern medical science also relies on observable and verifiable facts. Quantum theory incorporates energy, motion, and subatomic particle interaction that can push medicine into a magical realm that we cannot typically see nor capture. The world of quantum mechanics opens Pandora's box of medical healing possibilities. For most classically trained medical practitioners, quanta are well-beyond the scope of their training. The observable requirement of modern medicine and the intimidating nature of quanta make doctors wary and skeptical of its capabilities.

Fleming's Warning

While quantum theorists were devising the commonly taught Copenhagen interpretation to express the meaning of quantum mechanics, Alexander Fleming, a bacteriologist, neared his discovery of penicillin.

During World War I, Fleming served in a wound-research laboratory, led by Sir Almroth Wright, a pioneer in vaccine therapy. He observed soldiers die from uncontrollable infections and demonstrated that the antiseptics used to treat the combat wounds were not strong enough to kill anaerobic bacteria in jagged injuries. He was intrigued by the antibacterial powers of pus and the damage antiseptics caused to white blood corpuscles (leukocytes). Returning to his laboratory and motivated by his war experience, he used his vaccine experience to find a substance strong enough to kill bacteria. Within a few years, he discovered lysozyme, a protein with powerful antibacterial properties. Humans naturally produce lysozyme in the nasal and tear ducts mucous membranes, blood serum, saliva, milk, and a

ANTISEPTIC SPRAY

Clean skin, scrapes, cuts, toys, and other hard objects

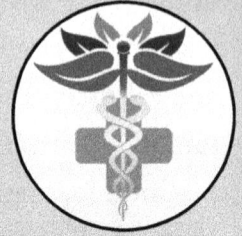

Ingredients

4 oz rose water or distilled water
3/4 cup lavender flower infusion
3/4 cup thyme leaf infusion
1 tbsp tea tree tincture

Directions

Mix ingredients in a spray bottle

Shake well before using

---

wide variety of other fluids. According to Fleming (1945), a small drop of lysozyme could clear harmless, airborne bacteria in a few seconds. Unfortunately, it had no practical effect on humans because it did not have any impact on disease-causing bacteria.

These experiments prepared Fleming for his next discovery. He placed several agar dishes of Staphylococcus (gram-positive bacteria) on a laboratory workbench to observe changes. Inspecting the plates required exposure to the air. During one of the inspections, Fleming noticed mold contamination. Viewing the specimen under the microscope, he reported a ring that prevented bacteria from growing and caused cell destruction (lysis). This discovery led to the launch of pharmaceutical antibiotics with the substance Fleming named penicillin, the world's first antibiotic that saved its first patient in 1942 (Newman, 2011).

During Fleming's 1945 Nobel Prize lecture, he gave only one warning about penicillin. In his laboratory, underdosing microbes failed to kill them completely. This failure led to bacteria quickly becoming resistant to penicillin. At the end of his speech, Fleming hypothetically illustrated his point, "Mr. X. has a sore throat. He buys some penicillin and gives himself, not enough to kill the streptococci but enough to educate them to resist penicillin. He then infects his wife. Mrs. X gets pneumonia and is treated with penicillin. As the streptococci are now resistant to penicillin, the treatment fails. Mrs. X dies. Who is primarily responsible for Mrs. X's death? Why Mr. X, whose negligent use of penicillin, changed the nature of the microbe. Moral: If you use penicillin, use enough."

Rise of Resistance

The discovery of penicillin was one of the greatest achievements of the twentieth century. Antibiotics increased the survival rates of infected people and saved millions of lives around the world. Life expectancy in the United States increased by eight years within three decades (Spellberg & Gilbert, 2014). Understandably, people believed antibiotics were a miracle cure.

Unfortunately, medical scientists, experts, and practitioners failed to heed Fleming's warning in practice. Antibiotics were quickly overused, misused, and under prescribed. Clinicians did not lack an understanding of the advice. Medical writings of the time prove a thorough understanding of the warning. Despite the warning, clinicians followed the rational use principal published in a 1952 issue of The Lancet, "use the new drug while it still acts" (as cited in Condrau & Kirk, 2011). Within four years of penicillin's mass release, there were reports of resistance. Penicillin resistance became a significant clinical issue within a decade (Spellberg & Gilbert, 2014).

COLD & FLU SOAK
Keep away from direct sunlight and children

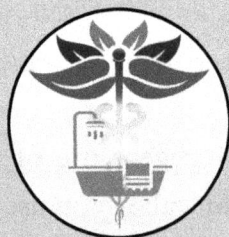

Ingredients

1 part yarrow leaf/flower
1 part linden leaf/flower
1 part peppermint leaf
2-5 drops ginger essential oil (optional)

Directions

Mix all herbs
Add one cup of the herbal blend in a cheesecloth or muslin bag
Draw a hot bath and leave herbal blend bag in while the tub fills
Let the bath cool
Remove the herbal blend bag before getting in the tub
Store herbal blend in a tightly-closed jar

Ginger essential oil creates a more in-depth and warmer detox

Rose hydrosol (1/2 cup) can be a cooling addition

Penicillin resistance boosted clinical microbiology, initiated the development of semi-synthetic antibiotics, and boosted the popularity of broad-spectrum antibiotics (Gradmann, 2016). Methicillin, the first semi-synthetic penicillin-related antibiotic treatment, arrived in 1959 (Davies & Davies, 2010). These advancements once again led the mainstream back to an over-reliance on antibiotics. In 1969, the US Surgeon General, William Stewart, told the US Congress: "We can close the books on infectious diseases" (as cited in van der Meer, 2013).

While antibiotics were publicly heralded, infectious disease experts warned at a 1965 roundtable that another round of resistance was about to occur. The pipeline of discoveries and replacement drugs had dwindled. In response, pharmaceutical companies attempted to restore potency by slightly altering the formulas (Condrau & Kirk, 2011; Spellberg & Gilbert, 2014).

Superbugs

As Fleming, and later bacteriologists, understood, bacteria are highly sophisticated. Microbials are capable of adapting, communicating, and collaborating. In the 1970s, most of the population, even medical professionals, believed we outwitted the single-celled microorganisms once again. Disastrously, they were wrong.

Medical innovation in the war on harmful microbes has left humans in dire straits. "The use of antibiotics is the single most important factor leading to antibiotic resistance around the world" (Centers for Disease Control and Prevention, 2013, p. 11). Throughout the decades, humankind has staggeringly set ourselves up to fail. Some hospitals in the 1960s followed a cross-contamination technique that called for spraying methicillin into the air to prevent methicillin-resistant Staphylococcus aureus (MRSA) infections (Newsom, 2004). Nevertheless, MRSA still plagues hospital wards. A recent study found one-fifth of tested objects in hospital rooms had "superbugs," antibiotic-resistant microbes, on them (Michigan Medicine - University of Michigan, 2019). Antibiotics used in the food supply chain created a feedback loop. Livestock manure contains 70-90% of unchanged or active antibiotics. Typically, manure is repurposed into fertilizer, thus spreading antibiotics throughout the soil and water supply (Massé, Saady, & Gilbert, 2014). Additionally, any medicines remaining in the livestock can then pass on to the human when consumed. Fifty years into the antibiotic revolution, a study found up to 50% of antibiotic prescriptions were not needed, or inaccurately dosed (Ventola, 2015). Our eradication efforts backfired because, at each step, we handed microbes our battle plan, and they used it to adapt and survive.

The war of superbugs and "super drugs" that began in the 1970s with a MRSA epidemic is still a global epidemic, according to the National Institutes of Health (2018). Antibiotics lost the war and major research financiers have surrendered. Pharmaceutical companies were the primary funders of antimicrobial research. In the United States, these companies consider antibiotics a market failure and not worthy of research and development financing. Five years after the CDC released Antibiotic Resistant Threats in the United States (2013), the Food and Drug Administration (FDA) announced its Strategic Approach for Combating Antimicrobial Resistance. In a speech by the Commissioner of Food and Drugs, he confirmed, "pharmaceutical companies have, for the most part, exited from antibiotic research" (Gottlieb, 2018).

The general population has its back against the wall. Antimicrobial resistance has been a well documented public health crisis for over twenty years. The developmental pipeline has long since dried up. Without a clear path to profit, regulators, hospitals, and companies have only nibbled at the problem. Their inactive approach spurred creative solutions to what the Centers for Disease Control and Prevention (2013) calls "one of the biggest public health challenges of our time."

Throughout 2019, there were numerous mass media news stories about potential antibiotic replacements. However, most are years away from clinical trials, which makes them even further removed from public use. Each of these solutions could be the answer or a stopgap. It is too early to determine what will happen. However, humankind does not have the time to find out. A World Health Organization ("WHO") report released in April 2019 says, "unless the world acts urgently, antimicrobial resistance will have disastrous impact within a generation." Without urgent action, drug-resistant diseases could cause "ten million deaths globally per year by 2050." WHO estimates that uncontrolled antimicrobial resistance could impact global markets similar to the 2008 global financial crisis, impact food supply, and create a greater inequity around the world.

Antibiotics were developed to fight acute bacterial infections. We now understand that long-term use of antibiotics on chronic diseases exacerbates resistance and creates additional issues for the patient (Jernberg, Lofmark, Edlund, & Jansson, 2010). Misprescribing antibiotics to chronically ill patients rapidly advanced bacterial resistance. In this chronic subset of patients, microbes fundamentally transform on a cellular level. Quorum-sensing bacteria build a protective biofilm shell that makes the entire community of microbes unrecognizable to the majority of antibiotics.

As a medical community, we need to provide viable treatment options for chronic illness and genetically susceptible patients.

Antifungals

Antifungal medications never reached the success of antibiotics, nor were they praised for their healing powers. Scientists have struggled to develop non-toxic antifungal therapies ever since Candida albicans, pathogenic yeast, was classed as a fatal disease in the 17th century. Elizabeth Lee Hazen, a microbiologist, became inspired by Fleming's penicillin discovery in 1944. She began collecting disease-causing specimens from around the world. Within four years, Hazen moved antifungal development the farthest it had ever been (Science History Institute, 2017).

Hundreds of soil tested samples successfully killed fungi. Nearly all of them were also highly toxic to animals. Interestingly enough, Hazen found one specimen in her friend's garden that killed fungi and was safe for animals. The Candida antifungal treatment, Nystatin, entered the market in the 1950s as Mycostatin (Espinell-Ingroff, 2013). Nystatin remains on the World Health Organization's List of Essential Medicines (2019).

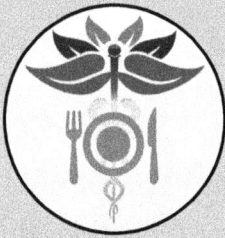

EASILY IMPROVE NUTRITIONAL VALUE

Increase organic consumption: decrease absorbed chemicals and trans fats by reducing or eliminating processed foods, artificial colors, and flavors

Minimize bovine dairy: lower mucus formation; replace it with probiotic-rich goat or sheep milk yogurt and camel milk

Reduce intake of simple sugars (soda and juice): sugar depresses immune function and aids microbial overgrowth; the fiber in fruits and vegetables slows natural sugar absorption into the bloodstream

Eliminate or rotate food allergens: even subtle food allergies (gluten, dairy, eggs, corn, and soy) and food sensitivities can cause low-level inflammation and may exacerbate seasonal allergies

Broader spectrum antifungal agents became available in the late 1960s, with the introduction of Amphotericin B to treat serious infections. However, this drug was known for its side effects, including nephrotoxicity. Azoles, a new class of antifungals, arrived in the 1980s (Maertens, 2004). Despite the azoles' superiority over the previous generation of drugs, this class also exhibited suboptimal activity. The fungus quickly developed resistance, and the antifungal had hazardous interactions with other medications.

These pitfalls lead to the development of analogs through the turn of the 21st century (Kontoyiannis & Lewis, 2014). The new generation of antifungals appeared promising because of a higher potency against fungus, particularly against aspergilli, a mold species. However, they still contained significant limitations due to drug interactions.

MARCoNS (multiple antibiotic-resistant coagulase-negative staphylococci) testing on biotoxin illness patients between 2002 and 2018 showed a dramatic rise in antifungal resistance, according to a 2019 study by Shoemaker, Lark, and Ryan. Indiscriminate use of antifungal nasal sprays in patients also taking antibiotics declined the overall effectiveness of treatment. The nasal spray used to treat MARCoNS and biofilm before 2015 stopped working after introducing azoles to a patient's protocol. Additionally, brain imaging with NeuroQuant MRI revealed a more significant percentage of atrophied gray matter in patients treated with antifungal nasal sprays.

Practitioners need to understand the subtleties of each antifungal and the hazards they pose for chronic and immunocompromised patients. The CDC (2018) issued the warning, "if people with weakened immune systems breathe in antifungal-resistant Aspergillus spores, then they could develop infections that are difficult to treat." Potentially exacerbating the issue, environmental factors partially drive patient acquired antifungal resistance, including azole fungicides used to treat crops.

Herbicides

Modern farming practices further compound the issues faced by chronically ill patients. Humans rely on their gastrointestinal tract and its microbiome for nutrients. Glyphosate is a broad-spectrum systemic herbicide sprayed on plants, parks, schools, pavements, grass, playgrounds, and crops.

Since the introduction of the herbicide, glyphosate, in the 1970s, farming practices dramatically changed. After the discovery that sodium salt variant in glyphosate regulates plant growth, farmers began using it to ripen and rapidly dry crops for early harvesting. Subsequently, the crops started to die from herbicide exposure. Genetically modified seeds were developed to make crops resistant to glyphosate effects. In the United States, there are over 750 products containing glyphosate, and experts expect the market to increase 5-6.8% by 2024 (Global Market Insights, 2019; Mordor Intelligence, n.d.).

Glyphosate disrupts human gut amino acid and cytochrome P450 (CYP) enzyme production (Samsel & Seneff, 2013). Humans use amino acids to produce proteins for life-sustaining functions including, breaking down food and repairing tissue. CYP metabolizes and detoxifies xenobiotics (drugs, food additives, and environmental pollutants) from a cellular level. Interference with the CYP gene could result in epigenetic changes leading to unknown responses to drug therapies (Tang & Chen, 2015).

Research found glyphosate residue on Western diet staples, such as sugar, corn, soy, wheat, and several other food products, including water, wine, and beer (Samsel & Seneff, 2013; Cook, 2019). Over time, the damaging effects of glyphosate could render gut bacteria useless and cellular systems throughout the body inflamed. Studies show that the build-up of glyphosate causes problems in the liver, kidneys, reproductive organs, brain, and methylation pathways (Samsel & Seneff, 2013).

Consequently, the amount of glyphosate on Western diet foods could be directly associated with the rise in gastrointestinal disorders, gluten intolerance, obesity, diabetes, heart disease, depression, autism, infertility, cancer, and Alzheimer's disease. At the introduction of glyphosate, it was determined that it was safe for human consumption because it solely disrupted the shikimate pathway in plants. Humans and animals do not contain shikimate pathways; therefore, according to herbicide producers, it cannot harm them. However, the microorganisms residing in human and animal intestinal tracts do have shikimate

SIMPLE CHANGES TO STRENGTHEN THE BODY

Increase antioxidant-rich foods: eating a variety of colorful fruits and vegetables lowers overall systemic inflammation

Gently stimulate the liver and healthy digestion: add bitter and sour flavors; drink warm lemon water in the morning; add bitter greens (arugula, watercress, and dandelions) to salads

Quercetin (plant pigment) reduces allergies, benefits mast cells, and lowers stress: add apples, onions, green tea, rose, nettle, grapes, tomatoes, leafy greens, and berries to meals

Local honey eases allergies: blend local honey with turmeric, sage, or rose (children under the age of two should not be given honey)

Omega-3 oil-based fats decrease systemic inflammation: add flax oil to salad dressing, or ground nuts and seeds (flax, chia, or hemp) as meal toppings

pathways (Hashimoto et al., 2012). The symbiotic nature of gut bacteria and its host aids digestion, synthesizes vitamins, detoxifies xenobiotics, and participates in immune system homeostasis and gastrointestinal tract permeability (Littman & Pamer, 2011). It is reasonable to suspect that glyphosate contributes to human diseases and conditions.

The documented long-term effects of glyphosate and its ability to induce disease are particularly troublesome for those genetically susceptible to environmental toxins (Samsel & Seneff, 2013).

Microbial Intelligence

Contrary to popular opinion, humans did not become resistant to antibiotics. Bacteria learned to become antibiotic-resistant by inheriting their mother's genes and copying resistance knowledge from nearby microbes (National Institutes of Health, 2018). They have survived billions of years and endured extreme environments. Swift evolution and evasion techniques come with each new generation, which can begin every twenty minutes.

Microorganisms use several antibiotic evasion tactics. Antimicrobials kill bacteria by passing through the cell membrane during nutrient intake. Bacteria can alter the permeability of their cell membranes or change their internal structure to shut down this invasion and prevent the antibiotic from binding. Germs also incorporate a variety of efflux pumps in their systems. These pumps immediately eject antimicrobials by identifying one or multiple structurally dissimilar antibiotic compounds (Webber, 2002; Soto, 2013).

The prolific researcher, J.W. Costerton, irritated the microbiology community in 1978 with a new perspective on surface growth microbes, which he called biofilm. Single-celled bacteria collaborate to build complex, extracellular protective matrices (biofilm) that prevent antibiotic detection (Newman, 2011). Biofilm in the nares of biotoxin illness patients aids immune system dysfunction by protecting MARCoNS and allowing the bacteria to thrive. The importance of biofilm and its ability to block antibiotics was not entirely accepted by the empirical medical community until the National Institutes of Health announced, "Biofilms are medically important, accounting for over 80% of microbial infections in the body" (National Institutes of Health, 2002, p. 1).

Biofilms exhibit different phenotypes and physiology than planktonic cells in their singular form (Donlan & Costerton, 2002). The exact mechanism to form biofilm is unknown. However, indiscriminate use of antibiotics provided an opportunity for antibiotic-resistant microbial pathogens to collaborate. Quorum-sensing bacteria can detect cellular density thresholds and release signals to induce gene expressions in nearby species. Research continues on the ongoing signaling within biofilm polymicrobial communities (Berndtson, 2013). Studies identified a four-step process to biofilm formation: adherence, accumulation, maturation, and detachment.

When participating microbes sense a quorum, they trigger the production of an autoinducer molecule. Proteins release extracellular DNA (eDNA), which has been proven to be an essential adherence/aggression factor in biofilm formation (Qin et al., 2007; Rice et al., 2007). Approximately 80% of biotoxin illness and chronic inflammatory response syndrome (CIRS) patients who have low melanocyte-stimulating hormone (MSH) also have MARCoNS (Shoemaker & Katz, 2013).

METHYLATION

Methylation is a crucial aspect of nutrition and detoxification. However, my recommendation is not to attempt methylation until the inflammation is under control, unless absolutely necessary, and under the guidance of an experienced practitioner.

Low MSH creates an opportunity for MARCoNS to build biofilm in the naturally occurring mucous secretions of the sinus cavities. The biofilm creates a protective shell allowing antibiotic-resistant staph to survive, evade immune system detection, and cause a perpetual cascade of system dysfunction.

Normal MSH levels strengthen the blood-brain barrier (BBB)

and help to reduce brain inflammation. Anatomically, the proximity of the sinuses to brain tissues creates an opportunity for bacterial toxins to penetrate a weakened BBB. Biofilm bacteria compound MSH deficiency by producing exotoxins A and B, which cleave MSH. Specialized MRI NeuroQuant brain imaging scans showed crucial neurological changes in gray and white matter areas of CIRS-WDB (chronic inflammatory response syndrome-water-damaged building) patient brains.

Finding MARCoNS in the nares of children increases the probability that their brain develops abnormally. These structural and functional changes directly correlate to immune suppression. Brain changes may be caused by genetics, lifestyle, or environment, but it is usually a combination of all three.

Epigenetics

Humans have about 37 trillion cells containing DNA. A single strand of DNA can carry over 20,000 genes tightly packed and organized into gene regulation structural units, known as histones. The intracellular sequence of DNA bases (A, C, T, and G) make up the genotype, or blueprints used to produce body regulating proteins.

When the body needs a protein, it creates an RNA transcript, a copy of the genotype. During transcription, epigenetics, a natural gene expression mechanism, decides if a gene is available or "expressed," by turning it on.

DNA and histones, collectively called chromatin, regulate gene expression, DNA replication, prevent DNA damage, and reinforce the DNA during cell division. A variety of factors, including disease, lifestyle, and environment, can influence epigenetics and gene expression without altering the DNA sequence (Kanherkar, Bhatia-Dey, & Csoka, 2014). The most common location for modifications is on histone tails.

All the chemical compounds added to a person's DNA or genome are called the epigenome. The chemical compounds are not a part of the original DNA sequence, but are on or attached to the DNA. A chemical compound added to a single gene can regulate or change its activity. Environmental influences such as diet, pollutants, pesticides, herbicides, and mycotoxins can impact the epigenome (Ji & Khurana Hershey, 2012).

Disrupted gene expressions underlie many human diseases. Research finds epigenetic errors occurring in several conditions, including pediatric disorders, cancers, immune disorders, neuropsychiatric disorders, autism spectrum disorders, and degenerative disorders (Ledon-Rettig, Richards, & Martin, 2012; Margaret McCarthy & Nugent, 2015). Evidence also suggests that environmental factors in early human development can influence adult susceptibility to chronic diseases.

Epigenetic toxins can take complete control of gene expression and thus gene availability. As cells divide, the changes can pass on to the next cell generation (Radtke et al., 2011; Wei, Schatten, & Sun, 2014). Some environmental effects may also pass on to future generations (Jirtle & Skinner, 2007).

Major epigenetic changes include histone modification, chromatin remodeling, non-coding RNA mechanism, and DNA methylation. The most broadly understood mechanism is DNA methylation, a biomarker for some diseases (Bommarito & Fry, 2019). Studies show that methylation, the addition of a methyl (CH3) group to affect gene expression, may play a significant role in long-term memory function. Methylation correlates with chromatin conformation and catalyzes DNA methyltransferases (DNMTs), a key player in silencing transcriptions (Jin, Li, & Robertson, 2011).

A recent Harvard University study (Knapton, 2019) found a "master control gene" within non-coding DNA that may allow controlled regeneration throughout the body. The scientists were able to control activation of the early growth response (EGR) to turn regeneration on and off in three-banded panther worms. They also discovered that DNA unfolds during regeneration, which allows new areas to activate.

Biotoxin illness is a transcriptomic illness. The human leukocyte antigen – DR isotype (HLA-DR) gene causes abnormal gene expression that renders the acquired immune system useless against biotoxins. The recent development of Genomic Expression: Inflammation Explained (GENIE), a gene expression assay for metabolic testing of chronic fatiguing illnesses, will help practitioners confirm differential gene expression to improve bio-individualized treatment plans.

COLD AND FLU SUPPORT

Drink 3-4 cups throughout the day

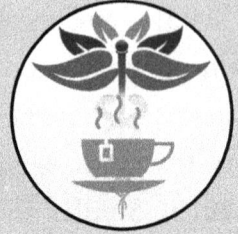

Ingredients

2 parts elderberries
1 cup water
2 parts echinacea root or leaves
2 parts calendula petals
1 part rose hips
1 part turmeric powder
1 part orange peel
1/2 part ginger root
(or 1 part fresh ginger root)
1/4 part cinnamon chips

Directions

Add elderberries to water and bring to simmer for 10 minutes

Turn off heat, add the rest of the herbs, and steep for 10 minutes

Strain into a mug

HLA Gene

The human leukocyte antigen (HLA) system found on the surface of every cell in the body is responsible for regulating the immune system. HLA genes fine-tune the adaptive immune system, help differentiate between pathogens and body tissue, and encode major histocompatibility complex (MHC) proteins.

There are three HLA MHC classes located on the sixth chromosome. Class I (A, B, and C) are responsible for attracting the invader and calling killer T-cells to destroy it. Class II (HLA - DP, DM, DO, DQ, and DR) stimulates the multiplication of helper T-cells (CD4+), causing invader antibody production. Class III encodes components of the complement system (C4a and C3a).

HLA genes are highly polymorphic, which means that they have many different alleles. Most chromosomes contain a coupling of alleles, one from the father and the other from the mother providing a haplotype. Fifty-four major HLA haplotypes assess risks and possible inflammatory responses.

About 25% of the population carry HLA-DR haplotypes that render their body incapable of natural immune system detoxification. The HLA by PCR blood test at LabCorp is a preliminary diagnostic tool (see Part 3: Finding a Diagnosis). The results on sections DRB1, DQ, DRB3, DRB4, and DRB5 are used to identify an individual's toxin susceptibility. Six of the HLA-DR haplotype sequences relate directly to biotoxin illness and one specifically to MARCoNS (Shoemaker, Heyman, Mancia, & Ryan, 2017).

Chronically ill patients who see short-term gains, no gain, plateau, or regress on conventional therapies should test for HLA-DR susceptibility. An inability to progress could indicate that the body has a high toxin load.

Quantum Medicine

Modern allopathic medicine is based on Newtonian physics and scientific materialism, creating anomalies and unaddressed paradoxes when confronted with the subatomic particles. Complex cases perplex some classically trained physicians because medical schools teach based on incomplete ideas. Carlo Rubbia, who shared the Nobel Prize in Physics in 1984, said, "matter is one billionth part of reality."

Quantum medicine uses scientific findings in physics, particularly quantum physics, for therapy. Natural medicine and innate plant intelligence can provide concrete tools for designing patient-centered, biologically individualized healing environments that support whole health. Merging quantum biology and quantum physics bestows cutting-edge and highly effective clinical tools that enhance patient outcomes.

Practicing quantum medicine means considering the whole health of the patient. A practitioner needs to empower the patient to shape their future while acting with compassion to cultivate a meaningful and productive transformational clinical relationship. As Philippus Aureolus Paracelsus, a Swiss physician and pioneer of the Renaissance medical revolution, once said, "The noblest foundation for medicine is love. It is love that teaches the art of healing. Without true love, healing cannot be born." Formulating a treatment plan within the primacy of consciousness, the practice of medicine transitions to being genuinely holistic. Typically, patients reciprocate and demonstrate their trust and acceptance of whole health healing by seeking support, guidance, and community resources to align themselves with core treatment compliance for successful outcomes.

Herbal Medicine

Natural medicine is a distinct system of primary health care that emphasizes prevention and the self-healing process through the use of natural therapies. The roots of naturopathic medicine date back to the 1890s. At the turn of the twenty-first century, a consumer movement to solve the healthcare puzzle granted a resurgence of naturopathic medicine.

Herbal medicine, also called botanical medicine or phytomedicine, refers to the art and science of using a plant's seeds, berries, roots, leaves, bark, flowers, and other natural substances for therapeutic medicinal purposes. Herbalism is one of the world's oldest healing arts dating back thousands of years in India and China, where herbal remedies treated a wide variety of diseases and disorders. Advances in science and clinical research pushed improvements in herbal medicine quality control, enabling clinically proven benefits.

According to the World Health Organization, over 80% of the world's population relies on herbs as their primary modality for the treatment of disease. Approximately 25% of all currently used pharmaceuticals, including aspirin, have their origins in plants (Nirmal et al., 2013). Herbal therapy can be a valuable, natural, complementary therapy for patients who are on drug therapies or as an alternative to over-the-counter treatments for children and adults. Modern formulations of natural medicines include herbs in pill or granulated form. Herbalism has a long and revered history treating both internal and external complaints.

BioNexus Health

BioNexus Health Clinic (BNH) is dedicated to scientifically formulated, naturopathic treatment options for adults, children, and families dealing with biotoxin illness, chronic inflammatory response syndrome (CIRS), autism spectrum disorders, Lyme disease, other tick-borne diseases, PANS/ PANDAS, and other chronic neurological diseases.

We believe it is the responsibility of clinicians to expand the limitations of conventional medicine's standard symptom versus illness checklist. A presenting symptom should be a clue that there is an underlying problem. Managing complicated cases requires understanding the possible explanations of confounding presentations and where it could originate. Navigating protocols for complex multisymptom conditions is a challenge for any practitioner. A chronic inflammatory response syndrome (CIRS) or MARCoNS diagnosis demands creative problem-solving to create a health plan for sensitive patients.

The BioNexus Approach was born out of necessity. My son's body, particularly his gut, was ravaged by allopathic medication. He needed an all-natural, plant-based protocol. The patients who come into BNH have been sick for several years and typically tried all the available treatment options. Some traveled the world seeking innovative solutions while spending a small fortune with every attempt at healing. Most arrive with severe histamine and mast cell issues making medicine selection, dosing, and tolerance levels a treacherous road to navigate. It took thousands of hours of research and many rounds of trial and error to find the plant-based options to treat environmentally acquired neuroinflammation.

Sensitive patients tend to gain more issues while taking allopathic pharmaceutical treatments. Many BNH patients fall into this subset, which poses an intriguing clinical challenge requiring a creative and effective solution to stop the low MSH cycle that causes the cascade of other issues. Formulating an effective herbal solution necessitated blending Ayurvedic medicine with the wisdom of western herbalism. The final formulas needed to meet two criteria: be entirely plant-based and effective at pediatric doses.

BioNexus Herbals are a unique range of small-batch proprietary herbal formulations developed for BNH patients. The herbs are sustainable, biodynamic, organic or wildcrafted, and consciously harvested. Even our most severely depleted patients benefit from our plant-based and highly customized treatment regimens.

There is a great need for practitioners who look at the full 360 and are capable of diagnosing and treating biotoxin illness as awareness of the disease spreads around the world. Outside the U.S., herbal medicine is not as stigmatized, and most of our international patients seek and prefer an herbal approach.

BITES & STINGS

Homeopathic options are available in pellets and liquid. If using a liquid, spray directly onto the bites and stings—otherwise, 5 pellets under the tongue 3x per day

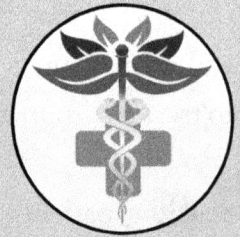

BioNexus Herbals Formula 4 IBT

Mix one dropper in any organic clay powder to form a paste and apply on the bite or sting *(see BNH Bite-Site Protocol in the BioNexus Herbals section of Part 4: Prepping the Approach)*

Homeopathic Options

Ledum 30C
Any puncture wound or jellyfish sting; the bite may feel cool

Apis 30C
Bee stings or insect bites; stinging pain that feels better to the touch

Aconite 30C
Feeling fearful or anxious; immediately after being bitten or stung

Cantharis 30C
Intense burning pain, redness, inflammation, or blistering

Hypericum 30C
Bite or sting in a nerve-rich area; feeling numbness, tingling, or shooting pain

GLYCERITE ALCOHOL-FREE

Popular herbs: ginger, burdock root, turmeric, dandelion, cleavers, chamomile

Instructions

In a jar, mix 1 part distilled water and 3 parts organic vegetable glycerine

Shake to combine liquids

Chiffonade or mince dried herb

In a different jar, fill 1/2 with the dried herb (2/3, if using fresh a herb)

Add liquid mixture to herb jar

Label jar with date, the ratio of water to glycerine, and herbs

Agitate jar daily for 4-6 weeks

Use cheesecloth to strain the liquid into a new jar

If finely chopped or powder herbs were used,
double filter (or use a coffee filter)
to remove all botanical material

Label new jar with date, the ratio of water to glycerine, and herbs

PART I

THE BIOTOXIN PATHWAY

"All truth passes through three stages. First, it is ridiculed. Second, it is violently opposed. Third, it is accepted as being self-evident."
—Arthur Schopenhauer (1788–1860)

Biotoxin illness is a highly complex, multisystem, and multi-stage disease. Patients diagnosed with chronic inflammatory response syndrome (CIRS) have severe multisystem dysfunction. Part 1: The Biotoxin Pathway presents simplified and pertinent information on each stage identified in Dr. Shoemaker's body of work and research. I recommend practitioners explore the disease more in-depth on survivingmold.com, a veritable treasure trove of evidence-based and peer-reviewed scientific information.

According to a 2013 Occupational Safety and Health Administration (OSHA) report, more than a quarter (25%) of all buildings in the United States are water-damaged (WDB). Faulty construction in new builds can be just as moldy as centuries-old buildings. Mold can grow in any building, at any given time, age and cleanliness are ancillary factors to consider when inspecting for water damage and mold. After natural disasters, building owners routinely visually inspect damaged areas. However, mold may find the right blend of moisture and humidity in inconspicuous areas too. Hidden spaces like crawl spaces, under sinks, attics, and behind walls pose more risk because they are harder to inspect.

The Environmental Relative Moldiness Index (ERMI) test has become the standard for most professionally trained mold inspectors. Samples need to be collected in all spaces and compared to an exterior sample for quality results. Frequently, due to a variety of factors, including cost, the sampling size does not reflect total square footage of a building, which leads to inaccurate results. An improperly administered test could result in a false-negative. If mold is present, at some point, a building occupant may see or smell mold. Usually, visually apparent mold has already circulated in the air and into the body of a mold susceptible person. Discovering mold at this late stage, in most cases, means that a fourth of the population has experienced puzzling and complex symptoms from their reactions to the mold, biotoxins, and their byproducts resulting in sickness.

A functional innate immune system efficiently removes mold and other toxins from the body. However, roughly a fourth of the population carries an HLA-DR haplotype making them genetically incapable of natural immune system detoxification (Shoemaker, 2010; Berry, 2014). The human leukocyte antigen (HLA) system is an integral part of disease defense. On the surface of every cell in the body, HLA genes are responsible for regulating the immune system and fine-tuning the adaptive immune system. They help differentiate between pathogens and tissue, and encoding major histocompatibility complex (MHC) proteins. There are 54 major HLA haplotypes. Each consists of HLA alleles used to assess risks and possible inflammatory responses. Seven of these haplotype sequences relate directly to biotoxin illness and two to post-Lyme disease (Shoemaker, Heyman, Mancia, & Ryan, 2017).

Chronically ill patients who see short-term gains, no gain, plateau, or regress on allopathic therapies should test for biotoxin illness. Their inability to progress could be an indicator that they are genetically susceptible to biotoxins and carrying a high toxin load that the body cannot discharge.

Stage 1: Biotoxin Effects

Pfiesteria, ciguatera, water-damaged buildings, blue-green algae, spider bites, red tide, and tick-borne diseases, especially Lyme disease spread and release tiny chemicals known as biotoxins. The small size of biotoxins allows them to pass between cells and through cell membranes that are unreachable by bigger toxins. Biotoxins crossing into the brain or across intestinal cell walls lay the groundwork for stage one, biotoxin effects, a complex cascade of cellular-level biochemical events across several systems leading to system-wide inflammation in genetically susceptible individuals.

The immune system of biotoxin illness patients is genetically incapable of correctly identifying biotoxins. Therefore the innate and adaptive immune systems also fail to expel the chemicals from the body. Unimpeded and untreated, biotoxins recirculate throughout bodily systems, potentially indefinitely, continuously triggering immune responses. An overactive innate immune system compounds system inflammation leading to dysregulation in several bodily systems, which could result in a CIRS diagnosis.

Part 2: Affected Systems goes more in-depth into the immune system and neurological components of biotoxin illness.

In addition to inflammation, CIRS patients also have high levels of transforming growth factor (TGF-beta1), a cytokine that affects growth and rapid reproduction of cell types. TGF-beta1 turns on differential gene activation enabling epigenetic mechanisms to express "bad genes." In immunocompromised people, especially those with biotoxin illness and autoimmune diseases, elevated TGF-beta1 levels are highly toxic.

BioNexus Health Clinic patients typically experience detoxification challenges from a variety of toxins, including biotoxins. The body detoxifies itself by binding and removing toxins through various system pathways, including nervous, vascular, lymphatic, and digestive. Practitioners should familiarize themselves with how the body detoxifies itself through these pathways and incorporate them into a thorough patient evaluation.

Nervous System Pathway

Neurons absorb toxins through the spinal cord or brainstem and send them to the brain. Biotoxins can also affect nerve cell function. The visual contrast sensitivity test (see Part 3: Finding a Diagnosis) provides additional information.

Vascular System Pathway

The portal vein takes in toxins and keeps them sequestered in a loop between the liver, gastrointestinal tract, gallbladder, spleen, and pancreas.

Lymphatic System Pathway

The thoracic duct, the largest lymphatic vessel, transports toxins to the left subclavian vein. The subclavian vein carries lymph, the fluid formed by body tissues. The thoracic duct also drains into the internal jugular vein, which transports toxins into the brain.

Digestive System Pathway

Bowel bacteria and tissues of the intestinal tract uptake roving toxins causing massive gut inflammation that may appear as classic Crohn's and colitis.

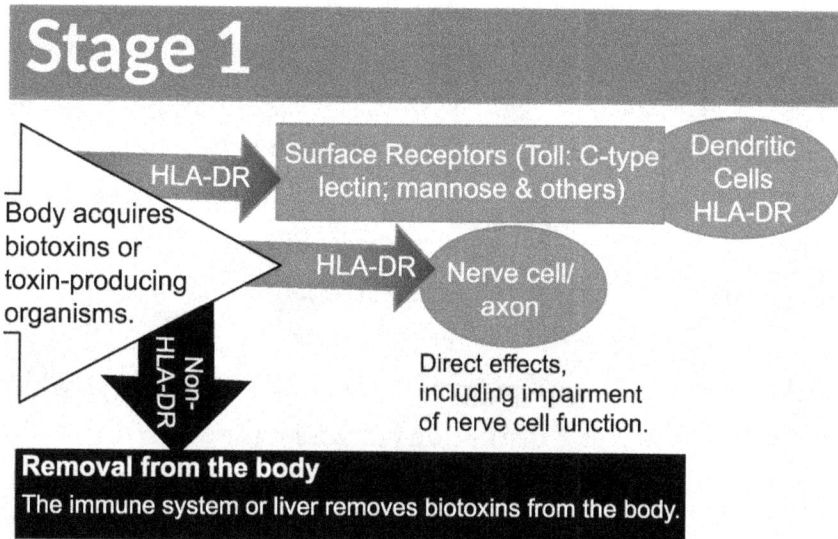

Figure 1. Stage 1: Biotoxin Effects. Adapted from R.C. Shoemaker, 2011.

Stage 2: Cytokine Effects

Stage two, cytokine effects, involves an immune system communication messenger known as a cytokine. Cells secrete cytokines into several substances, such as interferon, interleukin, and growth factors, to affect inflammation regulation. As a messenger, cytokines send modulation signals to other cells. The message generates the intensity and duration of the immune system response for itself, nearby cells, and sometimes a distant cell. A notified cell alters its function by either upregulating or downregulating cytokines.

During the first stage of biotoxin illness, there is already an upregulation and release of cytokines. Upregulation contributes to the production of more receptor blocking cytokines that release matrix metallopeptidase 9 (MMP-9) into the blood. Normal levels of MMP-9 repair and replace tissue. In an upregulated system, unnecessary inflammatory elements exacerbate inflammation in tissue, including the brain, muscle, lungs, and joints. MMP-9 is an essential marker for biotoxin illness to identify patients progressing towards chronic inflammatory response syndrome (CIRS).

Furthermore, biotoxins piggyback on MMP-9 delivery, which can cause further disruption across the systems. The upregulation of cytokines may also cause leptin receptor binding provoking hypothalamic dysregulation and heavily influencing body weight. A blockage forces the metabolism to become inactive and eventually induces a dramatic decrease in the alpha-melanocyte-stimulating hormone (MSH).

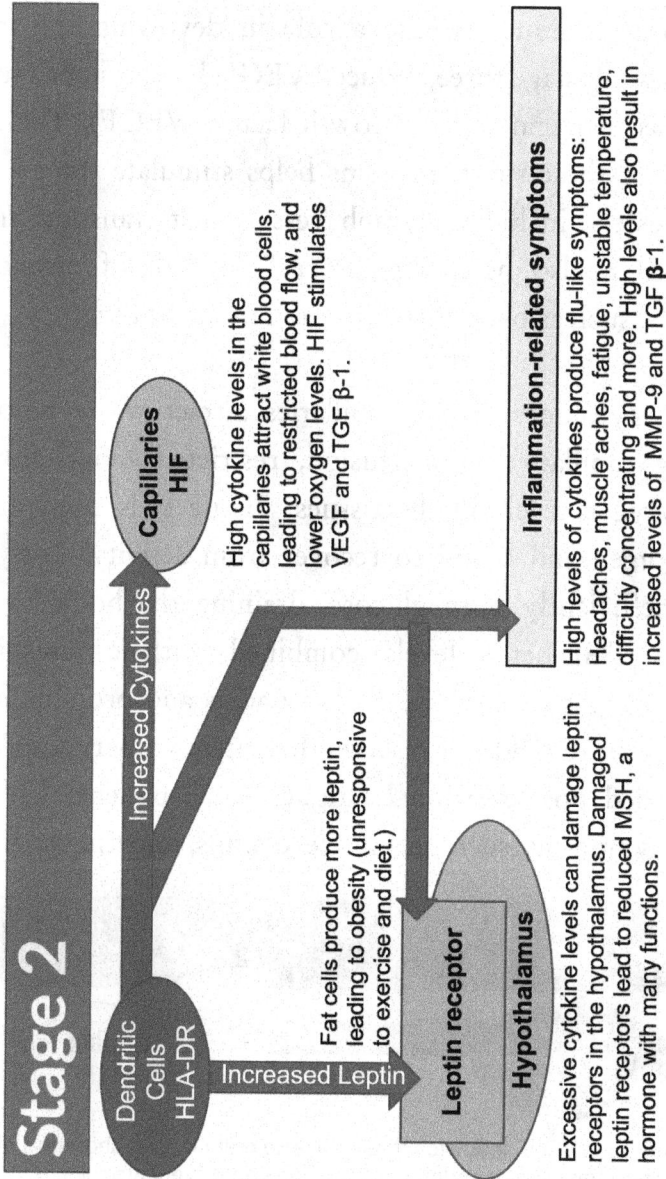

Figure 2. Stage 2: Cytokine Effects. Adapted from R.C. Shoemaker, 2011.

Stage 3: Reduced VEGF

Cytokines continue to play a role in devolving the immune system during stage three, reduced VEGF, by causing a reduction in the vascular endothelial growth factor (VEGF). The normal function of these signal proteins helps stimulate the growth of blood vessels, including lymph vessels that transport immune cells. VEGF also helps regulate cell growth of physiological functions, such as bone formation and tissue healing.

Elevated cytokines in the capillaries attract white blood cells inducing capillary hypoperfusion, restricted blood flow, and lower oxygen levels in the tissues. Tissue cells need nutrients from oxygen and blood to recover from activity. Low VEGF levels inefficiently burn glucose, draining the body's reserves. Elevated TGF-beta1 levels combined with diminishing fat reserves trigger the burning of fatty acids and proteins for fuel. As the body rebuilds its reserve, the patient experiences a phase of extended post-exertional fatigue. Some patients have more fatigue symptoms such as muscle cramps, shortness of breath,

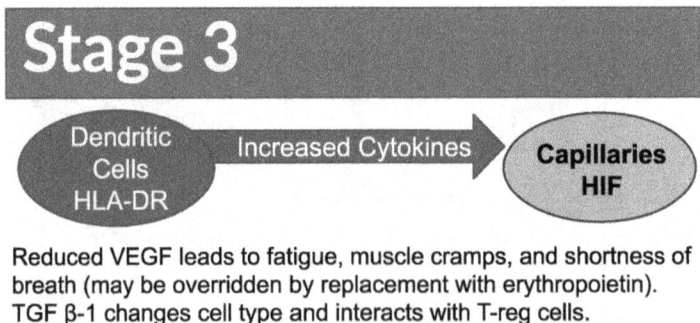

Stage 3

Dendritic Cells HLA-DR → Increased Cytokines → Capillaries HIF

Reduced VEGF leads to fatigue, muscle cramps, and shortness of breath (may be overridden by replacement with erythropoietin). TGF β-1 changes cell type and interacts with T-reg cells.

Figure 3. Stage 3: Reduced VEGF. Adapted from R.C. Shoemaker, 2011.

and mental confusion. Exceptional recovery periods might cause the patient to gain weight, even if the person eats less and exercises more.

Stage 4: Immune System Effects

Biotoxin illness becomes very serious in stage four, immune system effects. The patient experiences a severe and rapid onset of various symptoms. They are most likely receiving frequent treatments that have little to no effect. Some patients lose a lot of weight because they are not eating, leaving their nutrition in the gutter. Stage four adversely affects the pediatric endocrine system. Children often experience growth delays or may stop growing altogether. Some children may gain weight without changing their diet or eating habits.

When patients arrive at BioNexus Health Clinic in stage four, they typically take multiple pharmaceutical medications to balance and counter-balance their symptoms and side effects. The medication compensation commonly suppresses some symptoms but highlights others without directly addressing the underlying cause. Most of these patients spend years, even decades, without achieving any path to wellness. In all of our cases, biotoxins overloaded patients' systems, continuously adding to their toxin load multiplying their symptoms.

In our autism spectrum disorder patients, the pediatric cases were generally exposed and re-exposed to mold in their

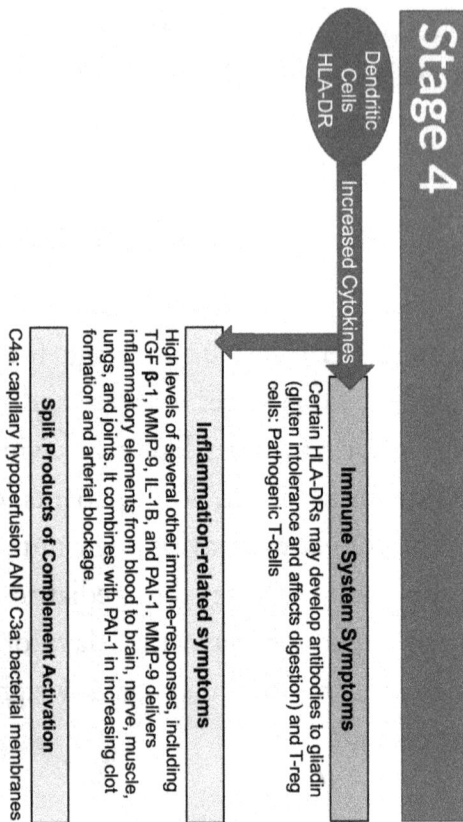

Figure 4. Stage 4: Immune System Effects. Adapted from R.C. Shoemaker, 2011.

residence, ABA (applied behavior analysis) therapy center, physical therapy office, and school. Autistic children spend hours in these locations. Genetically susceptible patients ride a roller coaster of emotions, behaviors, and symptoms triggered by mold.

The dysregulation of the immune response ultimately devolves in stage four, setting the stage for multiple opportunities for misdiagnoses. The impaired immune system begins producing antibodies enabling gluten sensitivity, ulcerative colitis, blood clotting, and other apparent symptoms. The immune system most commonly creates antibodies to actin, cardiolipin, myelin basic protein, and gliadin.

Actin, a critical player in cellular function, helps maintain cell shape, cell motility, and transcription regulation. It is also integral in several biological processes, including muscle contraction. In addition to moving limbs, organs, including the liver and heart, require muscle contraction to work.

Cardiolipin proteins are found in the mitochondrial membranes. Mitochondrial functions account for more than 90% of the energy organs need to function. Cardiolipin helps to convert energy and aids in respiration. Cardiolipin autoantibodies affect blood clotting and are commonly found in autoimmune diseases. These autoantibodies can lead to coagulation abnormalities when left untreated and may cause a lot of damage.

Myelin basic protein (MBP) helps protect the nerves. The protein plays a part in myelination, which is the production of myelin. Myelin is the fatty-white substance that surrounds some nerve cells and protects the electrical pulses of the nervous system. When antibodies occur, the protection around electrical pulses diminish and may cause communication issues between the brain and the rest of the body. These antibodies are commonly associated with multiple sclerosis (MS).

Gliadin proteins are commonly found in wheat, rye, barley, and oats. When the body creates an antibody to gliadin, it is unable to make enzymes to digest gliadin. Anti-gliadin attacks tissue transglutaminase enzymes resulting in volatile inflammatory processes and release of proinflammatory histamine, leukotrienes, prostaglandins, and cytokines. In extreme cases, it causes celiac disease. In minor cases, the result is non-celiac gluten sensitivity (NCGS). Both disorders cause gastrointestinal symptoms like constipation, cramping, and diarrhea, and may contribute to headaches, fatigue, and joint pain.

Biotoxin illness differs from allergies. Genetically-susceptible innate immune responses are not dose-dependent. Whereas allergic reactions are dose-dependent. For example, consuming gluten typically triggers allergies in proportion to the amount consumed. A little gluten amounts to a little bit of a bellyache. When biotoxin illness patients trigger anti-gliadin by eating a little gluten, the body reacts with substantial lower abdomen pain and a cascade of other issues.

During stage four, antineutrophil cytoplasmic antibodies (ANCA) production also increases. ANCAs are natural autoantibodies used by the immune system to regulate itself. High levels often indicate disease and are commonly associated with autoimmune diseases.

The most devastating component of immune system effects occurs in the complement system. Complement proteins (C4a and C3a) help the innate immune system fight off infection by reacting with one another to induce inflammation. If there are too many complements, it may trigger allergic reactions or cause tissue damage. Biotoxin illness commonly causes destructive chronic complement system activation resulting in elevated levels of complement C4a.

Stage 5: Low MSH

The pineal gland produces melatonin, the counter hormone to cortisol, a stress hormone. When a person's stress level increases, the production of these hormones becomes unbalanced, and the body produces less melatonin leading to insomnia and poor restorative sleep.

Alpha melanocyte-stimulating hormone (MSH) mentioned in stage two, is a stimulating hormone peptide produced in the pituitary gland. MSH controls several factors in the hypothalamus, hippocampus, cerebral cortex, spinal cord, and other regions of the brain. From these areas, MSH influences behavioral activity, memory, and attention.

In stage five, low MSH, the reduced MSH production causes more immune dysregulation that leads to malabsorption, or leaky gut. After the white blood cells lose regulation of the cytokine response, the body becomes exceptionally vulnerable to opportunistic infections like Lyme disease, PANS, parasites, and other diseases. Recovering from co-infections at this stage is also significantly reduced.

Decreased MSH suppresses endorphins causing chronic, severe, and often unusual pain in biotoxin illness patients. Patients may also complain about sleep problems, headaches, muscle aches, unstable temperature regulation, and difficulty concentrating.

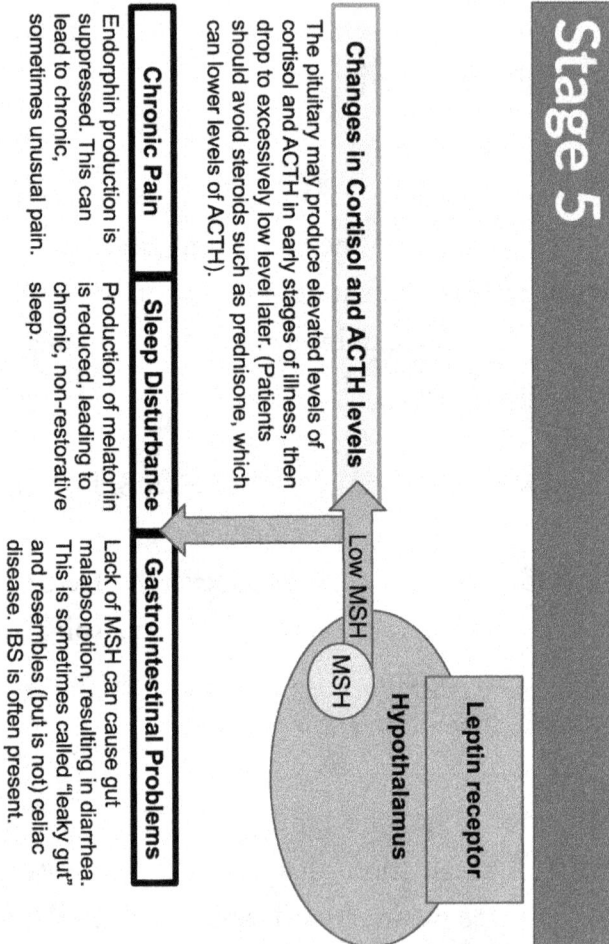

Stage 5

Changes in Cortisol and ACTH levels

The pituitary may produce elevated levels of cortisol and ACTH in early stages of illness, then drop to excessively low level later. (Patients should avoid steroids such as prednisone, which can lower levels of ACTH).

Chronic Pain	Sleep Disturbance	Gastrointestinal Problems
Endorphin production is suppressed. This can lead to chronic, sometimes unusual pain.	Production of melatonin is reduced, leading to chronic, non-restorative sleep.	Lack of MSH can cause gut malabsorption, resulting in diarrhea. This is sometimes called "leaky gut" and resembles (but is not) celiac disease. IBS is often present.

Low MSH

MSH

Hypothalamus

Leptin receptor

Figure 5. Stage 5: Low MSH. Adapted from R.C. Shoemaker, 2011.

*A **Clinical Note*** about "dramatic" children or those who slam body parts against things (ex. flapping hands and head butting walls). Most people feel slight pain when mildly injured. The pain subsides because endorphins rush in to block the pain. A patient with low MSH levels experience greater pain because of suppressed endorphin production. If an immunocompromised child screams, cries, or acts "dramatic" about their pain, it might be genuine pain. The child might have low MSH and is experiencing extreme pain. This is especially true for pediatric patients with chronic pain or inflammatory diseases.

Stage 6: MARCoNS

Coagulase-negative staphylococci (CoNS) are gram-positive bacteria with over 40 species that are mostly harmless and found on the skin and in mucous membranes. Multiple antibiotic-resistant coagulase-negative staphylococci (MARCoNS) are usually found deep in the nasal cavities and are evidence of stage six of biotoxin illness.

Methicillin-resistant Staph aureus (MRSA) has plagued the medical world for decades. Yet, MRSA is only resistant to methicillin, a semisynthetic penicillin-related antibiotic. A MARCoNS positive nasal swab indicates two or more antibiotic-resistant coagulase-negative staph bacteria in the nares. Unlike Staph aureus, MARCoNS sits silently under a biofilm (see Biofilm in the Appendix). The bacteria are protected from the immune system and regularly cause destructive multisystem dysregulation.

Normal MSH levels protect the mucous membranes from MARCoNS colonization. Stage six biotoxin illness patients already have low MSH levels due to fungal exposure, chronic Lyme disease, or CIRS creating an opportunity for a thriving MARCoNS colonization. The result is a perfect storm of possible infection and low MSH levels.

MARCoNS send hemolysin proteins into the bloodstream causing constant cytokine attacks (Shoemaker, 2010). The bacterial cells also secrete highly potent exotoxins A and B that cleave alpha-MSH, ensuring further MSH level depletion (Shoemaker, 2011).

Patients treated with antibiotics for more than one month are more likely to have MARCoNS and even lower MSH levels. Eighty percent of CIRS patients test positive for MARCoNS. Their genetically compromised immune system prevents their body from using its adaptive system, eventually causing adrenal fatigue. A cascade of issues set in, including hormone imbalances, mood swings, alternating diarrhea and constipation, leaky gut, and poor sleep. Lower antidiuretic hormone (ADH) and plasma

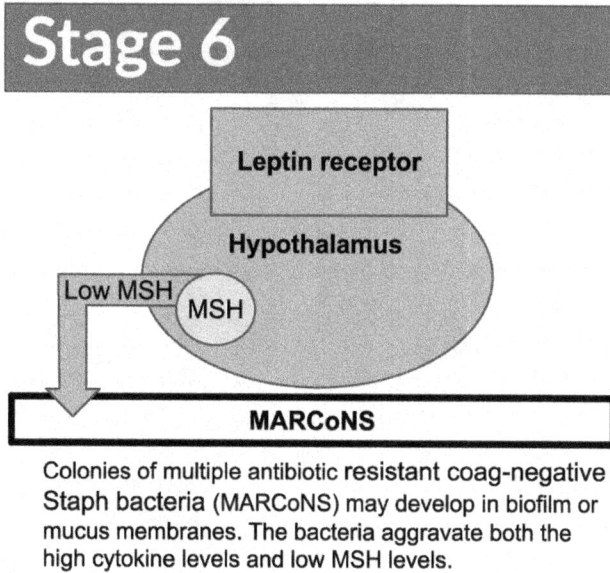

Figure 6. Stage 6: MARCoNS. Adapted from R.C. Shoemaker, 2011.

osmolality production create more salt on the skin causing static shocks, frequent urination, and chronic dehydration. Additionally, consistently low MSH levels increase cytokine production and fewer T-regulatory cells presenting as body aches, debilitating and unrecoverable exhaustion, chronic pain, and other chronic fatigue symptoms.

While MARCoNS most predominantly reside in the nasal cavity, it does not typically cause symptoms associated with sinus issues like a runny nose, facial pain, or sinusitis. In some patients, the same species of MARCoNS found in their nasal passages were found in their jawbones and dental work. Additional testing on pet canines was also positive for MARCoNS. These findings are being studied and explored.

Stage 7

Leptin receptor

Hypothalamus

MSH   VIP   AVP

Low MSH

Reduced Androgens

Reduced MSH can cause the pituitary to lower its production of sex hormones.

Reduced ADH

Reduced MSH can cause the pituitary to produce lower levels of antidiuretic hormone (ADH), leading to thirst, frequent urination, and susceptibility to shocks from static electricity.

Changes in Cortisol and ACTH levels

The pituitary may produce elevated levels of cortisol and ACTH in early stages of illness, then drop to excessively low level later. (Patients should avoid steroids such as prednisone, which can lower levels of ACTH).

Prolonged Illness

White blood cells lose regulation of cytokine response, so that recovery from other illnesses, including infections diseases, may be slowed.

Chronic Pain

Endorphin production is suppressed. This can lead to chronic, sometimes unusual pain.

Sleep Disturbance

Production of melatonin is reduced, leading to chronic, non-restorative sleep.

Gastrointestinal Problems

Lack of MSH can cause gut malabsorption, resulting in diarrhea. This is sometimes called "leaky gut" and resembles (but is not) celiac disease. IBS is often present.

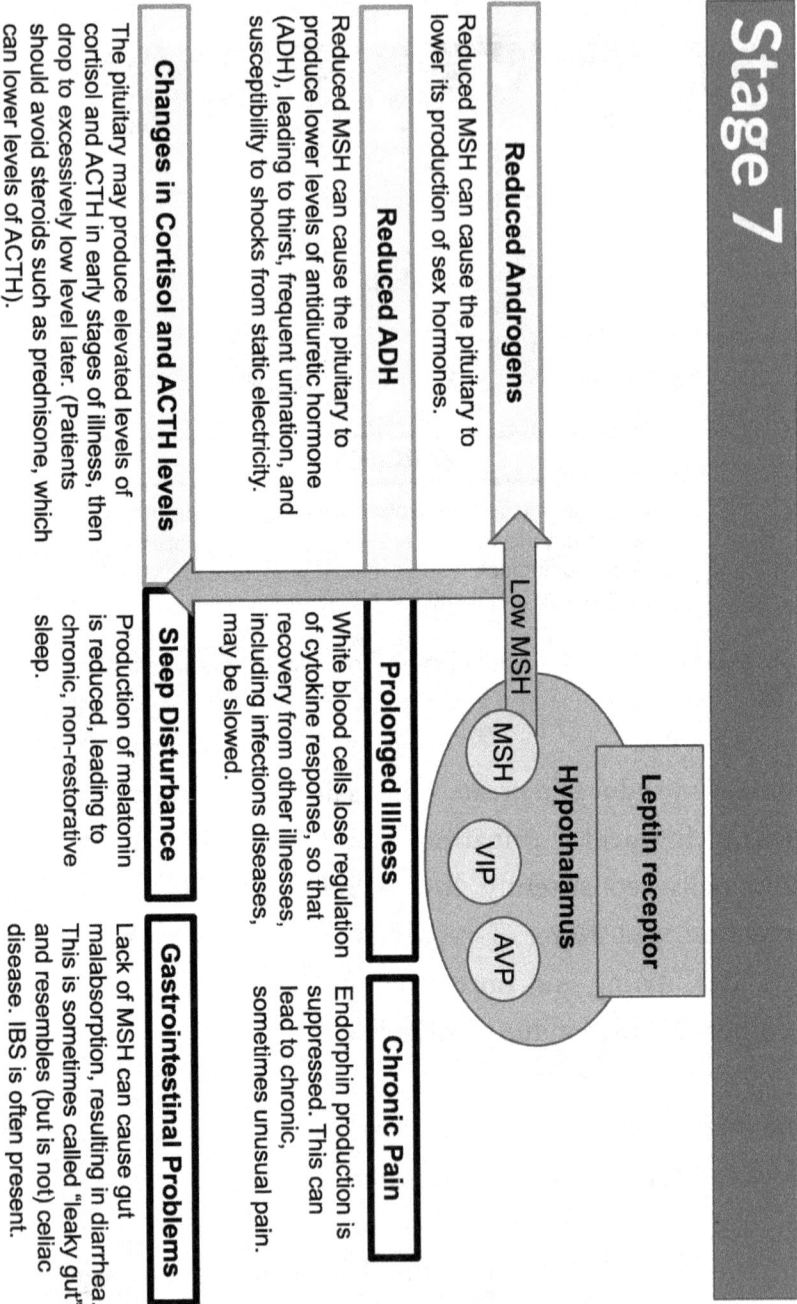

Figure 7. Stage 7: Pituitary Hormone Effects. Adapted from R.C. Shoemaker, 2011.

Stage 7: Pituitary Hormone Effects

Depleted MSH leads to deficient antidiuretic hormone (ADH) levels in stage seven, pituitary hormone effects. This deficiency causes lower blood volume, neurally mediated hypotension (NMH), and down-regulate sex hormones. The pituitary gland attempted to balance the change by initially upregulating cortisol and ACTH. As the disease progresses, the body cannot sustain the artificial production plummeting both cortisol and ACTH to abnormally low or low-normal ranges.

CIRS

Chronic inflammatory response syndrome (CIRS) is an ongoing dysregulation of the innate immune response, which is a deficiency of regulatory neuropeptides MSH and vasoactive intestinal polypeptide (VIP). MSH and VIP regulate several functions within the body. Dr. Shoemaker found these markers in more than 90% of patients in his initial studies.

CIRS patients often suffer from memory loss, inattention, easy confusion, difficulty assimilating new information, frequent trouble finding words while speaking, tremors, mood swings, sleep disturbances, and disorientation. Most CIRS patients have some degree of "brain fog," ranging from mild to debilitating.

A patient can live with biotoxin illness their entire life and may not notice it. Chronic exposure to biotoxins causes dysfunction in the immune and endocrine systems and metabolic issues. Patients experience uncontrollable infections, frequent illnesses, immune suppression, allergy/ sensitivity upregulation, multiple hormone dysregulation, and oxidative stress. A triggered response more often than not develops into CIRS in genetically susceptible individuals.

Patients presenting with prolonged or chronic environmental-related issues are most likely a CIRS candidate. The case definition of CIRS is a chronic, progressive multisymptom, multisystem illness caused by exposure to biotoxins (Shoemaker, R. C., Heyman, Mancia, & Ryan, 2017). A CIRS diagnosis requires a practical diagnostic approach that includes genetic predisposition, biomarkers, and symptom clusters following Dr. Ritchie Shoemaker's strict criteria (see Part 3: Finding a Diagnosis).

The Biotoxin Pathway

In HLA-DR genetically susceptible people, biotoxins bind to pattern receptors, causing continuing, unregulated production of cytokines.

Body acquires biotoxins or toxin-producing organisms.

HLA-DR → Surface Receptors (Toll; C-type lectin; mannose & others)

HLA-DR → Dendritic Cells HLA-DR → Increased Cytokines

HLA-DR → Nerve cell/axon

Non-HLA-DR

Direct effects, including impairment of nerve cell function.

Removal from the body
The immune system or liver removes biotoxins from the body.

Increased Leptin

Fat cells produce more leptin, leading to obesity (unresponsive to exercise and diet.)

Leptin receptor

Excessive cytokine levels can damage leptin receptors in the hypothalamus. Damaged leptin receptors lead to reduced MSH, a hormone with many functions.

Hypothalamus

Low MSH — MSH / VIP / AVP

MARCoNS

Colonies of multiple antibiotic resistant coag-negative Staph bacteria (MARCoNS) may develop in biofilm or mucus membranes. The bacteria aggravate both the high cytokine levels and low MSH levels.

Capillaries HIF

High cytokine levels in the capillaries attract white blood cells, leading to restricted blood flow, and lower oxygen levels. HIF stimulates VEGF and TGF β-1. Reduced VEGF leads to fatigue, muscle cramps, and shortness of breath (may be overridden by replacement with erythropoietin). TGF β-1 changes cell type and interacts with T-reg cells.

Immune System Symptoms

Certain HLA-DRs may develop antibodies to gliadin (gluten intolerance and affects digestion) and T-reg cells: Pathogenic T-cells

Inflammation-related symptoms

High levels of cytokines produce flu-like symptoms: Headaches, muscle aches, fatigue, unstable temperature, difficulty concentrating and more. High levels also result in increased levels of several other immune-responses, including TGF β-1, MMP-9, IL-1B, and PAI-1. MMP-9 delivers inflammatory elements from blood to brain, nerve, muscle, lungs, and joints. It combines with PAI-1 in increasing clot formation and arterial blockage.

Split Products of Complement Activation

C4a: capillary hypoperfusion AND C3a: bacterial membranes

Reduced Androgens

Reduced MSH can cause the pituitary to lower its production of sex hormones.

Reduced ADH

Reduced MSH can cause the pituitary to produce lower levels of antidiuretic hormone (ADH), leading to thirst, frequent urination, and susceptibility to shocks from static electricity.

Changes in Cortisol and ACTH levels

The pituitary may produce elevated levels of cortisol and ACTH in early stages of illness, then drop to excessively low level later. (Patients should avoid steroids such as prednisone, which can lower levels of ACTH).

Gastrointestinal Problems

Lack of MSH can cause gut malabsorption, resulting in diarrhea. This is sometimes called "leaky gut" and resembles (but is not) celiac disease. IBS is often present.

Prolonged Illness

White blood cells lose regulation of cytokine response, so that recovery from other illnesses, including infections diseases, may be slowed.

Sleep Disturbance

Production of melatonin is reduced, leading to chronic, non-restorative sleep.

Chronic Pain

Endorphin production is suppressed. This can lead to chronic, sometimes unusual pain.

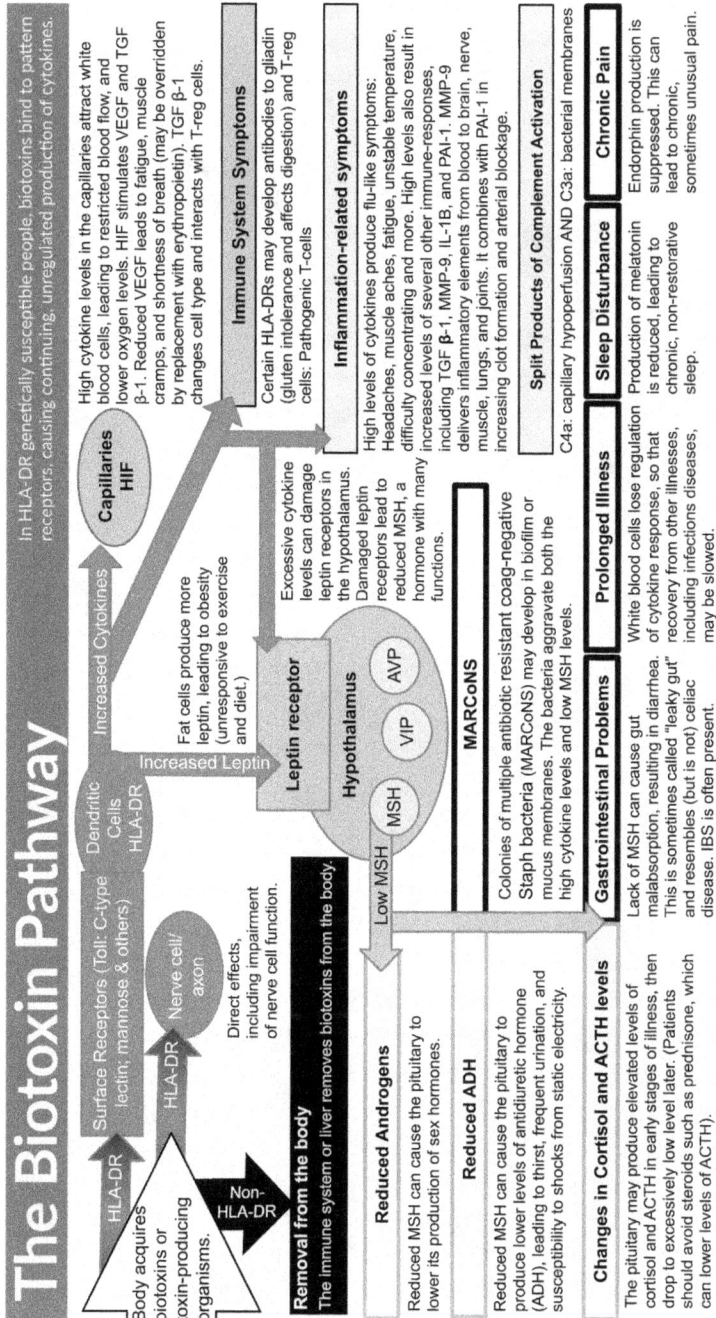

Figure 8. All seven stages of biotoxin illness. Adapted from R.C. Shoemaker, 2011.

PART 2

AFFECTED SYSTEMS

"It is far more important to know what person the disease has than what disease the person has."
—Hippocrates of Cos (c. 460 BC–c. 370 BC)

CIRS patients typically have a weakened blood-brain barrier due to the inflammatory processes, and commonly report various cognitive and executive function challenges. Dr. Shoemaker's NeuroQuant, a specialized brain MRI software, studies found statistically significant brain structure proportion differences in several areas of the brain: caudate nucleus, pallidum, left amygdala, parenchyma, ventricles, and right forebrain.

NeuroQuant research articles are available on PubMed and Dr. Shoemaker's website for those interested in additional information.

The human brain and function are explored in relative depth to give the reader some perspective on the brain changes and challenges seen in CIRS patients. Anyone with an in-depth understanding of the immune system and neurology can probably use this part as a reference to implement the BioNexus Approach to biotoxin illness.

Immune System

The immune system contains two points of attack for foreign invaders (pathogens). The first defense, known as the innate immune system, is the inborn system. This innate system acts as the gatekeeper and guardian to the rest of the body. The pathogen fighters, including antimicrobial proteins (broad-spectrum fighters); inflammatory responses; and phagocytic cells (white blood cells - lymphocytes, macrophages, mastocytes, and basophils) rove the skin, secretions, and mucous membranes to protect the body. When the innate immune system identifies and tags a pathogen, it provides a non-specific and rapid response to the infected area using a variety of methods to expel the toxin from the body.

Mast cells (mastocytes), rich in histamine and heparin, patrol the mucous membranes, skin, gut, lungs, connective tissue, and bloodstream. They act as mini-factories producing large quantities of cytokines and chemicals that can change blood flow and shift body fluids. Mast cells are the immune system's multipliers and can become dangerous for mold/ biotoxin illness patients (Shoemaker, Schaller, & Schmidt, 2005). Severe CIRS cases at BioNexus Health Clinic typically suffer from Mast Cell Activation Syndrome (MCAS) and require sensitive approaches to their care (see MCAS sections throughout the book).

If the initial innate responses are unable to eradicate the pathogen, then the immune system sends in the secondary, specific response utilizing the acquired immune system. This response is a learned defense system that the body has acquired from a previous infection. The body has the ability to store how it previously destroyed an invader and release specific antibodies to fight off the re-infection. As an example, most people only acquire varicella (chickenpox) once. That is because the body's acquired immunity recorded antibodies that defeated the pathogen. When a person is re-exposed to chickenpox, the body sends in its innate fighters. After this attack fails, the body sends in the specific response antibodies to expel the chickenpox from the body. Flu shots are a medically manufactured example of our acquired immune system. Small doses of the expected flu strains are injected into the body. This dose allows a healthy person to identify and "tag" the pathogen to develop antibodies. As flu season begins, those re-exposed to the flu strains delivered in the shot will most likely be able to fight the pathogens and remain in good health.

If a person receives a flu shot, yet still comes down with the flu, there are two potential reasons. The obvious reason is that the person became infected with a new strain of influenza, which was not included in the flu shot or previously acquired by the person. The second reason is that their body's acquired immune system is not functioning correctly. In regards to biotoxins, Dr. Shoemaker, in his book, Surviving Mold (2010), discusses a segment of the population who go through a circular non-diminishing relapse process when they are exposed to biotoxins because of their genetically impaired acquired immunity.

Those with biotoxin illness are more likely to have genetically defective acquired immunity. This subset of the population has a biological marker on chromosome 6 in the Human Leukocyte Antigen complex known as HLA-DR. HLA genes are found on the surface of every cell in the body to help the immune system identify foreign antigens and ignites the process for antibody production (Steere et al., 2006). In the HLA-DR population, there is an inability to produce specific protective antibodies. Without antibodies, the immune system sends the wrong signals that lead to a cascade of inflammatory responses (Shoemaker, 2010).

Low melanocyte-stimulating hormone (MSH) causes dys-regulation across several systems. The presence of multiple antibiotic-resistant coagulase-negative staphylococci (MARCoNS) only serves to send the body into further disruption creating an inability to function and regulate appropriately. This disruption has dramatic effects on the immune system. To survive, MARCoNS consume the natural sources the body utilizes to defend itself. MARCoNS release hemolysins (small proteins) into the blood that destroy red blood cells. The iron from the red blood cells provides a food source for the bacteria. When the hemolysins release into the bloodstream, it also creates an additional storm of cytokine production, leading to further inflammation. MARCoNS produced exotoxins A and B (ETA and ETB) cleave alpha-melanocyte-stimulating hormone (alpha-MSH), an endogenous neuropeptide hormone regulating immune cell activity, rendering it useless (Rago et al., 2000; Taylor, 2013).

The Brain

A cursory understanding of brain anatomy and neuroanatomy, particularly the subcortical structures, is needed to help navigate the symptoms, diagnoses, and treatment of this complex multisystem, multi-symptom illness. Abnormalities in the CIRS brain cause a cascade of health issues throughout the body.

The body's central processor, the brain, controls the majority of its functions. It innately controls all of the vital minutiae like balancing melatonin and cortisol to regulate sleep, controlling body temperature, and sending messages of hunger and thirst. The brain operates twenty-four hours a day, consciously and subconsciously ensuring homeostasis. The hidden assistant manages higher brain functions like thoughts, memories, behaviors, moods, communication, and decision making. The spinal cord (the "messenger") and the brain combine to compose the central nervous system (CNS). Together, they coordinate activity across the body. All of the CNS processing occurs in the brain.

The cerebrum's neuroanatomical structures organize the CNS. It encompasses the inner nerve fibers ("white matter") that connect to the nerve cells in the cerebral cortex ("gray matter"), subcortical structures of the limbic system (amygdala, hippocampus, hypothalamus, and thalamus) and basal ganglia.

Anatomically, there are three major brain regions: hindbrain, midbrain, and forebrain. The hindbrain is subdivided into sub-regions that regulates autonomic functions, relays sensory information, maintains balance, and coordinates movement. Movement is controlled by the midbrain, where visual and auditory data is also processed. The midbrain and hindbrain make up the brainstem.

The cerebellum ("little brain") resides wholly in the hindbrain. Nerve fibers ("white matter") are covered by a thin layer of cerebral cortex ("gray matter") that controls muscle tone, equilibrium, balance, and movement coordination. The neuron filled area processes data and relays information for motor control. The cerebellum contains two hemispheres and three lobes (anterior, posterior, and flocculonodular) to process the information received from the central nervous system and brain. Damage to the cerebellum or its nerves could result in speech difficulties, lack of eye movement control, balance control issues, and an inability to perform accurate movements.

A large bundle of nerve fiber tracts, called the cerebral peduncle, in the anterior portion of the midbrain connects the hindbrain to the forebrain. The tegmentum structure of the cerebral peduncle contains a nerve cluster in the brainstem that relays motor and sensory signals to the brain. The neurotransmitter dopamine is produced within the substantia nigra. The midbrain also contains the cerebral aqueduct, a canal that connects the third ventricle to the fourth ventricle.

The forebrain, the most prominent brain region, is subdivided into the telencephalon and diencephalon regions. There are four lobes (temporal, occipital, parietal, and frontal), the basal ganglia, and parts of the limbic system (amygdala and hippocampus) that make up the telencephalon region. The forebrain lobes are responsible for processing sensory information, controlling motor function, and performing high-level tasks like problem-solving and reasoning.

The diencephalon region connects the endocrine system to the central nervous system to regulate autonomic, endocrine, and motor functions; and contributes to sensory perception. The hypothalamus and thalamus (parts of the limbic system), and the pineal gland are a part of the diencephalon subdivision.

White Matter

Nerve fibers make up the white matter of the brain. These fibers, nerve cell axons, connect the cerebral cortex ("gray matter") to different areas of the brain and spinal cord. Lipids and proteins form a myelin sheath, an insulating coat around the nerve fibers, making the brain appear white.

Loss of the myelin sheath causes neurological issues and disrupts nerve transmission. Inflammation, immune disorders, and nutritional deficiencies can also occur from damage to the myelin sheath.

Cerebral Cortex

The cerebral cortex ("gray matter") is a thin layer of tissue that covers the brain surface of the cerebrum and cerebellum. It's commonly referred to as gray matter because the uninsulated (lacking myelin sheath) nerves appear gray against the white matter.

The gray matter is the most complex and developed part of the brain. Anatomically it is within the forebrain and responsible for several functions including, language, thinking, and perception. These functions are managed in the lobes. The brain is also divided in the center from front to back, creating the brain hemispheres. Each of the lobes contains a left and right side that correspond to the brain hemispheres.

Cerebral Hemispheres

In most people, the left side of the brain is the logic center and controls the right side of the body. It is here that analytic thought, language, reasoning, math, science, and writing occur.

The right side of the brain controls the left side of the body and is responsible for artistic and creative endeavors. The right side spurs the imagination, intuition, insight, music, art, and holistic thought. It is also the emotion center.

Figure 9. Cerebrum: white matter, cerebral cortex ("gray matter"), amygdala, hippocampus, hypothalamus, thalamus, and basal ganglia.

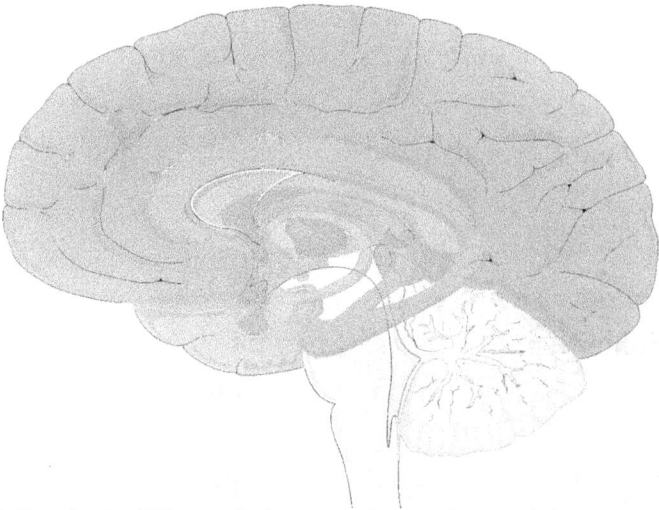

Figure 10. Forebrain: Telencephalon - cerebrum, frontal lobe, parietal lobe, temporal lobe, occipital lobe, basal ganglia, lateral ventricles, and limbic system's amygdala and hippocampus.

Diencephalon - pituitary gland, pineal gland, third ventricle, and limbic system's hypothalamus and thalamus.

The brain's other two regions (midbrain and hindbrain) and subcortical structures also contain left and right hemispheres to network for higher-level functions like reasoning and problem-solving. This is also the reason the forebrain lobes are referred to in the plural. For example, there is both a left and right frontal lobe, collectively called frontal lobes.

Frontal Lobes

The frontal lobes' two subdivisions [prefrontal cortex and motor cortex (primary motor cortex and premotor cortex)] control decision-making, problem-solving, movement, and planning. Complex cognitive processes (memory, planning, reasoning, and problem-solving) are managed by the prefrontal cortex. It helps to curb negative impulses, organize events, maintain goals, and it forms an individual's personality. The motor cortex controls voluntary and directed muscle movements, including the hands and face.

Inflammation or damage to the frontal lobes can cause apathy, lack of inhibition, diminished fine motor skills like speech and language processing, difficulties thinking or temporarily retaining information, changes in personality, paralysis, and a lack of facial expression, including Broca's aphasia (Huang, 2017).

Temporal Lobes

The temporal lobes house long-term memories, process auditory information sent by the sensory pathway, and convert it into an emotional meaning, including the ability to understand speech. The temporal lobes contain two parts of the limbic system (amygdala and hippocampus), which plays a vital role in the CIRS brain.

Damage to the temporal lobes drastically impairs word memory and language comprehension (Huang, 2017).

Parietal Lobes

The neurons in the parietal lobes receive sensory information from the thalamus. The somatosensory cortex within it uses touch input to identify objects, understand spatial relationships, and determine pain and temperature (Kandel, Schwartz, & Jessell, 1991). The parietal lobes coordinate with the appropriate area of the brain for further actions like a response, visuospatial navigation, language processing, and coordination (Huang, 2017).

The Parietal lobes also aid in cognition, speech, visual perception, reading, writing, and math computation. Damage within the lobes may cause deficiencies in writing, reading, recall of names for everyday items, an inability to properly move the

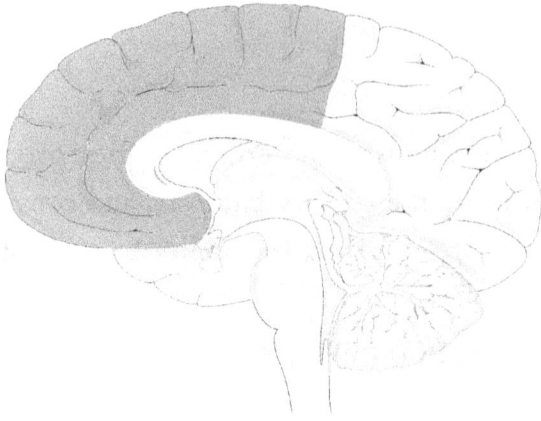

Figure 11. Frontal Lobes: prefrontal cortex and motor cortex.

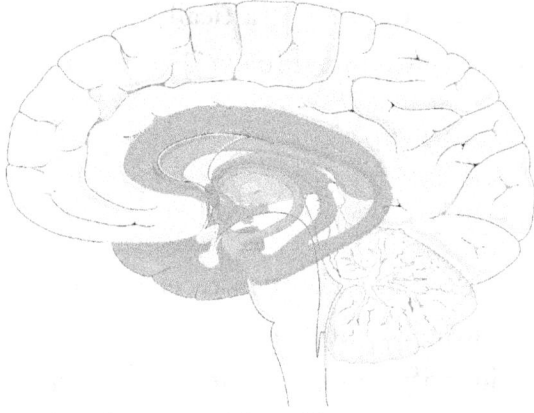

Figure 12. Temporal Lobes: amygdala and hippocampus.

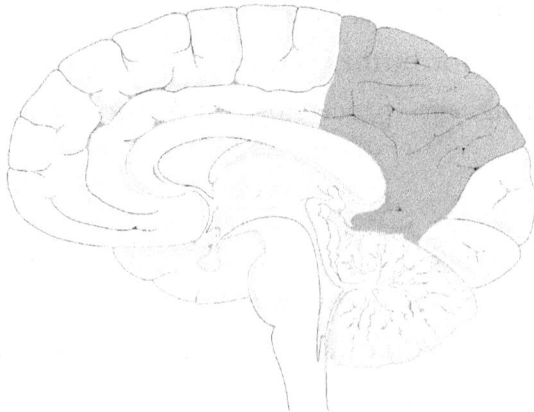

Figure 13. Parietal Lobes: somatosensory cortex.

tongue or lips to speak, distinguishing between different types of touch, attention disorders, an inability to perform or create order to complex tasks (Norris, 2017; Huang, 2017), and reduced body awareness. The symptoms can help identify left and/ or right hemisphere damage (Kimera, 1977).

Occipital Lobes

Visual information received from the sensory pathway is identified as colors, objects, words, shapes, and other visual perceptions. The information received passes to the parietal and temporal lobes for further understanding. The occipital lobes work in tandem with other lobes to perform tasks that require multiple senses like hand-eye coordination.

Located at the back of the brain, the occipital lobes are not prone to injury. Any significant damage may result in visual defects,

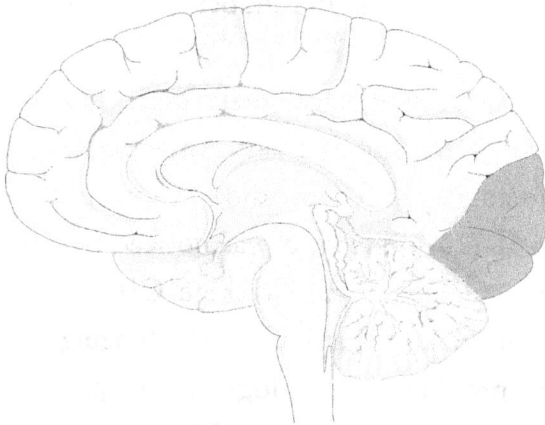

Figure 14. Occipital Lobes: coordinates with other lobes to understand sensory information.

including vision loss, hallucinations, perception, and an inability to identify words and colors (Benarroch, Westmoreland, Daube, Reagan, & Sandok, 1999). Vision loss may also occur in patches, blind spots, or by hemisphere (Kandel, Schwartz, & Jessell, 1991).

Limbic System

Located in the middle of the brain, under the cerebral cortex and at the top of the brain stem is the limbic system. It plays a role in emotions and motivations, including survival, eating, and sex. The limbic structures play a clinical role in the CIRS.

The limbic system is a complex set of structures from different areas of the brain. The forebrain telencephalon contributes the amygdala and hippocampus, and the diencephalon subdivision contributes the thalamus and hypothalamus. These structures influence the peripheral nervous system (counterpart to the central nervous system) and the endocrine system.

The **amygdala** is the brain's fear analyzer. It controls the way the body emotionally reacts to an event. Amygdala inflammation has been linked to anxiety and depression (Mehta et al., 2018). In the Shoemaker et al. (2014) study, it was noticed the left hemisphere amygdala was enlarged in the average CIRS brain. While the specific functions of each amygdala are still being studied, the left is believed to provide a more logical perception to emotional information (Gläscher & Adolphs, 2003). A study by Hardee,

Thompson, and Puce (2008) also found patients with a damaged left hemisphere amygdala had greater deficits in recognizing fear in other people's eyes.

The **hippocampus** helps to store long-term memories and is responsible for noting the location of people and objects. Natural stem cells generate new neurons here through a process known as neurogenesis. This process is associated with cognitive and emotional functions (Vasic & Schmidt, 2017). Inflammation decreased neurogenesis, and structural changes in the hippocampus lead to cognitive deficits and impairments, as well as psychiatric disorders (Green & Nolan, 2014).

Located in the diencephalon subdivision of the forebrain, the **hypothalamus** controls autonomic functions of the peripheral

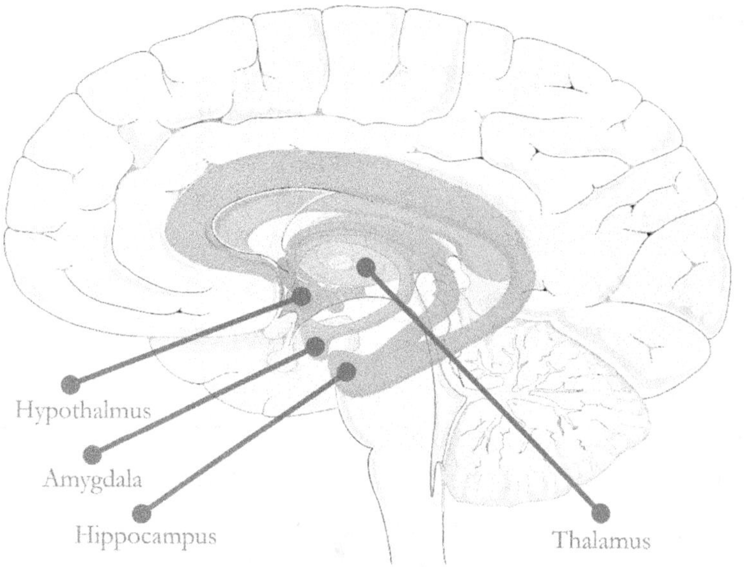

Figure 15. Limbic System: amygdala, hippocampus, hypothalamus, and thalamus.

nervous system and maintains equilibrium in the endocrine and nervous system by monitoring and adjusting physiological processes. The hypothalamus produces hormones that influence puberty, growth, and sex drive; regulates appetite, stress, water levels, and blood pressure; and it also influences metabolism and body temperature. Dysfunction, injury, or inflammation in the hypothalamus results in abnormal organ function and causes irregular body temperature, water balance, sleep cycles, and weight control (Cai & Liu, 2011; Valdearcos, Xu, & Koliwad, 2015; Le Thuc et al., 2017). It may also influence the pituitary gland's control of the thyroid gland, adrenal glands, and gonads.

Within the parietal lobe, the **thalamus** (mass of gray matter) identifies information sent by the sensory pathway and the peripheral nervous system in the brain stem. Nerves connect the thalamus to the cerebral cortex and hippocampus to relay the information to the appropriate lobe for further processing. Damage to the thalamus causes various cascading physiological malfunctions, including vision, sleep disorders, excessive pain, loss of sensation, memory problems, and chronic fatigue (Nakatomi et al., 2014).

Basal Ganglia

Deep in the cerebral hemispheres is a group of nuclei that are collectively known as the basal ganglia. These nuclei primarily provide the cerebral cortex with a feedback loop of increased or decreased motor function. Parts of the basal ganglia form side feedback loops that are believed to be involved with learning, cognition, and emotion (Stocco, Lebiere, & Anderson, 2010; Weyhenmeyer & Gallman, 2007). In the CIRS brain, the most affected structures are the caudate nucleus and globus pallidus (also part of pallidum with ventral pallidum) (Shoemaker et al., 2014).

Primarily located in the frontal lobe, the C-shaped caudate nuclei curves in the temporal lobe at the amygdala. Each hemisphere of the brain contains a nucleus that plays a vital role in learning and decision making (Lewis, Dove, Robbins, Barker, & Owen, 2004; Knierim, 1997), and is important to executive cognitive function,

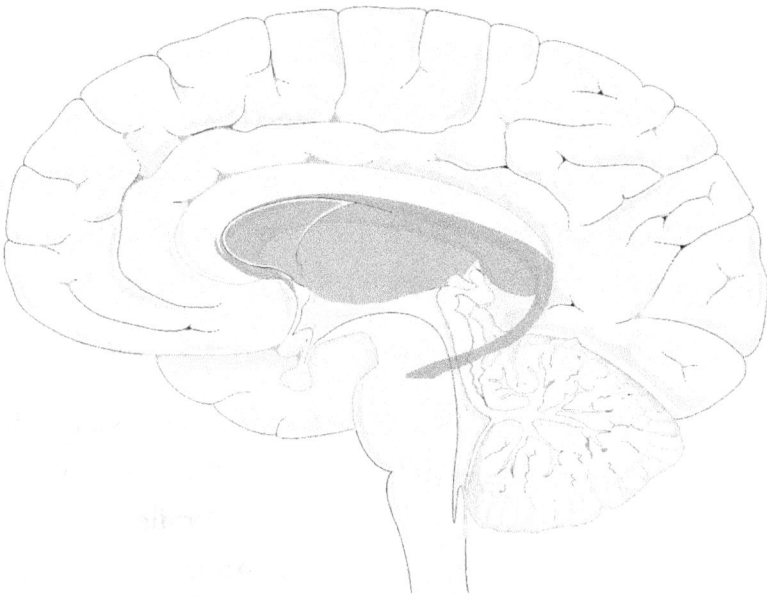

Figure 16. Basal Ganglia: Striatum (Caudate and Putamen), Ventral Striatum, Pallidum (Globus Pallidus and Ventral Pallidum), Substantia Nigra, Subthalamic Nucleus.

motor processing, and planning. It influences unconscious and long-term memory storage, associative and procedural learning, and inhibitory control to act as an evaluation processor.

If you imagine a funnel, the caudate nucleus fills the top third, while the globus pallidus fills the remainder. The external (lateral) rests near the caudate, and the internal (medial) segment sits on the other side. Like the caudate nucleus, each hemisphere of the brain has a globus pallidus. The ventral pallidum's output nucleus fibers project to thalamic nuclei and combine with the globus pallidus to form the pallidum. Together they relay neural visual emotional expression to and from the inferior prefrontal cortex as a part of the limbic loop (Koob, Moal, & Thompson, 2010).

The basal ganglia contain two distinct transmission pathways from the cerebral cortex that have an equalizing effect on the thalamic structures. The feedback loop closes when results arrive back in the cerebral cortex. The pathways are known as direct and indirect. The direct pathway works to excite the cortex, while the indirect pathway inhibits it. The caudate nuclei represent a part of the first synapse in both pathways receiving axons of spinal cord motor neurons (afferent nerve fibers) from the various areas of the cerebral cortex. The internal globus pallidus is also a part of both pathways, while the external (middle) is only a part of the indirect pathway. It's generally believed the pathways work to create a balance for an appropriate motor response (Knierim, 1997).

Prior experiences passed through the caudate nucleus are used to influence goal-directed actions, decision making, and planning (Grahn, Parkinson, and Owen, 2008; Wan et al., 2012). Several neurological disorders are a result of damage to the basal ganglia, including Parkinson's disease and Huntington's disease. A 2006 study by Voelbel, Bates, Buckman, Pandina, & Hendren found lesions in the caudate nucleus lead to impairments in problem-solving, mental flexibility, learning, attention, and short-term and long-term memory. While the caudate nuclei have yet to be fully understood, it's long been believed the left caudate works with the thalamus to learn communication skills. O'Dwyer et al. (2016) found that decreased volume in the left caudate is associated with autism spectrum disorder. Brain specialists hypothesize the development of obsessive-compulsive disorder (OCD) is an uncontrolled transmission of worry and concern from the basal ganglia transmission loop to the orbitofrontal cortex via the thalamus. A study by Hansen, Hasselbalch, Law, and Bolwig (2002) supported that the caudate plays an important role in the development of OCD.

Pituitary Gland

Known as the "Master Gland," the pituitary gland controls several important bodily functions as a part of the endocrine system. It's also a part of the forebrain diencephalon subdivision, and functionally and structurally connected to the hypothalamus (limbic system). Located in the middle of the base of brain, the pituitary gland translates messages from the nervous system into endocrine hormones.

Endocrine hormones regulate growth and endocrine function, as well as stimulate other endocrine glands, muscles, and kidneys. The adrenocorticotropin (ACTH) hormone stimulates the adrenal glands to produce cortisol, a stress hormone that regulates metabolism and immune response. The antidiuretic hormone (ADH) hormone helps to maintain water balance. Low ADH leads to thirst, frequent urination, low blood volume, neurally-mediated hypotension (NMH), and static electric shocks.

Insufficient hormone production creates deficiencies of brain hormones and downstream hormonal factories like the thyroid gland, adrenal gland, and gonads. Eighty percent of CIRS patients suffer from low melanocyte-stimulating hormone

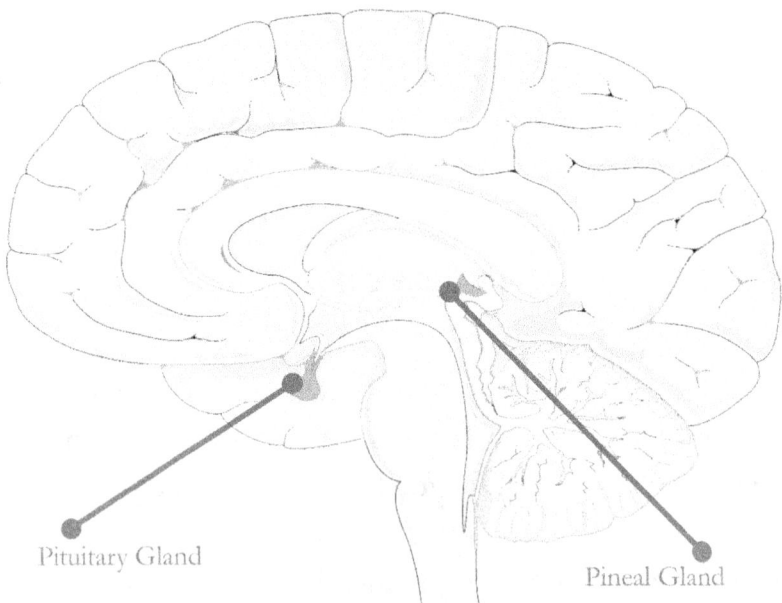

Pituitary Gland

Pineal Gland

Figure 17. Pituitary Gland and Pineal Gland: center of the brain between the brain's cerebral hemispheres.

(MSH), which is primarily made in the hypothalamus and partially in the pituitary gland. MSH regulates inflammation and immunity, yet has cascading effects: pituitary hormone production, limbic system regulation, circadian rhythms, and weight and pain perception (Shoemaker, Heyman, Mancia, & Ryan, 2017). The skin, blood, respiratory system, and gastrointestinal tract are "patrolled" by MSH. A deficiency of MSH leads to leaky gut, a breakdown of the intestinal barriers (Beck & Schachtrup, 2011).

Pineal Gland

In the center of the brain, between the two hemispheres, sits the pineal gland that is attached to the third ventricle. The pineal gland, hypothalamus, and thalamus comprise the forebrain diencephalon structure.

A part of the endocrine system, the pineal gland produces melatonin, which affects sleep cycles and sexual development. It also connects the nervous system to the endocrine system, converting nerve signals sent by the sympathetic system, a part of the peripheral nervous system, into hormone signals. The pineal gland is comprised of glial cells from the nervous system and pinealocytes.

Melatonin produced in the pineal gland is regulated by the hypothalamus, which directs production based on the light signals received from the eye's retina. Darkness increases melatonin production sent into the third ventricle's cerebrospinal fluid and then moves into the blood to promote sleep.

In children, melatonin production also impacts reproductive system development, a component of the endocrine system. Reduced melatonin levels impede the pituitary hormone gonadotropins that stimulate the release of sex hormones in the gonads, the male and female reproductive organs. Low melatonin reduces estrogen levels in females and testosterone production in males. In both cases, hypogonadism may occur and result in delayed puberty or failure to produce sex hormones due to the damage to the pituitary gland or hypothalamus (Ali & Donohoue, 2016; Kansra & Donohoue, 2016). Excessive melatonin levels may cause precocious puberty. Girls who begin puberty before age eight and boys before age nine are considered to be in precocious puberty. Their bones and muscles rapidly grow, and the body may begin reproduction development (Berberoglu, 2009). Dysfunction in a child's endocrine system may also cause children to be shorter than the average adult. These children tend to stop growing earlier than the average child. Traumatic brain injury has been linked as a cause of precocious puberty, although the exact mechanisms have yet to be determined (Reifschneider, Auble, & Rose, 2015; Shaul, Towbin, & Chernausek, 1985).

Insufficient melatonin production, in children and adults, may result in anxiety, insomnia, menopause, hypothyroidism (low thyroid hormone production), or intestinal hyperactivity. High melatonin production causes abnormal adrenal and thyroid gland function, low blood pressure, or seasonal affective disorder (SAD), also known as the "winter blues."

Brain Ventricles

The hollow spaces in the brain are called ventricles. They are filled with cerebrospinal fluid and connected by larger channels and small pores, called foramina. The ventricles provide a pathway for the cerebrospinal fluid to move throughout the central nervous system (brain, spinal cord, and networked neurons), protect the brain and spinal cord from trauma, and provide nutrients to the structures of the central nervous system. According to the volumetric MRI study using NeuroQuant by Shoemaker et al. (2014), CIRS patients showed generalized shrinking of the brain ventricles.

There is one lateral ventricle in each brain hemisphere of the cerebrum. Shaped like a horn, they span through all four cerebral cortex lobes (frontal, parietal, temporal, and occipital) with the central area located in the parietal lobe. Both lateral ventricles connect to the third ventricle.

In a narrow cavity in the middle of the forebrain diencephalon structure sits the third ventricle. It is formed by and connected to several structures important to CIRS, including the thalami. The hypothalamus (limbic structure) form part of its base. The right and left thalamus (limbic structure) make up its lateral walls. White matter (nerve fibers) form a portion of the anterior wall.

ESSENTIAL OIL BATHS

Essential oils are extremely powerful; hydrate with electrolytes and minerals <u>before and after</u>

Dilute Essential Oils

Dilution with carrier oil is very important; please refer to the General Essential Oils Dilution Chart in Part 4: Prepping the Approach

Preferred Essential Oils

Ginger: For a deeper detox

Jasmine: Helps dry, sensitive skin and soothes emotions

Lemon & Sweet Orange: Benefits oily skin and creates a happy, uplifting mood (do not use within an hour of sun exposure)

Lavender & Ylang-ylang: Benefits all skin types and calms the nervous system

Parsley: For improved drainage

Hot Basic Detox Bath

1 cup baking soda
1 cup Epsom salts
1-2 tsp diluted preferred essential oils (eucalyptus or rosemary are also good options for a detox bath)

Soak for 20 minutes or less

The posterior wall is partly formed by the pineal gland. Bands of gray matter cross over it, connecting the right and left thalamus. In addition to the third ventricle linking to the pineal gland, endocrine system, and limbic system structures, it also connects to the fourth ventricle.

The fourth ventricle begins at the brain stem and encases the spinal cord. It is the central aqueduct for transporting cerebrospinal fluid that began in the lateral ventricles. The fluid is responsible for moving metabolic waste, antibodies, chemicals, and pathological products away from the brain and down to the lumbar region. The volume of cerebrospinal fluid depends on several factors, including brain inflammation—the fluid acts as a volumetric equalizer. If the brain volume decreases, then the ventricles and amount of cerebrospinal fluid increase; conversely, if the amount of blood or tissue increases in the brain, then the cerebrospinal fluid decreases its volume. Brain inflammation causes the ventricles to decrease in volume, whereas brain atrophy causes an increase.

The purpose of the Shoemaker et al. (2014) MRI NeuroQuant study was to look at the volume of the brain in chronic inflammatory response syndrome (CIRS) patients. In the study, they compared the mean volumes of structures of CIRS-WDB patients against controls. A generalized pattern was observed. An enlargement of the brain parenchyma (functional tissue) structures showed coincident decrease of the brain ventricles and cerebrospinal fluid volume.

Blood-Brain Barrier

The brain is protected from toxins and pathogens in the bloodstream by the selective blood-brain barrier. Lining the inside of the brain's blood vessels are endothelial cells. These cells create a nearly impermeable boundary between the bloodstream and the brain. Cells on both sides of the blood-brain barrier signal when to allow or block molecules through the barrier.

Brain infections, inflammatory stressors, and tiny ruptures in the blood vessels can wear down or break the barrier. This weakness may allow toxins and pathogens direct access to the brain. A compromised blood-brain barrier has been associated with or shown to precede neurodegenerative diseases. In the case of

FEVER REDUCING TEA

Tasty option for both children and adults to help sweat out and reduce fevers

Ingredients

1 part catnip leaf
1 part elderflower
1 part spearmint leaf

Optional

Ginger, turmeric, and honey
5 drops - Homeopathic Aconite 30 C
5 drops - Belladonna 12C

multiple sclerosis, too many white blood cells enter the brain and attack the myelin that protects the white matter nerve cells. The 2014 Shoemaker et al. MRI NeuroQuant study found chronic volumetric abnormalities and inflammatory markers (blood levels of TGF-beta1, C4a, MMP9, and VEGF) increase permeability and integrity of the blood-brain barrier (Shoemaker & House, 2006).

MARCoNS Toxins

Approximately 67% of CIRS patients lack normal regulation of ACTH and cortisol. This is due in part to MARCoNS cleaving MSH when it releases exotoxin A and B, and the constant feedback loop created by hormone dysregulation (Shoemaker, Heyman, Mancia, & Ryan, 2017).

MARCoNS releases exotoxins A and B. Exotoxin A is known to be made by coagulase-positive Staph aureus and are also found in MARCoNS isolates. Studies have shown each of these toxins has potent and severe effects on the immune system. More research is needed; however, in MARCoNS, the most devastating effect is the cleaving of alpha-MSH.

Alpha-MSH is an important mediator within the immunosuppressive ocular micro-environment. Cleaving of alpha-MSH impairs its contribution to promoting induction of mucosa surfaces (CD4+CD25++) regulatory T cell. Thus, lowering T cell production (Taylor, 2007). This becomes important for the complement system, which is also affected by MARCoNS.

Proopiomelanocortin (POMC)-derived peptides are responsible for regulating appetite suppression, body weight, and energy balance in the melanocortin system.

CASTOR OIL PACK
Do not share castor oil packs; compostable

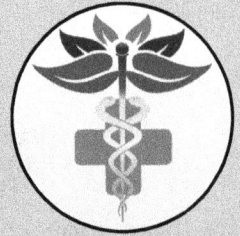

Cut enough flannel to cover the desired area

Place flannel in an oven-safe glass (or enamel) pan

Fill the pan with high-quality castor oil, covering the flannel (approximately 2-8 oz)

Turn the oven on to the lowest heat and warm the flannel; not hot

Place the warmed flannel pieces on the desired area

Cover the flannel with a heavy piece of cloth (old sweater, wool, etc.)

Use a hot water bottle wrapped in an old towel to retain heat

Lie down and rest for at least an hour

Refrigerate castor oil flannel in a glass container
Suitable for approximately twenty uses

POMC prohormone processing involves proteolytic cleaving by prohormone converting enzyme 1 (PC1) and prohormone converting enzyme 2 (PC2). PC2 stimulates food intake (Mountjoy et al., 2018), while PC1's post-translational processing of ACTH1-39 to ACTH1-13 produces endogenous alpha-MSH that significantly reduces food intake (Gumbiner, 2001; Millington, Tung, Hewson, O'Rahilly, & Dickson, 2001).

Loss of restful sleep and disruption to the circadian rhythms are the dominant features of inflammatory illnesses. When energy molecule (ATP) production plummets, biotoxin illness patients are left feeling fatigued after attempting normal activities. Their recovery process is frequently extended from a few minutes to several days due to a mitochondrial break down of glucose.

Hemolysins

Study of the lethal effects of hemolysins ramped up in the late 1920s after 21 children were inoculated with diphtheria toxin-antitoxin in Australia. Within 48 hours, 12 of the children were dead. This tragic event created mass awareness of the toxic and potentially invasive properties of staphylococci (Wiseman, 1975).

The first mechanism MARCoNS deploys is the release of hemolysins, a protein chain of 22 amino acids that form "tetramers," a four-member matrix of hemolysins (alpha, beta, gamma, and delta). The primary function of these proteins is to find nutrients for bacterial growth and survival. The HLA gene encodes alpha-hemolysin (Gray & Kehoe, 1984).

After secretion, alpha-hemolysins seek to integrate into the membrane of a target cell, forming cylindrical heptamers in the cell membrane. The toxin monomer binds and incorporates into the cell membrane (Belmonte et al., 1987; Mellor, Thomas, & Sansom, 1988), creating a pore. The toxin has numerous effects on the cell, including osmotic swelling that causes a breakdown of cell integrity (Dinges, Orwin, & Schlievert, 2000).

In the bloodstream, the immune system identifies alpha-hemolysin as foreign invaders, setting off cytokine production, damage to the leptin receptors, and a further reduction in MSH production.

The hemolysins persistently seek to steal iron from red blood cells to feed the bacteria. Hemolysins also release exotoxins that seek to destroy alpha-MSH, which again further perpetuates the low MSH cycle.

MOOD TEA

Drink 3-4 cups throughout the day

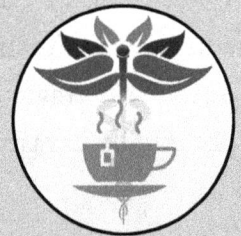

Ingredients

3 parts lemon balm leaves
2 parts St. John's wort
  flower and leaf
2 parts milky oat tops
2 parts spearmint leaves
1 part linden leaf & flower

Directions

Steep 1-2 tablespoons of tea blend per cup of water for 10-15 minutes

Add honey to sweeten

Optional squirt of lemon and zest

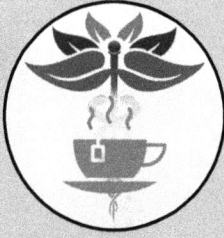

BOOST RESPIRATORY IMMUNITY TEAS

One

Prepare ginger and tulsi tea
Add 1/2 dropper: reishi, astragalus, and licorice tinctures
Drink 1/2 - 1 cup; 2 - 3x per day

Do not use licorice for extended periods

Synergistic Essential Oils in Diffuser:
Equal parts: frankincense, ravensara, palo santo, and orange

Two

4 tbsp astragalus root
Simmer in 4 cups water for at least 15 minutes
Add 1 tablespoon cardamom seeds and steep
Fill 1/2 - 1 cup and add 1/2 dropper Chaga tincture
Drink 2 - 4x per day

Synergistic Essential Oils in Diffuser:
Equal parts: lemon balm, lavender, geranium, and eucalyptus

PART 3

FINDING A DIAGNOSIS

"When most physicians look for evidence of inflammation they order standard tests such as C-reactive protein (CRP) and erythrocyte sedimentation rate (ESR). Since these are the tests most physicians are familiar with for detecting inflammation, most physicians miss CIRS. Furthermore, many physicians are trained in a one-system specialty. As a multisystem illness, CIRS is hiding in broad daylight."

—Scott McMahon, MD (2018)

The case definition of chronic inflammatory syndrome (CIRS) is a chronic, progressive multi-symptom, multisystem illness caused by exposure to biotoxins. Dr. Shoemaker divides the diagnosis into three criteria tiers:

Tier 1: History
Tier 2: Laboratory Tests
Tier 3: Response to Treatment

Assess every patient as an individual because biotoxin illness presents in a multitude of ways. Every patient has their own set of symptoms that require a bio-individualized protocol. Symptom presentation may even change over time and may demand a tweak to the protocol.

Toxins come from a variety of sources, including various types of mold and bacteria. Their effects on the health of the patient can range wildly, adding to the complexity of the diagnostic challenge because toxins can act synergistically and reshape their impact at any given moment.

Genetic susceptibility to mold negatively affects the immune system. A patient with a dysfunctional system can develop additional toxic sensitivities that will compound health issues. Despite overall system complexity and unique presentations, there are defined symptom clusters that, once identified, make a diagnosis reasonably straightforward.

Finding a diagnosis explains the key elements of Dr. Shoemaker's CIRS diagnosis criteria. A patient must meet the requirements of a tier before progressing to the next one. Anyone with an in-depth understanding of Dr. Shoemaker's diagnosis criteria for CIRS may reference this section to craft their BioNexus Approach for treatment and laboratory testing.

Symptoms

The thirteen lists of biotoxin illness symptoms (see right and following pages) on the following pages have been divided into general categories to help practitioners navigate the various affected systems. These categories differ from the CIRS symptom clusters in the CIRS tiered criteria. Many patients will exhibit several of the symptoms, while others might have only a few. A tiny number will have all the symptoms.

Anergy
BioNexus Health Clinic patients typically present three different immune reactions: anergy, allergy, and autoimmunity.

AUTONOMIC SYMPTOMS

- Abnormal body temperature
- Capillary hypoperfusion
- CCVSI
- Delayed recovery
- Hypotension
- Increased pulmonary artery pressure
- Night sweats or increased sweating
- Pulmonary anomalies
- Tachycardia
- Tics: Vocal or motor
- Trouble standing or sitting (orthostatic intolerance)

BODY SYMPTOMS

- Appear stiff when moving around
- Arthritis
- Cold/clammy feet and hands
- Dizziness
- Fainting when standing
- Hair loss
- Hyper-flexibility
- Marfanoid habitus
- Muscle cramps
- Poor balance
- Shoulder muscle or grip weakness
- Skin: Pallor, flushing, red sclera, rashes (mold facies), keratosis, rosacea, raynaud's disease, edema, easy bruising
- Slow wound healing
- Tender abdomen, soft tissue tenderness
- Tumors
- Unsteady gait
- Vertigo
- Weight: Overweight or unusual weight change

Anergy is the lack of an immune response. It prevents the innate immune system from doing its job and creates an opportunity for infection overrun.

Several parents of BioNexus Health Clinic's pediatric patients think the lack of fevers is a sign of a healthy child. It is actually the opposite. A functional immune system produces a fever to fight off infections like the common cold, sinus infections, and ear infections. Never running a fever is a warning sign of possible immune dysfunction.

Tier 1: History

A thorough evaluation includes a laborious history, past medical records, symptoms, and a physical exam. An extensive physical examination aids in identifying several factors of Tier 1 and could provide clues to specific bodily dysfunction. As a practitioner moves through each of the tiers of diagnosis, the goal is to rule out biotoxin illness. Tier structure helps practitioners avoid unnecessary testing.

Exposure

Potential exposure to biotoxins needs to be confirmed. Explore the patient's history to discover if they have been exposed to water-damaged buildings, Lyme disease, other tick-borne infections, spider bites, or exposed to ciguatera.

BEHAVIORAL SYMPTOMS

- Abnormally tardy
- Anger episodes
- Anxiety
- Bipolar or manic episodes
- Brain fog
- Decreased empathy
- Decreased sociability
- Depression
- Inability to process interpersonal trauma or pain
- Inappropriate or poor responses to stress
- Irritability
- Isolation from friends or feel that friends are enemies
- Low or loss of self-confidence
- Mood swings
- Narcissism
- OCD
- PANS/ PANDAS
- Poor sleep or sleep disturbance
- Romanticizing suicide
- Suicidal thoughts

COGNITIVE SYMPTOMS

- Appetite swings
- Blood sugar issues
- Confusion
- Constipation
- Decreased learning ability
- Diarrhea
- Difficulty organizing information
- Difficulty concentrating
- Difficulty processing instructions or treatment plans
- Digestive symptoms
- Disorientation in familiar places
- Excessive thirst
- Forgetful
- Frequent urination
- Heartburn
- Insomnia
- Irritable bowels
- Issues with executive function
- Liver problems
- Metallic taste
- Nausea
- Poor short term memory
- Poor word recall
- Trouble with math or remembering numbers
- Quick to frustration and overwhelm

Explore all the buildings a patient visits during history assessment. Any structure may be the source or contributing trigger. Also, consider vehicles, mobile homes, and other possible causes of exposure. Water-damaged buildings host a myriad of different toxins, including:

- mold (toxic metabolic fragments and filaments);
- microbial growth (bacteria, fungi, mycobacteria, and actinomycetes); and
- inflammagens (mannans, beta-glucans, hemolysins, proteinases).

Furthermore, practitioners need to consider other underlying causes, such as Lyme disease. Dr. Shoemaker's research shows 21% of the population is genetically susceptible to post-Lyme syndrome on the HLA gene. Borrelia burgdorferi (Lyme disease) produces biotoxins, and genetically susceptible people are less responsive to traditional antibiotic treatment.

Assess a patient's exposure to neurotoxin producing invertebrate species, including dinoflagellates (red tide and ciguatera), cyanobacteria (freshwater blue-green algae Cylindrospermopsis and Microcystis), and Pfiesteria-associated Possible Estuary Associated Syndrome (PEAS).

The rule of thumb is to consider anything that produces neurological and/or biological toxins. Additionally, if a patient presents with multisystem or confounding symptoms, biotoxin illness should be considered.

ELECTRICAL SYMPTOMS

- Convulsions
- Seizures
- Static shock

- Tremors, fidgeting, muscle
  jerks or twitches

ENDOCRINE SYMPTOMS

- Atypical hypothyroidism
- Decreased testosterone
- Low DHEA level

- Low growth hormone level
- Poor growth
- Weak adrenal function

HEARING SYMPTOMS

- Decreased ability in active
  listening
- Hearing loss

- Sensitivity to sound
- Tinnitus

ENVIRONMENTAL EXPOSURES QUESTIONNAIRE

The environmental exposures questionnaire helps practitioners navigate the various possible sources of exposure

1. Do you have exposure to the interior of a water-damaged building and/or microbial growth?
   a. Do you have samples/evidence of spore or genus and species of fungus? (air test, ERMI test, etc.)
   b. Is there visible microbial growth (mold)?
   c. Is there a presence of musty smells?

2. Do you remember a tick bite occurring before your illness beginning?
   a. Did you have an unexpected rash after the bite?
   b. Did you experience a flu-like illness after the bite?

3. Have you had a brown recluse or another poisonous spider bite?
   a. Did you experience a flu-like illness after the bite?

4. Did you become ill after eating fish?

5. Did you become ill after exposure to a fresh body of water?

6. Did you become ill after exposure to the ocean during a "Red Tide" or another type of bloom?

7. Did you become ill after exposure to an estuary fish kill?

8. Did you become ill after exposure to a closed shell fish bed area?

IMMUNE SYSTEM

- Chronic lymph node swelling
- Chronic lymph node pain
- Increased infections
- Frequent colds
- Never experiences colds or the flu

PAIN SYMPTOMS

- Abdominal pain
- Body aches
- Burning
- Fibromyalgia
- Headaches
- Ice-pick pain
- Itching
- Joint pain
- Migraines
- Morning muscle or joint stiffness
- Muscle cramps
- Numbness in limbs
- Pain or tingling: abdominal, arm, back, chest, chronic, cycles, feet, hip, joint, legs, lungs, sinus, vulvar
- Skin sensitivity

REPRODUCTIVE SYMPTOMS

- Decreased libido
- Endometriosis
- Erectile dysfunction
- Hormone imbalances
- Infertility
- Vulvar pain or tingling
- Yeast or bacterial infections

Differential Diagnoses

Practitioners need to rule out other possible diagnoses. Many patients will have a history of at least one diagnosis. Consider that the patient may have received a misdiagnosis if the patient fails to respond to treatment, plateaued during treatment, or regressed post-treatment. It is also common for patients to receive a diagnosis and still have unexplained symptoms that do not fit their diagnosis.

Patients diagnosed with a wide variety of diseases routinely find their conditions improve after receiving a biotoxin illness or CIRS diagnosis and treatment. Too many of these patients were never tested for inflammatory markers or dysregulation. A collection of blood tests stood between perpetual disease and a path to a healthier life. See Clinical Note: Diagnoses Where CIRS Might Be The Root Cause for common misdiagnoses received by biotoxin illness/ CIRS patients who improved or lost symptoms during treatment.

Clinical Cluster Questionnaire

The clinical cluster questionnaire was determined by statisticians to maximize accuracy. There are 37 CIRS symptoms grouped into eight organ system categories and 13 symptom clusters (See Figure 18). Each cluster contains one to five symptoms.

RESPIRATORY SYMPTOMS

- Asthma
- Chronic cough
- Inability to speak loudly
- Nasal congestion
- Nasal or vocal polyps or nodules
- Sinus infections
- Shortness of breath or exercise intolerance
- Sleep apnea
- Stuffy nose

SENSITIVITY SYMPTOMS

- Alcohol
- Chemical
- EMF
- Foods: dairy, gluten, meat, seafood, or new intolerances
- Light, sound, touch
- Medication

VISION SYMPTOMS

- Blurred vision
- Burning eyes
- Low visual contract sensitivity (VCS)
- Poor night vision
- Red eyes
- Tearing

Children typically complain about one continuing symptom

Symptom Organ System Categories

- General symptoms
- Muscles
- Neurological
- Respiratory
- Cognitive
- Eyes
- Gastrointestinal
- General fatigue and weakness

If the patient confirms the symptom for more than two weeks, then the response is "Y" for yes or "N" for no. A yes answer to at least one symptom in a cluster equals one point. Otherwise, the cluster result is zero.

A CIRS diagnosis requires adults to present symptoms in at least eight clusters (8 points), whereas pediatric patients only need six points.

Patients meeting the criteria move on to Tier 2: Laboratory Tests.

SYMPTOM CLUSTERS	Y or N	1 if ≥ Y
Fatigue		
Weakness		
Decreased assimilation of new knowledge		
Aches		
Headache		
Light sensitivity		
Memory impairment		
Decreased word finding		
Difficulty concentrating		
Joint pain		
A.M. stiffness		
Cramps		
Tingling		
Tremors		
Unusual pain		
Unusual skin sensitivity		
Shortness of breath		
Sinus congestion		
Cough		
Excessive thirst		
Confusion		
Appetite swings		
Difficulty regulating body temperature		
Increased urinary function		
Red eyes		
Blurred vision		
Sweats (night)		
Mood swings		
Ice-pick pain		
Abdominal pain		
Diarrhea		
Numbness		
Tearing of eyes		
Disorientation		
Metallic taste		
Static shocks		
Vertigo		
TOTAL POINTS		

Figure 18. Clinical Cluster Questionnaire. R.C. Shoemaker, 2012.

DIAGNOSES WHERE CIRS MIGHT BE THE ROOT CAUSE

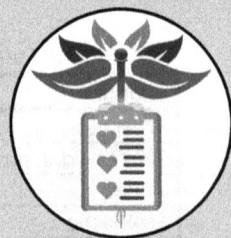

ADD/ ADHD

Allergy

Anxiety

Arthritis

ASD / Asperger's

Asthma

Autoimmune disease

Bell's palsy

Bipolar

Celiac disease

Chronic fatigue syndrome

Crohn's and colitis/
   Ulcerative colitis

Depression

Dermographism

Diabetes - Type 1

Edema

Endometriosis

Erectile dysfunction

Fibromyalgia

Grave's disease

Hypotension

Irritable bowel syndrome

Keratosis

Lupus

Marfanoid habitus

Multiple sclerosis

Obesity

OCD

Parkinson's disease

Post-Lyme disease

PTSD

Raynaud's disease

Red sclera

Rheumatoid arthritis

Rosacea

Sensory processing disorder

Somatization

Stress

Tachycardia

Tinnitus

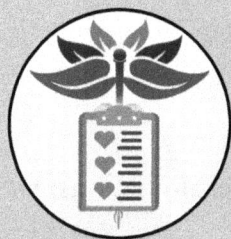

ADDITIONAL CLINICAL OBSERVATIONS

Parasites

- Aggravations around the full moon (bloating, etc.)
- Children crave foods that feed parasites (sugar, etc.)
- Discoloration around the mouth
- Elevated eosinophils and absolute eosinophils in CBC (10%)
- Fatigue
- Pimples within the hair
- Rashes on the chest, back, or neck
- Odd, aggressive, self-injurious behaviors

Pediatric CIRS

- Primary nocturnal enuresis
- Severe asthma
- Unexplained joint or muscle pains
- Chronic abdominal pains
- Chronic headache
- Fatigue
- Inattentiveness, ADD/ ADHD
- PANS

Viruses

- Cold sores or canker sores that are often cyclical
- Debilitating anxiety
- Enlarged lymph nodes
- Fatigue
- Tinnitus and noise sensitivity

Yeast

- Brain fog
- Concentration difficulties
- Fatigue
- Gas and bloating
- Headaches
- High pitched squealing
- Flushed cheeks
- Stimming in children
- Joint pain and morning stiffness
- Light sensitivity
- Memory loss
- Muscle aches and pain
- Numbness and tingling
- Rashes
- Shortness of breath
- Silliness
- Sinus congestion
- Skin sensitivity
- Stinky and sticky bowel movements
- Sugar cravings
- Vaginal or anal irritation/ itching/redness
- Weakness
- Weight loss-resistant lower abdomen
- White coating on the tongue

Tier 2: Laboratory Tests

The second tier for a CIRS diagnosis contains six examinations:

- visual contrast sensitivity test (VCS),
- human leukocyte antigen (HLA-DR),
- matrix-metallopeptidase 9 (MMP-9),
- adrenocorticotropic hormone (ACTH) and cortisol,
- vasopressin or antidiuretic hormone (ADH) and osmolality, and
- alpha-melanocyte-stimulating hormone (MSH).

A patient must be abnormal in at least three of these tests for a CIRS diagnosis.

Visual Contrast Sensitivity Test

The visual contrast sensitivity (VCS) test measures the patient's ability to see low contrast levels in each eye. Patients must have at least 20/50 vision on the near vision test card to qualify to use the VCS test with or without glasses. Practitioners may test only one eye if the patient's sight in the other eye is too weak. On a calibrated computer screen or with the VCS APTitude handheld kit, the patient is shown five sets of nine patterns. Patients indicate the pattern direction: left, up, right, or none. As the sets progress, the marks lighten, and bars move closer together to make each image harder to distinguish (See Figure 19).

VCS testing is not a diagnostic tool for any particular illness because there are several causes for a positive result. A positive result is an objective indicator of visual system dysfunction. A practitioner must assess the test result in tandem with clinical assessment and a review of laboratory results to determine the underlying cause.

According to Dr. Shoemaker, 92% of biotoxin illness patients fail the VCS test. There is a predictable decline in a patient's ability to see an edge, whereas control patients' decline was very rarely predictable. Biotoxin illness patients tend to have reduced blood flow, which lowers the oxygen levels in the optic nerves. Decreased oxygen in the eyes increases light sensitivity and diminishes night vision.

Test results plot all responses and analyze the contrast sensitivity in each eye (See Figure 20). Convert all five sets into columns. Contrast sensitivity is measured on the left axes and percentage of contrast on the right axes. The bottom axis specifies the test images spatial frequency of the parallel bars in cycles per degree (CPD). Higher spatial frequency means the parallel bars are closer together. The plot points represent the image's spatial frequency and contrast level, as well as the patient's response.

There are a few versions of the VCS test. We recommend using the VCS test provided on SurvivingMold.com or purchasing the VCS APTitude handheld kit from the same website.

Figure 19. Sample VCS Test: do not use for testing

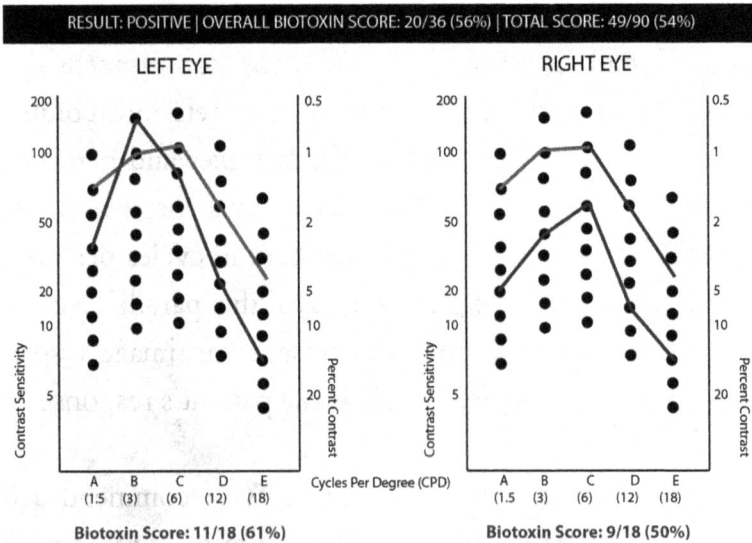

Figure 20. Sample VCS Test Results

According to research, a healthy patient places on or above the contrast sensitivity average. The patient's curve is created by connecting the highest correct responses in each column. If the patient's line dips below the average in any column, there is an underlying health issue. Possible nutritional deficiencies due to subpar absorption, poor digestion, or inadequate diet affecting the patent's health can be noted in columns A (1.5 CPD) and B (3 CPD). The underlying cause can be a gut imbalance, pancreatic insufficiency, increased intestinal permeability ("leaky gut"), exposure to toxic substances, and other underlying issues.

The primary biotoxin illness columns are C and D (6 and 12 CPD) and indicate neuropathology. Poor contrast function in these columns may indicate toxins produced by several species of mold, animal venom, Lyme disease and its co-infections, cyanobacteria, dinoflagellates, and others.

The far-right column (E/ 18 CPD), can be used to measure progress in biotoxin illness patients. During treatment, the spatial frequency at this contrast level usually improves faster than the other columns.

Patients in treatment may see lowered levels in columns D and E if they experience a detox Jarisch-Herxheimer reaction.

In the example, the patient's results show positive for possible biotoxin illness. The biotoxin illness columns (C and D) scored 11/18 (61%) in the left eye and 9/18 (50%) in the right eye. The patient should undergo further examination to conclusively determine if the patient's neurological issues and reduced oxygen levels in the optic nerve are a result of biotoxin illness or another underlying problem.

There is a 98% chance a patient has biotoxin illness if they also fit the CIRS cluster markers and test positive (fail) in one or both eyes. If a patient passes the test, there is still an eight percent chance that they are biotoxin susceptible. If a practitioner suspects biotoxin illness because of the patient's Tier 1 evaluation, yet test negative (pass) on the VCS test, it is still advisable to move on to inflammation and HLA testing.

HLA Genetic Testing

Human leukocyte antigen genes on chromosome six are found on the surface of nearly every cell in the body. These genes provide the instructions to create HLA complex proteins that help the immune system identify and remove proteins made by foreign invaders.

Ninety-three percent of those suffering from biotoxin illness carry one of the six HLA-DR haplotypes associated with elevated risk for CIRS (Shoemaker, Rash, & Simon, 2006; Shoemaker, 2010). There are 54 major HLA haplotypes, and each consists of HLA alleles used to assess the risks and possible inflammatory responses. Six of these haplotype sequences relate directly to biotoxin illness and one to MARCoNS (Shoemaker, Heyman, Mancia, & Ryan, 2017).

The HLA-DR haplotype 11-7-52B indicates susceptibility to MARCoNS. This haplotype is not one of the worst haplotypes for CIRS. However, over 80% of Dr. Ritchie C. Shoemaker's patients with low-MSH also had MARCoNS. Less than two percent of his patients with normal MSH had MARCoNS (Shoemaker, 2010).

The most dreaded haplotype, multi-susceptible, contains three possible results: 4-3-53, 11-3-52B, and 12-3-52B.

The HLA-DR by PCR blood test at Lab Corp determines a patient's HLA-DR haplotype. About 25% of the population will fall into a scale of susceptibility to toxins.

The results on sections DRB1, DQ, DRB3, DRB4, and DRB5 are used to determine where, or if, the patient falls on the susceptibility scale.

Shoemaker Rosetta Stone

The lab report numbers do not directly correlate to the susceptibility chart. Convert all the numbers using the Shoemaker "Rosetta Stone." Each report contains up to two digits for the sections DRB1, DQ, DRB3, DRB4, and DRB5. The numbers under each represent the gene alleles.

In a six-column Rosetta Stone conversion chart, add the patient's allele numbers in the rows labeled "Top Lab" and "Bottom Lab" (See Figures 21-23).

Rosetta Stone Conversion Rules

DRB1

1. The conversion requires two results.
2. If the lab report contains one number, then repeat the result in the other row.
3. If there is a 03 result, write 17 in the conversion row.
4. All other results do not need conversion, write the same number into the conversion row.

DQ

1. The conversion requires two results.
2. If the lab report contains one number, then repeat the result in the other row.
3. None of the lab results require conversion, write the same number into the conversion row.

DRB3

1. If the lab report contains zero numbers, then skip to DRB4.
2. If there is a 01 result, write 52A in the conversion row.
3. If there is a 02 result, write 52B in the conversion row.
4. If there is a 03 result, write 52C in the conversion row.

DRB4

1. If the lab report contains zero numbers, then skip to DRB5.
2. If there is a result, write 53 in the conversion row.

DRB5

1. If the lab report contains zero numbers, then you are done.
2. If there is a result, write 51 in the conversion row.

Use the Rosetta Stone rules to convert the patient's alleles.

Now you need to make a list of all the possible combinations. The haplotype combination chart will consistently have eight rows and eight possible combinations (See Figure 24).

The Rosetta Stone always provides two results for DRB1 and DQ. Merge the results for DRB3, DRB4, and DRB5 into one column. The patient will have zero, one, or two outcomes for this column.

Compare the haplotype combinations against the CIRS Associated HLA-DR Haplotypes chart to interpret the results (See Figure 25).

When comparing Figure 24 to Figure 35, the last variation matches multi-susceptibility (4-3-53). The other results do not match any of the CIRS haplotypes.

If your variation results have two matches and one of them indicates "no recognized significance," use the one with susceptibility. If they match two susceptibility levels, then use both.

Additionally, up to five percent of non-CIRS haplotypes can receive a CIRS diagnosis due to mold. This subset of patients will recover faster than their HLA-DR counterparts.

DRB1	03
	04
DQ	02
	03
DRB3	03
	—
DRB4	01
	—
DRB5	—
	—

Figure 21. Example HLA Result: do not use for testing

RESULTS	DRB1	DQ	DRB3	DRB4	DRB5
TOP LAB	03	02	03	01	
Conversion Top					
BOTTOM LAB	04	03			
Conversion Bottom					

Figure 22. Rosetta Stone Conversion Chart

RESULTS	DRB1	DQ	DRB3	DRB4	DRB5
TOP LAB	03	02	03	01	
Conversion Top	17	2	52C		
BOTTOM LAB	04	03			
Conversion Bottom	4	3		53	

Figure 23. Rosetta Stone Conversion Chart with Example

Haplotype Combination Rules

DRB1

1. Write the top result in the first four rows.
2. Write the bottom result in the last four rows.

DQ

1. Write the top result in the first two rows.
2. Write the bottom result in the third and fourth rows.
3. Write the top result in the fifth and sixth rows.
4. Write the bottom result in the seventh and eighth rows.

DRB3

1. If there are no results, skip.
2. Write the top result for each DRB1 and DQ combination.
3. Write the bottom for each DRB1 and DQ combination.

DRB4

1. If there are no results, skip.
2. Write the top result for each DRB1 and DQ combination.
3. Write the bottom for each DRB1 and DQ combination.

DRB5

1. If there are no results, skip.
2. Write the top result for each DRB1 and DQ combination.
3. Write the bottom for each DRB1 and DQ combination.

DRB1	DQ	DRB3, DRB4, or DRB5
17	2	52C
17	2	53
17	3	52C
17	3	53
4	2	52C
4	2	53
4	3	52C
4	3	53

Figure 24. Haplotype Combination Chart

	DRB1	DQ	DRB3	DRB4	DRB5
Multisusceptible	4	3		53	
	11/12	3	52B		
Mold	7	2/3		53	
	13	6	52A,B,C		
	17	2	52A		
	18*	4	52A		
Borrelia, post	15	6			51
Lyme syndrome	16	5			51
Dinoflagellates	4	7/8		53	
Multi Antibiotic Resistant Staph epidermidis (MARCoNS)	11	7	52B		
Low MSH	1	5			
Low-risk Mold	7	9		53	
	12	7	52B		
	9	3/9		53	
No recognized significance	8	3,4,6			

Figure 25. CIRS Associated HLA-DR Haplotypes

Diagnostic Lab Panel

In addition to the HLA-DR by PCR and VCS test, practitioners need to run a full panel of blood tests. The "Shoemaker Panel" tests provide valuable details on the patient's immune system. An accurate diagnosis requires all the lab results covered in this section.

According to Dr. Shoemaker, healthy control patients consistently show less than four abnormal labs, while biotoxin illness patients have four or more. A CIRS diagnosis requires five or more abnormal blood tests.

MSH

Low alpha-melanocyte-stimulating hormone (MSH) is a critical player in biotoxin illness. More than 95% of CIRS patients have decreased MSH. The MSH hormone regulates or catalyzes several essential functions. It is highly active in regulating pituitary functions and protecting cytokine responses in the gastrointestinal tract, skin, and nasal mucous membranes. A boss regulator, MSH, patrols several hormone pathways and controls the innate immune system responses, particularly inflammatory regulators. It controls several factors in the HPA axis, hippocampus, cerebral cortex, spinal cord, and other regions of the brain, influencing behavioral activity, memory, and attention. Synthesized in the hypothalamus, MSH affects melatonin, cortisol, ACTH, endorphins, sex hormones, and endocrine hormones.

For biotoxin illness patients, MSH protects the nare mucous membranes from the colonization of MARCoNS. An MSH deficiency enables bacteria to quorum, forming a protective biofilm barrier. The development of biofilm in the nares creates a perfect opportunity for toxins to deplete MSH levels further.

Initially, the body compensates for low MSH levels by increasing adrenocorticotropic hormone (ACTH) and cortisol. Eventually, the counterbalance causes adrenal fatigue, and the body stops rectifying the balance. The imbalance of MSH and ACTH launches a cascade of health issues, including hormone imbalances, mood swings, alternating diarrhea and constipation, leaky gut, and poor sleep.

Consistently low MSH levels lead to increased cytokine production and the lowering of T-regulatory cells. The dysregulation results in chronic pain, body aches, and debilitating and unrecoverable exhaustion. Patients may have chronic fatigue, inflammation, or an autoimmune disorder. Cytokines freely roam across the blood-brain barrier seeking compatible receptors. They commonly find receptors in the middle of the most important neuroregulatory pathway, the hypothalamus.

The proopiomelanocortin pathway (POMC) controls the post-translational processing of MSH from its leptin production (Böhm, Luger, Tobin, & García-Borrón, 2006). The POMC leptin fat cell molecules usually bind to receptors in the hypothalamus to activate leptin and the production of beta-endorphins and MSH. When cytokines bind before leptin, it leads to high leptin and low MSH levels.

If a patient receives an antibiotic treatment for more than one month, they are more likely to have MARCoNS and deficient MSH levels.

Hypothalamic-Pituitary Axis Function

ADH/ Osmolality

Antidiuretic hormone (ADH) controls the amount of water removed by the body. It's naturally produced by the hypothalamus and released by the pituitary gland. ADH binds to receptors in the kidneys and collecting ducts to reabsorb water. The ADH levels fall as the cells rehydrate.

Common symptoms of ADH dysregulation include frequent urination, dehydration, excessive thirst, and static electric shocks. When correcting ADH deficits, the patient may experience rapid weight gain and edema due to water retention.

The osmolality test measures the concentration of all chemical particles in the blood. It helps evaluate ADH function, water and electrolyte balance, and hydration status.

ADH production affects MSH and VIP levels in the hypothalamus. These three hormones significantly affect hypothalamic function. Reduced ADH and increased osmolality indicates low oxygen levels and VEG-F production. High osmolality causes the production and storage of ADH in the pituitary.

Biotoxin illness patients have production and regulation dysfunction. Most patients have low ADH and high osmolality levels. The lack of water increases headaches, and salt levels on the skin make patients more susceptible to static electric shocks. Eighty percent of CIRS patients have ADH/osmolality dysregulation with a noted increase in thirst and urination, according to Shoemaker data. In most cases, ADH/osmolality levels correct themselves after removing patients from exposure, and VCS and MARCoNS test negative.

ACTH/Cortisol

Adrenocorticotropic hormone (ACTH) synthesis occurs in corticotrophs of the anterior pituitary by proteolytic processing of the proopiomelanocortin (POMC). Alpha-melanocyte stimulating hormone (MSH) peptides derive from ACTH. ACTH has MSH-like activity. However, MSH does not have ACTH-like activity.

The breakdown of POMC causes cortisol to release in the cortex of the adrenal gland. Cortisol is known as the body's primary stress hormone and alarm clock. A person with normal circadian rhythms typically experiences their maximum cortisol levels around 6 AM, making levels higher in the morning than in the afternoon. That is why it's crucial to test the patient during the morning hours. Patients with insomnia triggered by mental or physiological stress have high levels of cortisol and dehydroepiandrosterone (DHEA) hormone, which synergistically rise during the night time. Over time DHEA levels may fall, resulting in lower cortisol levels. High levels of cortisol at night disrupts sleep and may lead to daytime fatigue. Prolonged insomnia and day time fatigue indicates dysregulation.

ACTH and cortisol are hypothalamic-pituitary-end organ dysfunction biomarkers, particularly adrenal gland regulation. Typically, ACTH and cortisol balance out. As one rises, the other falls. In the early stages of CIRS, they both might become elevated as the body compensates for the lack of MSH. This balance can limit symptoms. However, in later stages, both are usually low. As ACTH falls, symptoms become more apparent. Fifty percent of biotoxin illness patients with HPA axis dysregulation also have low MSH.

MMP-9

Matrix-metallopeptidase 9 (MMP-9) plays a vital role in inflammation, wound healing, tissue remodeling, and clearing pathogens from the ocular surface. Macrophages activate MMP-9 during the innate immune response to destroy the basement membrane of endothelial cells. Cytokines also become activated by MMP-9 to help the healing process. High MMP-9 is an excellent marker for hidden cytokine levels.

Continuously unregulated MMP-9 makes the basement membrane of endothelial cells and the blood-brain barrier porous. The porous barriers allow cytokines access to muscles, joints, lungs, brain, and the nervous system.

The constant remodeling of tissue leaves apparent tissue damage. The patients may experience arthritis, atherosclerosis, and cardiomyopathy. They may feel aches and pains in their muscles because high MMP-9 levels make the muscles and tissues very sensitive.

High levels of MMP-9 also correlate to a high toxin load, total cytokine load, indicate continuous exposure, and possibly cause Jarisch-Herxheimer reaction.

VIP

The vasoactive intestinal polypeptide (VIP), a neuroregulatory hormone/ cytokine and endocrine peptide is present in the gastrointestinal tract, lungs, thyroid, heart, kidneys, urinary bladder, gonads, brain, as well as peripheral and central nervous systems. It regulates peripheral cytokine responses, operates an array of cardiovascular functions, modulates endocrine activity, and controls inflammatory reactions. VIP relaxes smooth muscles in the airways and digestive system (lower esophageal sphincter, stomach, and gallbladder).

VIP production occurs in the gut, pancreas, and hypothalamus.

In the digestive system, it stimulates electrolytes and water secretion, inhibiting gastric acid secretion, and absorption of the intestinal lumen. Excessive VIP leads to watery diarrhea, loss of potassium, and possibly dehydration. In the cardiovascular system, VIP regulates pulmonary artery pressures, promotes local blood flow, stimulates contraction of the heart, and lowers blood pressure.

From the hypothalamus, VIP helps regulate the pituitary, modulates the circadian rhythm, and effects social behaviors. Prolactin secreted by the pituitary gland increases aggression.

In biotoxin illness patients, low VIP levels cause breathing trouble, particularly during exercise. According to Dr. Shoemaker, 100% of patients with multiple chemical sensitivity (MCS) also have decreased VIP. Correcting other dysfunction typically corrects VIP in most patients. The VIP treatment cannot be used on patients actively exposed to mold.

TGF-Beta1

Transforming growth factor beta-1 (TGF-beta1) produced by lymphocytes, macrophages, and dendritic cells are proteins with strong immunoregulatory properties. TGF-beta1 production is one of the immune system's first reactions after mold exposure. It suppresses T-regulatory (T-reg) cell activation, decreases T-reg proliferation and cytokine production, and reduces IL-1 receptors making cells less sensitive to other cytokines.

Concerning MARCoNS, TGF-beta1 has been linked to creating susceptibility for opportunistic infections (Letterio & Roberts, 1998). TGF-beta1 also plays an essential role in tissue repair and controls growth differentiation, activation, and death of immune cells, as well as T-regulatory cells found in the peripheral mucous surfaces (CD4+CD25++). Elevated TGF-beta1 typically displays with low CD4+CD25++ T-regulatory cells (Wan & Flavell, 2007), a contributing factor in the cyclical storm of MARCoNS and the cleaving of MSH.

The proteins help control cell proliferation (growth and division), differentiation (maturing to accomplish function), motility (movement), and apoptosis (self-destruction). Impaired T-regulatory cell function by TGF-beta1 contributes to both autoimmune activation and suppression. Its ability to act as an anti-inflammatory or pro-inflammatory cytokine on inflammatory cells makes TGF-beta1 an important fibrogenic factor in structural asthmatic airway changes. According to the Environmental Protection Agency (EPA), 21% of new asthma cases are due to exposure to water-damaged buildings.

At levels over five-thousand, TGF-beta1 can cause remodeling in the heart, central nervous system, liver, kidneys, and lungs. Patients with levels over ten-thousand can get pulmonary hypertension, tremors, interstitial lung disease, cognitive issues, and joint pain. TGF-beta1 causes toxicity in the hair follicles that can lead to hair loss that often occurs in large clumps.

C4a (and C3a)

A product of mannose-binding lectin pathways, C4a (complement system), an activation protein, is a part of the body's innate immune system. It helps phagocytic cells and antibodies remove toxins and infections from the body. High C4a levels are a biomarker for innate immune system overdrive due to pathogen burden.

Too many complement proteins cause them to react with one another, which induces inflammation. High levels can trigger allergic reactions or cause tissue damage. The innate immune system response to the complement system's warning of an allergen is to release histamine. This reaction can cause a devastating effect on the body when histamine is not needed. The body releases more mast cells, which activates even more exotoxins and creates an even friendlier environment for quorum bacteria. Mast cells also increase vascular permeability and cognitive dysfunction. The overall influx of changes can create a flurry of other autoimmune disorders, asthma, migraines, and other multi-symptom illnesses.

Elevated complement levels promote cell death. Complement proteins become active components when they split from their inactive form. This split promotes the membrane attack complex (MAC) immune response. MAC kills the outer layer of cells.

Biotoxin illness usually causes high levels of C4a and is a highly significant lab marker for the severity of biotoxin exposure.

When CIRS patients are re-exposed to biotoxins, they tend to get "sicker quicker." This phenomenon is caused by mannan-binding lectin serine protease 2 (MASP-2) cleaving C4a. As the patient's C4a level drops, their cognitive function improves. A patient with low MSH and C4a levels over 20,000 should not be in a home with an Environmental Relative Moldiness Index (ERMI) above negative one.

Complement C3a activates when complements C2a and C4a split to make C4b and C2a. The innate immune system only triggers C3a when it is presented with a bacterial cell membrane. Levels in biotoxin illness patients are typically low. If the patient has elevated levels, then Lyme disease and other tick-borne illnesses must be excluded or diagnosed. Levels rise within twelve hours of a tick bite.

Auto-Antibodies

Anticardiolipin/ Anti-gliadin Antibodies

Antibody proteins fight foreign invaders by creating immunity against the microorganism. They are the first line of defense against infections to help keep homeostasis of the immune system. Autoantibodies are antibodies that attack with self-antigens and comprise of nucleic acids, proteins, carbohydrates, lipids, or any combination of these. Several antibodies are useful biomarkers for disease and provide information about inflammation in patients.

Anticardiolipin antibodies (ACLA) IgA, IgM, and IgG are associated with collagen vascular diseases like lupus and scleroderma. ACLA autoantibodies disrupt blood vessel function and proteins, attempting to reach vessel walls.

Anti-gliadin antibodies (AGA) IgA, IgM, and IgG are useful markers for increased risk of autoimmunity and gastrointestinal permeability ("leaky gut"). These are produced in response to gliadin, a wheat storage protein. AGA antibodies are found in over 58% of CIRS pediatric patients.

Untreated patients with a negative AGA - IgA result does not rule out gluten-sensitive enteropathies. False-positives are possible because gastrointestinal disorders are known to induce the circulation of anti-gliadin antibodies.

Pregnant biotoxin illness patients with ACLA are at risk of fetal loss in the first trimester. The autoantibodies are found in over 33% of pediatric biotoxin-associated illness patients.

MARCoNS

Primarily found deep in the nares, Multiple Antibiotic Resistant Coagulase Negative Staphylococci (MARCoNS) builds a protective shell known as a biofilm. Symptoms of MARCoNS are not the same as those associated with a runny nose, facial pain, or sinusitis. MARCoNS dysregulates the immune system, aids in lower MSH levels, and causes issues across multiple systems.

Eighty percent of biotoxin illness, CIRS, and other chronic illness patients who have low MSH also test positive for MARCoNS. If the patient has been treated with antibiotics for more than one month, they are more likely to have MARCoNS and even lower MSH levels. Adrenal fatigue will continue until MARCoNS is eradicated.

In some patients, the same species of MARCoNS found in their nasal passages have also been found in their jawbones, dental work, and frequently their pet dog.

Pediatric Labs

The standard Shoemaker panel requires 22-32 vials of blood. Small children have a lower blood volume (~80 ml/kg). Therefore, practitioners need to be selective in which tests to run. HLA by PCR, ADH/osmolality, and ACTH/cortisol provide the best diagnostic indicators to decide on the best course of action for pediatric patients.

If all three tests return at normal levels, then do not pursue a biotoxin illness diagnosis. However, if one returns abnormal, then a biotoxin illness diagnosis requires further investigation.

Supportive Testing

Optionally, practitioners can run supportive testing labs to help identify issues and recognize a patient's progress. I also recommend repeating these tests during the first three steps of the BioNexus Approach to balance and tweak the bio-individualized protocol.

Non-Diagnostic Labs

Leptin

Leptin regulates the POMC pathway, then ultimately MSH and ADH levels. Low leptin levels contribute to low MSH, ADH, VIP, and ACTH.

High levels of the leptin hormone mean the body is holding onto fatty acids and storing fat, leading to weight gain. Standard approaches to weight loss will fail. Due to the inflammatory responses, patients with high leptin levels will be chronically tired, overweight, and in chronic pain.

If leptin receptors are disrupted, the test will show high leptin levels. Leptin outside of the brain binds to immune cells, which increases inflammatory cytokines.

VEGF

Vascular Endothelial Growth Factor (VEGF) dilates blood vessels and stimulates blood vessel growth. It restores oxygen to damaged tissues and restores blood circulation. Elevated levels increase innate immune system activation. As white blood cells accumulate and capillary blood flow is reduced, hypoxia occurs. Hypoxia stimulates the production of more VEGF.

In the early stages of biotoxin illness, the patient's body may compensate for hypoxia by increasing VEGF. In later stages, particularly in CIRS patients, inflammation and cytokine suppression tend to lead to decreased VEGF. Reduced VEGF causes capillary hypoperfusion, which in turn creates anaerobic mitochondrial metabolism that results in diminished muscle endurance. The patient experiences increased recovery time from physical activity, fatigue, muscle aches, shortness of breath, and brain fog. Low VEGF typically indicates low VO2 max levels.

Von Willebrand Factor

Von Willebrand disease is a rare mucocutaneous bleeding disorder. Biotoxin illness patients can acquire von Willebrand that causes them to develop thinner blood and possibly spontaneous bleeding due to elevated complement C4a levels. The severity of the bleeding varies considerably among patients. Most patients develop clotting abnormalities in the nose. Patients who acquire von Willebrand need to avoid re-exposure to mold and susceptible biotoxins. Complement C4a is the driving force behind patients feeling "sicker faster" after re-exposure.

Pulmonary Function

Patients with post-activity fatigue or abnormal shortness of breath require additional testing to identify possible causes. The patient may have acquired pulmonary hypertension, capillary hypoperfusion, or interstitial lung disease.

A differential diagnosis begins with a pulmonary function test. If the results require more testing, then the practitioner should move on to the VO2 max and stress echocardiogram tests.

VO2 Max

Use VO2 max testing only if the results from the pulmonary function test requires it.

Low VO2 max in a biotoxin illness patient typically means there is capillary hypoperfusion due to low VEGF, and not necessarily cardiopulmonary function. CIRS patients have a lower threshold for hypoxia due to high cytokine and low VEGF levels.

Stress Echocardiogram

Only continue with a stress echocardiogram if a patient's pulmonary function and VO2 max test results require it.

In healthy patients, arterial pressure (PA) response drops with exercise. PA may increase in CIRS patients. If the patient has high TGF-beta1 and low T-regulatory cells, then TGF-beta1 converts T-regulatory cells into pathogenic cells. High pressure at rest might also be possible in these patients.

At a baseline and after maximal exercise with a 90% of maximum predicted heart rate, measure pulmonary artery pressure through the Bernoulli equation.

Androgen Deficiency

Low VIP and inflammation can cause testosterone to convert to estrogen rapidly. An upregulated aromatase enzyme causes abnormal androgen levels. In this case, the patient will have elevated estrogen and low testosterone. Patients with testosterone dysregulation typically have low DHEA levels.

NeuroQuant

As mentioned in Part 2: Affect Systems, NeuroQuant is a software used in conjunction with an MRI. It analyzes the MRI results for brain volume and structure based on 11 different quantifiable brain areas. CIRS-WDB and CIRS-Lyme neuroborreliosis patients have specific pattern abnormalities.

Control patients in Dr. Shoemaker's research never had more than three points. In contrast, none of the CIRS patients had less than five points. Adequately treated patients demonstrate significant improvements (McMahon S., et al, 2016).

Tier 3: Response to Treatment

Once the patient begins treatment, repeated testing is vital to tracking their progress. Practitioners should expect to see changes in lab markers and clinical symptoms.

The Future

The Genomic Expression: Inflammation Explained (GENIE), developed by Dr. Shoemaker and based on the work of James Ryan, PhD is a gene expression assay performed on a single blood specimen for metabolic testing of chronic fatiguing illnesses. The test, released in 2019, is currently for "research use," which means only practitioners may order it.

The application of transcriptomics can be used to confirm differential gene expressions for cytokines, Lyme disease, coagulation, TGF-beta1, and mycotoxins on 173 genes to design bio-individualized therapies.

There are a select number of CIRS certified practitioners, including myself, enrolled in Dr. Shoemaker's GENIE interpretation and application training program. The goal is to have all CIRS certified practitioners GENIE literate.

NeuroQuant

Mold	1 Point	2 Points
Forebrain	≥ 31.9	≥ 32.5
Cortical Gray	≥ 16.3	≥17.0
Caudate Nuclei	≥ 0.255	≥ 0.235
Pallidum	≥ 0.07	≥ 0.08
Lyme	**1 Point**	**2 Points**
Putamer	≥ 0.345	≥ 0.335
Right Thalamus	≥ 0.58	≥ 0.60
	Atrophy	**Hypertrophy**
Forebrain	≥ 29.00	≥ 31.90
Cortical Gray	≥ 13.50	≥ 16.30
Hippocampus	≥ 0.255	≥ 0.31
Amygdala	≥ 0.10	≥ 0.14
Caudate Nuclei	≥ 0.255	≥ 0.30
Putamer	≥ 0.345	≥ 0.375
Pallidum	≥ 0.055	≥ 0.07
Thalamus	≥ 0.495	≥ 0.58
Cerebellum	≥ 3.5	≥ 4.55

NeuroQuant Results: CIRS ≥ 5 Points

CIRS-WDB Results

Increased forebrain parenchyma (eight of nine structures)
Increased cortical gray matter
Increased hippocampus (not included in criteria)
Increased pallidum
Increased amygdala
Decreased caudate nuclei (reversible with VIP treatment)
Decreased ventricles

CIRS-Lyme Neuroborreliosis Results

Small forebrain parenchyma
Small putamen
Large thalamus (isolated post gray matter change)
Large cerebellum

MSH Testing

MSH Draw Instructions: The specimen requires a Trasylol® kit. Use a chilled 6-mL lavender-top (EDTA) tube from the kit to collect 2 mL whole blood specimen.

MSH Lab: LabCorp only
MSH Normal Range: 35-81 pg/mL

ADH/Osmolality Testing

ADH: At least 2 mL of frozen plasma collected in a lavender-top (EDTA) tube.
Osmolality: At least 2 mL of serum or plasma collected in a red-top, gel-barrier, or green-top (heparin) tube. For pediatric patients, draw with a heel-stick for capillary.

ADH/Osmolality Lab: LabCorp or Quest
ADH Normal Range: 1.0-13.3 pg/mL
Osmolality Normal Range: 280-300 mOsm/kg

ADH/ Osmolality Normal Results:
—High ADH - High serum osmolality
—Low ADH - Low serum osmolality
ADH/ Osmolality Abnormal Result:
—Low ADH - High serum osmolality
ADH/ Osmolality Dysregulation:
—Absolute high: ADH > 13 or osmolality > 300
—Absolute low: ADH < 5 or osmolality < 275
—Relative: ADH > 4 when osmolality 275-278
—Relative: ADH < 2.2 when osmolality 292-300

ACTH/Cortisol Testing

ACTH Draw Instructions: Draw should occur between 7 AM and 10 AM. At least 0.8 mL of frozen plasma in an iced plastic or siliconized glass lavender (EDTA) tube.

Cortisol Draw Instructions: Draw after ACTH between 8 AM and 4 PM. At least 0.8 mL in a gel-barrier or red-top tube. Transfer serum to a plastic transport tube, if a red-top tube was used for draw.

ACTH/ Cortisol Lab: LabCorp or Quest

ACTH Normal Range: 8-37 pg/mL
Cortisol Normal Range:
—AM: 4.3-21.0 µg/dL
—PM: 3.1-16.7 µg/dL

ACTH/ Cortisol Dysregulation:
—Absolute high: ACTH > 45 or cortisol > 21
—Absolute low: ACTH < 5 or cortisol < 4
—Relative: ACTH > 15 when cortisol > 16
—Relative: ACTH < 10 when cortisol < 7

The recommended laboratories and test result ranges listed in this book are based on Dr. Shoemaker's recommendations. The lab result reference ranges may differ from laboratory ranges.

MMP-9 Testing

MMP-9 Draw Instructions: The blood draw requires a pre-chilled lavender tube. To prevent the release of MMP-9 into the blood cells within the specimen, the sample needs to be immediately centrifuged and frozen. A room temperature test tube can double or triple MMP-9 levels within 30 minutes.

MMP-9 Lab: LabCorp

MMP-9 Normal Range: 85-332 ng/ml

VIP Testing

Draw Instructions: Patient must fast for the eight hours before the blood draw. At least 1 mL of frozen plasma collected in a lavender-top (EDTA) tube.

VIP Lab: Quest

VIP Normal Range: 23.0-63.0 pg/mL

TGF-Beta1 Testing

Draw Instructions: At least 1 mL collected in a lavender-top (EDTA) tube. Double spin plasma to ensure all platelet contamination is gone. If the results are greater than 40,000, then the specimen was most likely mishandled.

TGF Beta-1 Lab: LabCorp or Quest

TGF Beta-1 Normal Range: 0 - 2,380 pg/mL
Symptoms Appear: > 5,000 pg/mL
Multisystem Symptoms: > 10,000 pg/mL

C4a/C3a Testing

C4a Draw Instructions: At least 1 mL of frozen plasma collected in a lavender-top (EDTA) tube. At least 0.5 mL for pediatric patients.
C3a Draw Instructions: Two collections in lavender-top (EDTA) tubes of at least 1 mL of frozen plasma.

C4a/ C3a Lab: Quest
—C4a Level RIA (not Futhan)
—C3a desArg Fragment

C4a/ C3a Normal Range: < 2830 ng/mL / < 940 ng/mL

ACLA and AGA Testing

Draw Instructions: At least 1 mL in a gel-barrier or red-top tube.

ACLA and AGA Lab: LabCorp or Quest

ACLA IgA Negative: < 12 GPL
ACLA IgG Negative: < 10 GPL
ACLA IgM Negative: < 9 GPL

AGA Normal Range: 0 - 19

MARCoNS Testing

Request an API Staph Isolate test kit from the lab. Follow all of the instructions.

Sit the patient with their head held erect with their chin parallel to the floor. Remove the blue top collection swab, insert it 2-3 inches into the left nostril, and rotate for 3-5 seconds. With the same swab repeat in the right nostril.

MARCoNS Lab: Microbiology DX

MARCoNS Positive Result: Resistance to two or more distinct antibiotic classes, plus biofilm.

Non-Diagnostic Labs

Lab: LabCorp or Quest; unless otherwise noted.

Leptin Male Normal Result: 0.5 - 13.8 ng/mL
Leptin Female Normal Result: 1.1-27.5 ng/mL

VEGF Normal Result: 31 - 86 pg/mL
The VEGF test is not a diagnostic tool. Practitioners should use it as a recovery marker.

VWF Lab: Quest
VWF Normal Result: By component
VWF Abnormal Result: Factor VIII, Ristocetin associated cofactor, or von Willebrand's antigen: > 50 or < 150 IU

Pulmonary Function Results: If results show restrictive patterns of respiratory difficulties with interstitial lung disease, then move on to a VO2 max test.

VO2 Max Normal Result: > 35
CIRS Result: < 20
Stage IV Cardiac Failure: 12-15

Stress Echocardiogram Results: Any rise in PA systolic pressure over 8 is abnormal. Result can be used as an indicator for VIP treatment to correct the irregularity.

Androgen Deficiency Normal Result: Based on age and gender.

Supportive Testing

Many patients are unable to complete the entire testing regimen due to personal finances or lack of testing in their country.

For BNH patients, we obtain informed consent, and proceed with their treatment based on detailed history, in depth clinical evaluation, and guided by whatever tests they are able to complete.

Hormonal Imbalance
Neurotransmitter Balance
Mitochondrial Function
Organic Acids Test (OAT)
Mycotoxins
Non-Metal Chemical Toxin Panel
Heavy Metals
Glyphosate
Methylation Sites (SNPS)

Pediatric Results

1 abnormal test; use clinical judgment
2-3 abnormal tests; do a full CIRS work up

Additional Testing

T-Regulatory Cells - CD4+, CD25+ and CD4+CD25+
Normal Result: > 18%

Erythrocyte Sedimentation Rate (ESR)
Normal Result: 0 - 30

C-reactive Protein (CRP)
Normal Result: 0 - 4.9 mg/L

Complete Blood Count (CBC)
Plasminogen Activator Inhibitor-1 (PAI-1)
Magnetic Resonance (MR) Spectroscopy
Cardiopulmonary Exercise Test (CPET)

PART 4

PREPPING THE APPROACH

"One of the greatest struggles naturopathic, integrative, and functional clinicians face is figuring out the best course of treatment for each patient. When a patient presents with perplexing symptoms and inconclusive test results, the task compounds itself. As practitioners, we need a variety of treatment options available when the science demands we see and address the full 360, often with an extraordinary approach."

—Jodie A. Dashore, PhD

The flexibility of the BioNexus Approach allows practitioners to create and customize bio-individualized protocols with their unique flair. This part of the book covers factors that are important to understand and consider before implementing the BioNexus Approach.

The medicinal recommendations in the BioNexus Approach are wholly plant-based alternatives to the treatment of biotoxin illness. A thorough understanding of herbs and their bio-chemical interactivity matters when treating genetically-susceptible, immunocompromised patients. All the herbal information in this section, including guidelines, preparations, and guides are to assist the reader in understanding the herbal protocols used at BioNexus Health Clinic.

Anyone deciding to treat patients or themselves with holistic or naturopathic methods should seek more specific information about herbs and individual circumstances, including speaking with their primary care physicians.

Herbal Preparations

Patients relatively new to herbal medicine generally research before deciding to choose alternative approaches. They arrive prepared to make life changes but usually cannot comprehend how much their life may need modification. New patients can quickly and easily become overwhelmed and stressed. At BioNexus Heath Clinic (BNH), we remind them that the changes we ask for are less stressful than their current hectic schedule of doctor and pharmacy visits. A holistic approach for chronic inflammatory response syndrome (CIRS) requests that a patient change the way they shop, consider ingredients, and find more time for relaxation. Incorporating herbs into their life will be different, but also progressively effortless. Patients become accustomed to shopping at organic stores, and some use gardening as a part of their stress-reduction strategy. Patients should be encouraged to view recovery as a new and positive adventure that does not end at yet another doctor's appointment.

People can integrate herbs into their lives as decoctions, meals, teas, baths, tinctures, and essential oils. There are eight primary herbal categories: anti-inflammatory, anti-microbial, digestive, immune, neurological, nutritive, supportive, and rejuvenative.

Prepare every herb for its purpose. Most anti-inflammatory herbs need to be mashed up and cooked. Fresh turmeric in a morning smoothie with lemongrass, kale, green apple, and celery, reduces swollen fingers and balances the mood. Patients can boil or pressure cook roots and bark (cinnamon) to make extracts. Fragrant dry or fresh herbs (lavender) may be crushed in a mortar and pestle but never boiled or pressure cooked.

Preparation Purpose
Baths: fresh or dried plant material in hot water for inhalations, steam, sauna, or bath

Decoctions - roots, barks, seeds, and forms other than aromatic leaves

Meals: fresh or dry herbs added to soups, stews, and sauces require very little cooking; roots and barks of traditional spices added to anything from cereal to curries; or fresh salad toppings

Tea: aromatic leaves and flowers; dried herbs produce stronger flavors and retain potency for 6 to 12 months

Tinctures: single remedies or in combinations; some herbs require specific dosages; can add to infused teas

Herbal Safety Guidelines

The herbs listed in this book are considered safe when used as suggested and prescribed by a qualified practitioner. A non-medical professional should not attempt to use the BioNexus Approach as a do-it-yourself program. Like pharmaceutical medications, herbs can also cause harm when misused.

Each patient requires a bio-individualized dosage determined by a qualified practitioner who practices naturopathic and functional medicine with a working knowledge of clinical herbalism. It is imperative that all recommendations in this book are considered for educational purposes only and not intended as a substitute for medical advice. A non-professional should consult a physician relating to health, diagnosis, treatment, and/or medical attention.

Herbs are powerful and available around the world. Some people can walk into their backyard, pull Japanese knotweed from the ground, and make a tincture. It is marvelous that our planet has given us access to healing plants, and it is even more remarkable that they are capable of evolving in their effectiveness. Informational sources like Stephen Harrod Buhner and Rosemary Gladstar's books are excellent resources to develop expertise about herbs and the intelligence of plants.

It is important to remember, herbs inherently contain more active ingredients than pharmaceutical drugs. The herbal ingredients work on several different biological levels and can affect a multitude of changes. Always consider the unique physiological factors in each patient. Without biochemical analysis, herbs can complicate treatment. Herbal medications also interact and can reduce the effectiveness of pharmaceutical medications. A chemical change within the body can be harmful and potentially dangerous. Anything in excess can also be hazardous. Professionally trained clinical herbalists are aware of herbal details that can interact with other treatment regimens and affect outcomes.

Herbal Introduction Period

As long as the BioNexus Approach and herbs are used responsibly and taken under the guidance of a clinical herbalist and primary physician, herbal medicine can be used throughout treatment and into maintenance without additional complications.

Medicinal herbs are processed into tinctures, capsules, and tablets. Follow the recommended dosage printed on the package or adhere to general herbal usage instructions.

If the patient has previously taken the prescribed herb, regularly takes herbal medicine, and is not on any pharmaceutical medication, then the patient may start at the recommended dosage. Otherwise, the patient requires an "herbal introduction" period, one week at the low or sensitive dose. After successfully introducing the herb to the patient's body, it is acceptable to increase the dosage and add another herb.

Common aromatic herbs (oregano, parsley, thyme, mint, etc.) usually do not require an introduction period.

The How Many Drops Per 1 oz Bottle? approximations chart on the following page, and the General Dosage and General Dilutions charts available in this Part can help make doses consistent. Always review product instructions against the charts for any variation.

How Many Drops Per 1 oz Bottle?
all measurements are approximate

1 oz bottles hold approximately 29.5 ml,
    7.4 teaspoons, 29.5 full droppers, and
    1,000-2,200 drops
10 ml water ~275 drops
10 ml alcohol extract ~440 drops
4 ml ~1 teaspoon
1 ml dropper ~1/4 teaspoon
Dropper from 1 oz bottle ~30 drops
Dropper from 2 oz bottle ~40 drops

HERBAL PREPARATIONS
General recipes

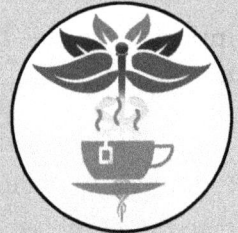

Decoctions

1 tsp to 1 tbsp of roots, bark,
seeds, berries, or mushrooms

Gently boil, then simmer for
20-40 minutes; cool and strain

1/4 tsp per cup hot water

Teas

1 tsp dry herb per cup hot water,
steeped for several minutes

Herbal Frequency

After the herbal introduction period, it is more important to increase herbal frequency than single dosages. If a patient experienced a Jarisch–Herxheimer reaction, this recommendation is especially true.

Instead of increasing a single dose from one drop per day to two drops per day, increase the frequency by prescribing one drop twice per day.

Taking an entire daily dose at once spikes the body's herb level. When the herb level drops off, the immune system lacks the support provided by the herb and diminishes its effectiveness. Whereas spreading the daily dose out over the day keeps the herbal levels high enough for it to perform effectively.

Frequency Is Better

One-Dose vs. Frequency
2 Drops vs. 1 Drop 2x Per Day
20 Drops vs. 6 Drops 3x Per Day
45 Drops vs. 15 Drops 3x Per Day

Adverse Reactions

If the patient develops severe flu-like symptoms: fever, chills, headaches, or muscle and joint pain, they need to discontinue the herbal protocol immediately. These symptoms are a sign of Jarisch–Herxheimer ("Herxheimer," "herxing," or "die-off") reactions. The symptoms are generally temporary and a sign that the antimicrobial action of the herbal medication are killing off bacteria. The die-off reaction occurs when the patient cannot clear the cytokines and dead bacteria fast enough. The toxin overload in the bloodstream disrupts the pH balance of the blood, which results in an acid imbalance impairing enzymes.

I encourage all practitioners to learn more about herxing and all its associated symptoms because the intensity of the response typically signifies the severity of the patient's infection and inflammation.

Patients experiencing any adverse reactions, side effects, or herxing reactions during herbal introduction or treatment should immediately discontinue the herbal protocol and notify their practitioner.

When a patient develops an adverse reaction to an herbal protocol, discontinue herbs for at least one day. If the patient reacts during the introduction phase, the patient should take a few days off. Reset the patient's dosage to the lowest level and, in some cases, restart with a slower schedule. Alternatively, the practitioner may need to re-examine the treatment plan and consider a different herb.

Pulse Therapy

Pulse therapy focuses on intermittent administration of the medication's frequency, intensity, and duration of doses. When transitioning a patient from pharmaceuticals to herbal medicines, it can be dangerous to stop the pharmaceutical treatment without tapering. Pulsing was a treatment strategy used at the turn of the century to combat antibiotic resistance (Roberts, Kruger, Paterson, & Lipman, 2008). The interval-based regimen has successfully treated non-bacterial diseases for decades and is mostly associated with steroid therapies (Isenberg, Morrow, & Snaith, 1982; Sinha & Bagga, 2008).

Pulsing decreases the potential of antibiotic-resistance without significantly increasing the patient's pathogen burden while transitioning a patient from conventional medicine to herbal medicine. According to mathematical models used by Baker, Ferrari, & Shea in Beyond Dose (2018), a range of dose concentrations help prevent resistance but need adequate management.

During the pulsing transitional phase, herbal treatment acts as a support mechanism to the active pharmaceutical ingredient, and bodily systems like the gut and immune system.

Pulse intervals are typically a week to a month. However, I've found that three and four days usually yields better results.

Pharmaceutical Interactions

Herbs interact with certain pharmaceutical medications. If a patient takes conventional medicine, avoid all herbs with established drug interactions (Kava, St. John's Wort, and Ginkgo biloba). Only add other herbs after careful consideration.

The herbs listed below are the most popular herbs with known interactions due to their overall effects. Ask patients if they use any of these herbs as over-the-counter supplements. Please do not consider the following list complete as it is best practice to understand the effects of herbs fully and know ways they may interfere with pharmaceutical drugs.

Examples of Pharmaceutical & Herb Interactions
Asian Ginseng: High risk (narrow therapeutic index) - blood pressure, diabetic medications, blood thinning; induces CYP3A4 enzyme metabolizing in the liver and possibly the GI tract

Black Cohosh: Low interaction - atorvastatin, acetaminophen, and alcohol

Cranberry: Low risk - anticoagulants

Echinacea: Low risk - slows caffeine breakdown; changes some drug metabolism in the liver

Evening Primrose: Low risk - a blood thinner; anti-seizure medication, ibuprofen, multivitamin, vitamins (b12, c, d3, and e)

Feverfew: Low risk - a blood thinner

Garlic: Low risk; extended use of extracts may reduce pharmaceutical efficacy and blood thinning

Ginger: Low risk - a blood thinner

Ginkgo Biloba: Low doses show no risk; higher doses may affect the pharmacokinetics

Green Tea: Low risk - pseudoephedrine

Goldenseal: High risk - inhibits CYP3A4 and CYP2D6 enzymes

Kava: Low risk - CNS depressants may experience increased drowsiness and motor reflexes; high risk - buprenorphine

---

WARNING

Avoid Kava when drinking alcohol

Melatonin: Low risk - anticoagulants, antihistamines, benzodiazepines, muscle relaxers, and opioid analgesics; kava, St. John's Wort, 5-HTP

Saw Palmetto: Low risk - blood thinning, estrogen, and oral contraceptives

St. John's Wort: High risk (narrow therapeutic index) - benzodiazepines, Coumadin, digoxin, cyclosporine (immunosuppressant), indinavir (antiretroviral), oral contraceptives, and more

Valerian: Low risk - antidepressants, muscle relaxants, pain killers, and sleep and anxiety medications

Yohimbe: Low risk - hypertension, angina pectoris, heart disease, dilates blood vessels; erectile dysfunction

Tinctures

The naturally occurring phytochemical, active ingredient in some herbs, is not water-soluble. Creating tinctures with phytochemical herbs requires medicinal-purpose alcohol to produce the highest quality medicinal compound. Herbal tinctures may use any spirit with an alcohol by volume (ABV) of at least forty percent. However, vodka is the most commonly used because of its neutral flavor.

The amount of alcohol used in tinctures is not enough to produce intoxicating effects. Nevertheless, people with alcohol sensitivity should use extracts instead of tinctures. Herbal extracts are typically manufactured with glycerine, water, vinegar, or menstruum, but are less concentrated than tinctures.

The alcohol in tinctures quickly evaporates during dosage preparation. After the patient prepares their herbal mixture, it should sit in the open air for twenty minutes before consumption to allow evaporation. Still, the open-air method may not be enough for a few patients, including pregnant women, children, elderly adults, and recovering alcoholics. For this subset of patients, add a small amount of distilled boiling water to the herbal mixture to accelerate evaporation.

Generally, it is never advisable to take more than forty-five drops of herbal tinctures per day. Consuming more than forty-five drops may cause impairment, intoxication, additive intoxication, or an overdose. It takes approximately 1,500ml of non-evaporated herbal tinctures for a patient to become intoxicated. Accidental intoxication due to overdose will require proper medical attention.

Herbs can also increase typical alcohol effects. Combining alcoholic beverages with herbs may reduce herbal effectiveness and interfere with absorption in the gastrointestinal tract. Some herbal combinations may have a more significant impact on the body, such as raising blood concentration to toxic levels, impair breathing, cause liver damage, and induce drowsiness.

Cultural Considerations
Most religions find the ABV of herbal tinctures to be acceptable. However, the source of the alcohol used in production may prevent tincture use. For example, some Islamic sects forbid

tinctures produced from wine alcohol (grapes, dates, and raisins), while permitting herbal medications made from grain alcohol.

Religions with Alcohol Restrictions: Jainism, Islam, Buddhism (discouraged), Hinduism (discouraged), Sikhism, Babi, Baha'i, and some Christian sects, including Mormonism and Jehovah's Witnesses.

Even if a faith allows medicinal or non-medicinal consumption, the individual might live an alcohol-free lifestyle. It is best practice to ask if the patient has an issue with an alcohol-based tincture.

General Tincture Dosage

The General Tincture Dosage chart in this Part shows the guidelines for herbal tinctures. Prepare herbal medicine for use by succussing (vigorously shaking) each tincture, then adding each herbal dose to a small glass with 1-2 oz. (30-60 ml) of distilled water.

After preparing the dose, the patient needs to wait at least twenty minutes to allow alcohol to evaporate. Ten minutes before consumption, the patient should eat. After taking the dose, the patient should not ingest any foods or drinks for an additional ten minutes.

Essential Oils

Essential oils, plant material (leaves, barks, and roots) extracts, have a long history of medicinal use. Commonly known essential oils include lavender, peppermint, wintergreen, sandalwood, sage, tea tree, and eucalyptus. The extraction method (distillation, extraction, maceration, enfleurage, et cetera) depends on the type of plant, the part that contains the oil, and its purpose. The pressure and temperature of the process affect the quality of the final product. The late master herbalist Michael Moore wrote in *Herbal Formulas For Clinic And Home* (1995), "I have always maintained that formulas are the least important part of herbalism," adding, "You can get the same effects from 100 different variations of various herbs. You need to know the craft well in order to get the same end result."

Due to the mainstream popularity of essential oils, it is vital to remind patients that they can be dangerous and poisonous if swallowed. If a person aspirates the oils, it could become pneumonia. Additionally, essential oils can interact with herbal and pharmaceutical medications. Essential oils should be treated like any other medicine and use them only as directed on the product packaging or by a professionally trained clinical herbalist.

Always dilute essential oils in a carrier oil before use. Applying essential oils directly on the skin may cause severe

GENERAL TINCTURE DOSAGE CHART

All the daily doses may all be prepared in the morning; refrigerate uncovered

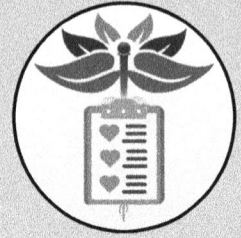

Adult
Homeopathic: 5 Drops

Tonifying: 10 Drops

Anti-Microbial/Therapeutic: 15 Drops

Pediatric
Dosage may vary depending on herbal extraction method or compounded formula. Children of the same age can vary greatly in weight. Adjust dosage accordingly or use alternative dosage method.

3-12 month: 1 part tincture diluted with 10 parts water; 1-2 <u>droppers</u> of tea or liquid several times per day

1-5 yrs: 1 part tincture diluted with 10 parts water; 1-2 <u>teaspoons</u> of tea or liquid several times per day

6-10 yrs: 1/4 - 1/3 of the adult dose

11-16 yrs: 1/2 of the adult dose

16-18 yrs: adult dose, but with caution and guidance

Alternative Pediatric Dosage

Child's imperial weight divided by 160 = D%

Do not exceed D% of the adult dose

Examples:

40 pounds (18.14 kilograms);
40/160 = 25%
or a quarter of the adult dose

90 pounds (40.82 kilograms);
90/160 = 56%
or about half of the adult dose

GENERAL ESSENTIAL OILS DILUTION CHART

Dilutions over 3% are for short term use only; over 10% for acute purposes

DILUTION & BEST USE	CARRIER OIL	DROPS
0.5% Sensitive/ Elderly	5 ml (1/6 oz, 1 tsp, 1-1/3 drams)	0.75
	10 ml (1/3 oz, 2 tsp, 2-2/3 drams)	1.5
	15 ml (1/2 oz, 3 tsp, 4 drams)	2.25
	30 ml (1 oz, 6 tsp, 8 drams)	4.5
1% Age 3 - 24 months; Face Creams	5 ml (1/6 oz, 1 tsp, 1-1/3 drams)	1.5
	10 ml (1/3 oz, 2 tsp, 2-2/3 drams)	3
	15 ml (1/2 oz, 3 tsp, 4 drams)	4.5
	30 ml (1 oz, 6 tsp, 8 drams)	9
2% Age 2 - 6 years	5 ml (1/6 oz, 1 tsp, 1-1/3 drams)	3
	10 ml (1/3 oz, 2 tsp, 2-2/3 drams)	6
	15 ml (1/2 oz, 3 tsp, 4 drams)	9
	30 ml (1 oz, 6 tsp, 8 drams)	18
5% Age 6-12 years; General Massage; Aromatherapy; Massage Oils	5 ml (1/6 oz, 1 tsp, 1-1/3 drams)	7.5
	10 ml (1/3 oz, 2 tsp, 2-2/3 drams)	15
	15 ml (1/2 oz, 3 tsp, 4 drams)	22
	30 ml (1 oz, 6 tsp, 8 drams)	45
10% Age 13+; Salve; Massage Treatment; Localized Treatment; Wound Healing	1 ml (1/3 oz, 1/5 tsp, 1/4 drams)	1
	5 ml (1/6 oz, 1 tsp, 1-1/3 drams)	15
	10 ml (1/3 oz, 2 tsp, 2-2/3 drams)	30
	15 ml (1/2 oz, 3 tsp, 4 drams)	44
	30 ml (1 oz, 6 tsp, 8 drams)	90
25% Muscular Aches and Pains; Acute Physical Pain; Trauma Injury	1 ml (1/3 oz, 1/5 tsp, 1/4 drams)	2.5
	5 ml (1/6 oz, 1 tsp, 1-1/3 drams)	37.5
	10 ml (1/3 oz, 2 tsp, 2-2/3 drams)	75
	15 ml (1/2 oz, 3 tsp, 4 drams)	110
	30 ml (1 oz, 6 tsp, 8 drams)	225

irritation, redness, or burning. Organic carrier oils (sesame, real extra virgin olive, or coconut) reduce absorption rates while preventing evaporation.

Cold expeller pressed essential oils retain fragile nutrients and are best used for aromatherapy. This method pierces and presses the plant to extract the oil. Then it is centrifuged to remove any solid pieces, and as the oil separates, it is siphoned off to another receptacle for processing and packaging.

Human Connection

Years ago, I attended a Stephen Harrod Buhner workshop, where he did a little experiment. He passed around food-grade hawthorn to everyone in the room. Hawthorn is excellent for the heart and opening up the heart chakra. It also smells terrible. Even bees avoid their flowers. Stephen was talking about consuming herbs, being contemplative, and grateful for its effects to allow your thoughts to enhance efficacy. Stephen said everyone who drank it smiled, making his point. Focusing on intent and grace can even turn the strong odor of hawthorn into a smile.

Consciousness also extends to harvesting and preparation. Take a moment to notice the color, fragrance, textures, and freshness of the herbs. Slowly sip herbal teas, inhale the aromas, and appreciate their flavors. Mentally connect with the herbs by thinking about their benefits and how they work. Gather

STANDARD DILUTION & MASSAGE BLEND

See General Essential Oils Dilution Chart in this section for more options and ratios

2.5 - 5% dilution

Example: 15 drops of essential oil per 10 ml of carrier oil.

sensory information about the taste and the smell. Be especially mindful of their energies, elements, and botanical intelligence. Afterward, notice the sensations created by the body, including digestion, appetite, energy, sleep, et cetera.

Over the centuries, herbs have been used in part and as a whole. Many factors determine the herbs' effectiveness and potency. Whole herbs contain many ingredients, and like other crops, are affected by the environment (climate, bugs, and soil quality), harvesting, and processing.

Medicinal herbs, when used under the guidance of a knowledgeable practitioner, can effectively treat various disease processes (Ekor, 2014). While scientists are unsure what makes some herbs work explicitly, there are proven ideas that might be able to explain how herbs produce results. It is believed that the synergy of all the herbs ingredients produces the most beneficial effect.

Quanta

Studies reveal that energy cannot divide infinitely. The tiniest amount of an interaction involving anything physical (entity or property) is called a "quantum." Quanta (plural of quantum) contain aspects of a particle and a wave. The smallest part of an electromagnetic field is a photon, a single quantum of light or radio wave.

At these small scales, the laws of quantum mechanics govern chemistry. Nanoscale biological systems exhibit strange and counterintuitive effects. Seth Lloyd (2011), Director of the Center for Extreme Quantum Information Theory, discusses the emergence of quantum coherence in a precise biological process. Quantum entanglement and coherence set the valence structure of atoms and form covalent bonds. Quantum mechanics parameterizes the chemical compounds and reactions.

Plant Biology

Throughout the early 20th century, Bengali biophysicist and botanist Sir Jagdish Chandra Bose, PhD pioneered plant biology. He studied their interaction with the environment and proved plants have a nervous system and express empathy. Plants adapt their behavior with purpose and in reaction to stimuli. Their electrical nervous system and tissues respond to sound, climate, seasons, and chemicals by transmitting information through their roots, stems, and leaves. In The Nervous Mechanism of Plants (1926), Bose details how plants are sensitive to heat, cold, light, noise, and various other external stimuli.

The basic principle of life is simple: CO_2 and water produce sugars (Miller, 2006). In a plant, when the chlorophyll inside a leaf captures a photon from the sun, it manufactures sugars (carbohydrates). When a person consumes food, the sugars break down and give off photons. Photons sustain life. All vitamins, nutrients, and sustenance, including sugar, carry light.

Ingesting intelligent photons provides more benefit than any amount of vitamin intake or a particular chemical form. Studies demonstrated the interconnectivity of plants, animals, and humans by measuring the emission from an isolated plant, animal, and human mitochondria (Meduski et al., 1974; Cercek & Cercek, 1979; Hideg et al., 1991; Hideg, 1993). The studies found that increased photon emission also increases oxygen free radical concentration and decreases environmental nitrogen consistent with the increased oxidative metabolism of wounded tissue during the repair phase. Photon emissions from injured plants and root tissue emanated from leukocytes inside animals (Salin & Bridges, 1981).

Additionally, there appears to be a correlation between singlet oxygen production, not related to chlorophyll or mitochondria, and increased photon emission (Slawinska, 1978; Slawinski et al., 1978; Tilbury & Quickenden, 1988; Voeikov et al., 1999). Recent theories of biophoton emission consider the possibility that this radiation helps regulate biological and biochemical functions within and between cells (Van Wijk, 2001).

Quantum Biology

Franck & Teller first hypothesized a quantum element for the migration and photochemical action in 1938. Developments in observational techniques have allowed more recent studies to evidence quantum mechanical effects on a range of biological processes that cannot be accounted for by Newtonian physics. Research from biophysicist Gregory Engel in 2011 revealed plants harvest almost 95% of its energy from sunlight. Photosynthetic organisms evolved antenna systems to optimize light collection using a fundamental principle of quantum computing, the exploration of a multiplicity (Horton, 2012). The antenna systems regulate light-harvesting efficiency in photosynthesis by rapidly directing energy from photon-sensitive molecules to the protein reaction centers without losing energy. The one-millisecond transfer exists in multiple places at once, achieving near-perfect efficiency. The exact mechanism of this near-instantaneous functional event remains a mystery (Biello, 2007).

German physician Dr. Bodo Koehler (2007), incorporates quantum physics and biology principles into modern integrative medicine, "in the organism, chemical processes are actually bio-informational processes. Molecules are formed from atoms by means of electron exchange, i.e., energetic processes. And we are thus already into quantum physics. No metabolic reaction in the organism can take place without the transfer of the relevant information."

Organs and their functions need to adapt to environmental changes to keep the body healthy. Accumulated energy information continually influences every system, toxin overload in regulatory systems stalls adaptation. Koehler (2020) teaches how the steep rise in environmental toxins and epigenetic triggers overhauled the clinical image of chronic disease. He says that healing is a process of consciousness. In chronic illness, the systems have "resigned" themselves to the fight. To heal, the patient needs to awaken their systems with a mindful willingness to change and recover. Dr. Koehler's bio-physical information therapy "The Four Poles Approach" derives from various indicators of environmental diseases, such as biotoxin illness.

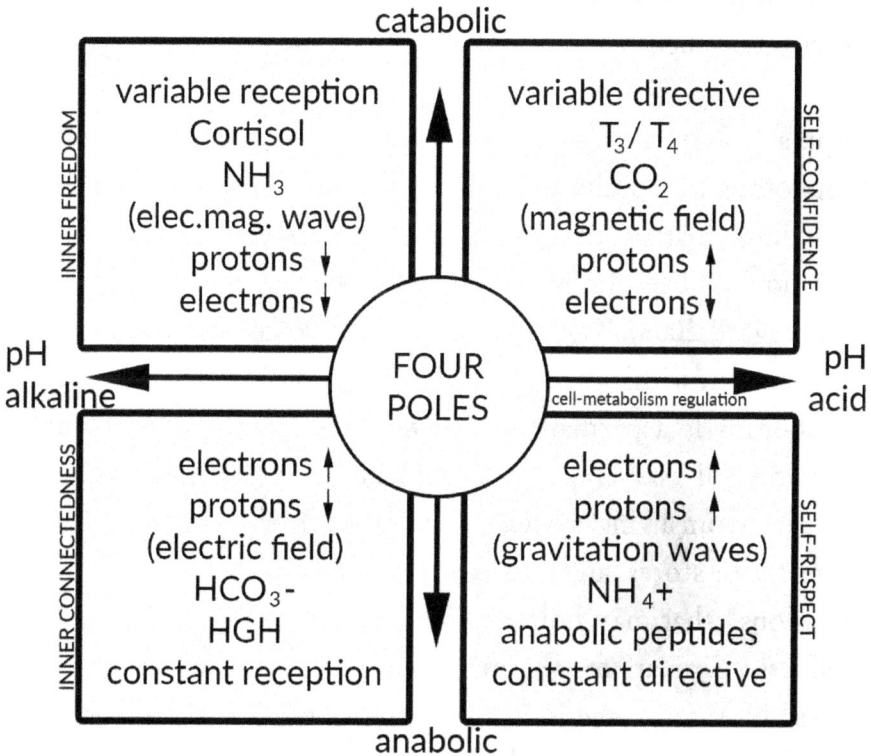

catabolic

INNER FREEDOM

variable reception
Cortisol
NH_3
(elec.mag. wave)
protons ↓
electrons ↓

SELF-CONFIDENCE

variable directive
T_3/ T_4
CO_2
(magnetic field)
protons ↑
electrons ↓

pH alkaline ← FOUR POLES

cell-metabolism regulation → pH acid

INNER CONNECTEDNESS

electrons ↑
protons ↓
(electric field)
HCO_3-
HGH
constant reception

SELF-RESPECT

electrons ↑
protons ↑
(gravitation waves)
NH_4+
anabolic peptides
contstant directive

anabolic

Figure 26. Biophysical Mechanics: Living Systems = Energy/Matter & Information. Compiled and adapted from "Integration instead of separation," by B Koehler, 2007

Biophoton Theory

In the 1970s, Dr. Fritz-Albert Popp, a German researcher, discovered wild plant foods were the most abundant food source of biophotons. Living cells emit a weak form of UV light producing a glow (photon radiation). Popp applied quantum optics to prove radiations (biophotons) were responsible for cellular communication. He co-developed a biophoton meter that detected plant cell emissions to confirm food quality. Popp found wild-organic food grown without human intervention emitted exponentially more biophotons than commercially grown food (Burroughes, 2013). Later studies found wildcrafted herbs retain their maximum biophoton value (Cousens, 2009).

Popp's (1984) research also confirmed every human cell emits biophotons that orchestrate all bodily processes, possess a semi-crystalline matrix, and have an ideal resonant frequency or vibration: "The human cell has an energetic structure" (McTaggart, 2008). The light particles have no mass, but transmit information within and between cells. Biological emission of biophotons is a permanent ultraweak (1-100 photons/sec/cm2) emission of coherent (phase-locked or frequency-locked) photons from living systems. His research shows that DNA in living cells stores and releases photons creating "biophotonic emissions" that may hold an essential key to illness, health, and wellness. Similar to thermal radiation and bioluminescence caused by radical reactions, the quantum biological phenomenon is a by-product of metabolism. Metabolic activities, without excitation or enhancement, constantly and spontaneously emit light from all systems. Popp demonstrated biophotonic emissions occur in the visible and UV part of the electromagnetic spectrum at ultra-low intensities (10-16 – 10-18 W/cm2). These ultraweak photon emissions originate from a relaxation of electronically excited states of the constituents of living cells.

Chlorophyll demonstrates fluorescence on plants placed in darkness. After a few minutes, it begins to decay and releases an ultraweak emission. Studies indicate that biologic processes increase oxidative metabolism producing singlet oxygen and other oxygen-related free radicals tend to correlate with measured biophoton emission (Salin and Bridges, 1981; Hideg, 1993).

Studies have shown that the coherent emission of bio-photons is connected to information and energy transfer processes and can have a critical influence on DNA function and gene regulation. "We are still on the threshold of fully understanding the complex relationship between light and life, but we can now say emphatically, that the function of our entire metabolism is dependent on light" (Popp as cited in Biontology Arizona, n.d.).

Synergy

Although plant constituents make up most modern medicines, a rift between chemical pharmacology and traditional herbalism developed. The separation grew stronger over time until recent

Popular Synergistic Herbs

Andrographis	Garlic
Ashwagandha	Ginger
Astragalus	Gotu Kola
Bacopa	Lemon Balm
Catnip	Licorice
Chamomile	Marshmallow
Cinnamon	Mints
Cramp Bark	Mullein
Dandelion	Plantain
Dill (Gripe Water)	Propolis
Echinacea	Thyme
Elderberry	Tulsi
Elderflowers	Turmeric
Eleuthero	Valerian
Eyebright	Wild Cherry Bark
Fennel	

interest in integrative medicine began to bridge the divide. One of the factors that contributed to the renewed interest in medicinal herbs is the growing awareness that isolated constituents extracted from herbal plants are often less active than the whole plant.

A living plant is a complex system with thousands of interacting chemicals, and many of them synergize – creating a more significant impact than the effect of consuming isolated components in single-molecule pharmaceuticals. The constituents of a whole plant, or whole plant extract, influence each other in several ways that affect their impact on the consumer. Buhner (2012) explains herbal synergy may be stabilizing, potentiating or enhancing, or modifying the effects of individual elements. Synergistic herbs can also make a constituent more water-soluble or protect it from stomach acids. Chemically isolated ingredients lose synergistic effects of whole plants producing radically different results.

Chinese Herbal Medicine

Medicinal plants contain hundreds of unique compounds. Traditionally, pharmaceutical companies isolate one active ingredient and synthetically reproduce it for mass consumption. Removing one compound eliminates the benefits of other compounds in the whole plant, which can reduce the effectiveness of the active ingredient.

Chinese herbal medicine has a long history of promoting the use of whole plants and the belief of synergy when herbs are combined to create intricate herbal formulas. Historically, empirical evidence of herbal reliability lacks considerably. However, several recent studies have demonstrated that whole herbs and synergistic formulas exceed the efficiency of single active ingredient medications (Leonard et al., 2002; Scholey & Kennedy, 2002; Lam, Seto, Kwan, Yeung, & Chan, 2006; Kong, Li, & Zhang, 2009; Zhang, Sun, & Wang, 2013).

Synergistic herbs and nutrients enhance the bioavailability of an active ingredient, reduce toxicity, and/or promote the therapeutic effects of another active ingredient. Synergy also applies when two herbs enhance each other for a composited result on a biological level. Conventional medicine over the past two decades has slowly moved away from the "one drug, target, one disease" approach to utilizing synergistic treatments for chronic illness (Zhou et al., 2016). Studies show that a multi-target treatment approach provides more significant therapeutic benefits for highly complex diseases, including chronic inflammation (Jukema & van der Hoorn, 2004; Weber & Noels, 2011).

Chinese herbal medicine formulations are known as "Fufang" and follow the "Peiwu," principal of compatibility. According to Peiwu, there are five herbal interdependencies to consider "Xiang Xu" (synergism), "Xiang Shi" (assisting), "Xiang Shu" and "Xiang Wei" (detoxification), "Xiang Wu" (antagonism), and "Xiang Fan" (rejection). A Fufang formulation under the composition guidance of Peiwu follows the "Jun-Chen-Zuo-Shi" (Emperor-Minister-Assistant-Courier) rule. The "Jun" herb is the main ingredient and typically contains a higher ratio to directly target the disease. "Chen" acts as the adjuvant to the Jun and enhances its therapeutic effects. A "Zuo" herb reduces side effects caused by the Jun and/or Chen. Finally, the "Shi" harmonizes the active ingredients and helps them achieve their goal.

Ayurvedic Medicine

The ancient herbal science of Ayurveda and its plant-based medicinal principles began as early as 6,000 BCE and written about in scientific scriptures, the *Vedas*, and the *Upanishads*. In the modern era, renowned master herbalists like David Crow, Rosemary Gladstar, Vasant Lad, Stephen Harrod Buhner, and others have passionately written and spoken about the medicinal and spiritual gifts of plants.

The ancient Ayurvedic medical works *Astanga Hridaya*, *Sushruta Samhita*, and *Caraka Samhita* were written in Sanskrit over 2,000 years ago. These three texts are collectively known as the *Great Trilogy*. In the fifth century, the trilogy was translated into Chinese, and by the Italian Renaissance, it had already been available in Persian and Arabic for several hundred years (Wujastyk, 2012; Selin, 2008). British physicians published articles about the ancient methods at the turn of the 19th century. Despite their interest, during England's occupation of India, Ayurveda was nearly lost to Western medicine. After India's independence, the Central Council of Indian Medicine Act of 1970 officially recognized Ayurveda, naturopathy, homeopathy, and yoga in the national healthcare system (World Health Organization, 2001).

According to the Ayurvedic tridosha homeostasis concept, health is a balancing act of the three constitutional identifiers ("doshas"): Vata, Pitta, and Kapha. Ayurvedic science offers unique therapeutic approaches to illness that incorporate dietary regulation, yoga, exercise, bodywork, detoxification, and psychological interventions that help achieve optimal wellness and immune balance. Modern clinical herbalism assessments are broadly inspired by and based on Ayurvedic tridosha science.

Understanding a body's tendencies is key to discovering the patient's energetic constitution. Adjusting diet and herbs based on an in-depth analysis can immensely benefit extreme gut sensitivities. Most people have a dominant dosha, but everyone has all the elements within them.

Vata (air and ether) - Dosha of Movement: Compared to the wind, Vatas tend to be light, have thin bones, and dry skin and hair. In life, they move and speak rapidly, and are often late and distracted. Vata constitutions can be creative and spontaneous but also plagued by anxiety and worry. When they are out of balance, Vatas tend toward digestive upset, lose weight, bloat, become constipated, and have weakened immune and nervous systems.

Vatas respond to warming and moistening herbs.

Pitta (fire and water) - Dosha of Transformation: Focused, energetic, and competitive, pittas tend to feel warm and have somewhat oily skin. In life, they tend to be Type A personalities, intelligent, competitive, and are overly intense problem-solvers. When out of balance, Pittas are more prone to heartburn,

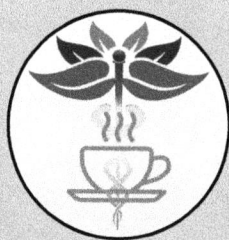

IMMUNE CIDER
Non-Traditional Version

Cider stimulates the appetite, soothes aches and pains, acts as an antibacterial and decongestant, and helps coughs and colds

Ingredients

1 quart organic apple cider vinegar containing "mother"
1/2 cup horseradish root grated
1/4 cup of garlic, chopped
1/4 cup of ginger, grated
2 tsp cayenne

3 tbsp raw honey
1/4 cup grated fresh turmeric
1 tsp ajwain seeds
20 drops tulsi glycerite
(or 20 fresh leaves)

Directions

Place all ingredients in a quart jar and cover with Apple Cider Vinegar

Tightly cover the jar

Steep for 4 weeks

Strain into a clean jar

Drink it straight or diluted in a bit of water or warm lemon tea

Start with 1 tsp to test tolerance level

Individual tolerance to the spicy heat will vary; experiment with quantity

diarrhea, upset stomachs, infections, skin problems, and deficiency in the liver, spleen, and blood.

Pittas benefit from cooling and drying herbs.

Kapha (water and earth) - Dosha of Structure And Stability:
Physically dense Kaphas tend to be cool, moist, and stocky. In life, they very grounded, nurturing, caring, trusted confidantes, loyal friends, and known for their stable personalities. When out of balance, Kaphas move slow; they are prone to weight gain, water retention, congestion, and weakened lungs and sinuses.

Kaphas find balance in drying, warming, and tonifying herbs.

In Ayurvedic practice, the concepts of Agni and Ama are opposites and a vital adjunct for digestion and metabolism issues in complex multisystem cases. The strength of Agni, heat of the body, represents overall health, whereas Ama brings toxic pathogenic mucus and waste to destroy Agni. Agni and Ama are especially helpful with body tonification and rejuvenation. Modern clinical herbalists find great value in including the tridosha system in their assessments.

Dr. Vasant Lad (2002) discusses the importance of the twenty attributes, an Ayurvedic qualitative physiological principle, and their effects on the doshas and everyday life that are the keys to healing. In daily life, we encounter these attributes in numerous scenarios, including relationships, environment, emotions, feelings, and symptoms. Awareness and observation of how these attributes affect the patient and correction of the opposing forces is a valuable tool in the arsenal of an experienced clinical herbalist. Incorporating the attributes into patient care enhances a client-centered outcome and homeostasis restoration. It can often be the critical difference between an inadequate response and a fresh reboot to a healthy life.

Twenty Attributes

Heavy – Light	Gross – Subtle	Soft – Hard
Oily – Dry	Cold – Hot	Dense – Liquid
Stable – Mobile	Slow – Sharp	Cloudy – Clear
Slimy – Rough		

BioNexus Herbals

The proprietary BioNexus Herbals were formulated by drawing on the wisdom of ancient Eastern medicine, modern Western herbalism, and the incredible power of quantum medicine. Formula 1 NSB (nasal spray broad-spectrum) developed out of several years of research into mycotoxins and the search for an herbal alternative to eradicate MARCoNS. Research and clinical experience enabled the creation of a full line of formulas and blends to help BioNexus Health Clinic patients heal, repair, and maintain their health. The herbs used in BioNexus Herbals are sustainably grown, biodynamic, organic or wildcrafted, consciously harvested, and handmade in exclusive small batches in our FDA registered cGMP (current Good Manufacturing Process) facility in the United States. The formulas are also gluten-free, vegan, and lab tested for purity.

MARCONS SUCCESS STORY

Hayley spent her first 22 days in the NICU diagnosed with hyperinsulinism and hypoglycemia. Her mother reported Hayley developed slowly but reasonably met milestones until the age of three, except for language. Hayley used two to three-word phrases to express hunger and most of her needs, but never spoke in full sentences nor initiated or held conversations. At daycare, she lost interest in social interaction, kept mostly to herself, and reduced eye contact. Hayley received an ASD diagnosis at 3.5 years of age.

A local holistic practitioner started Hayley on a comprehensive biomedical protocol consisting of dietary modifications and nutritional supplements. Hayley enrolled in a special needs pre-school program where she received occupational therapy, physical therapy, and speech therapy.

Described as an easy-going child, Hayley continued to keep mostly to herself, had no behavioral issues, and did not require any behavioral intervention. For the next two years, Hayley made progress and demonstrated improvements in gross motor skills, self-care, activities of daily living, and some growth in language. Her language developed into short phrases. She also expressed a renewed interest in playing with peers and participated in group activities. The improvements prompted her mother to look for innovative therapies.

Hayley's mother attended a national autism conference where she learned about mold, biotoxin illness, and the devastating effects of mycotoxins on the brain. Recalling two incidents of water damage in their house, she decided to explore it.

When Hayley arrived at BioNexus Health Clinic, she was a pleasure to meet. A well-behaved, quiet little girl with big brown eyes and a lovely smile. As a part of the initial consultation, her nares were swabbed for MARCoNS testing. The results tested positive as resistant to four antibiotics and a moderate amount of biofilm.

A part of her protocol included a low amylose anti-inflammatory diet and Formula 1 NSB therapy. Hayley was unable to tolerate the first trial spray. Diluting her dose to tolerable levels for two weeks helped acclimate her to the spray, then the dose was slowly built up to three times per day for each nostril.

Four months after starting the treatments, Hayley tested negative for MARCoNS. Her parents reported impressive progress, improvements in fine motor skills, handwriting, focus, and attention to detail. Hayley was happier, more energetic, and lost her seasonal allergies. Her teacher also recommended half-day mainstream schooling with neurotypical kids.

SUSTAINABLE & LIFE-ENHANCING

BIONEXUS

Drawing on the wisdom of ancient Eastern medicine, modern Western herbalism, and the incredible power of quantum medicine.

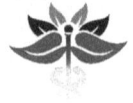

HERBALS & APOTHECARY

GLUTEN-FREE and VEGAN

"Look deep into nature, and you will understand everything better."

ALBERT EINSTEIN

All formulas and blends are lovingly handcrafted in small batches, never more than one gallon at a time, in old fashioned glass vats using artisanal methods, triple extraction techniques for maximum potency, and produced in an FDA registered facility using cGMP (current Good Manufacturing Process) practices in the United States.

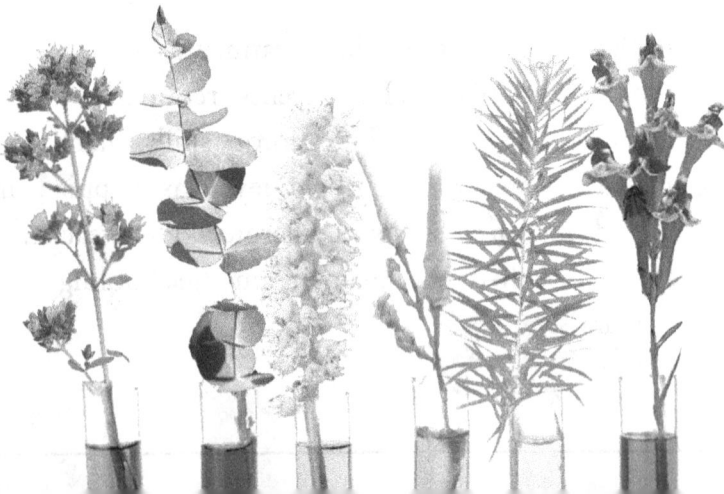

BioNexus Herbals were created to meet the unique needs of the our patient population. A large number of patients, including my son, Brian, just could not tolerate pharmaceuticals. I had to come up with an all-natural approach, which led me to the spectacular farm nestled in a fertile, lush green region of nearby Pennsylvania. With the genuinely gifted farmers onboard, the BioNexus apothecary was created. The rest, as they say, is history.

From seed to harvest, our biodynamic farm and apothecary is a labor of love. Our farmer and his wife are Yogis, trained herbalists, and passionate about their work with plants. Whether field grown or greenhouse sprouted, our spiritual herbal practices allow for conscious and respectful harvesting, including following the lunar cycles that optimize the herbal extracts' vitality and vibrance.

After two years in research and development, we began infusing the powerful rejuvenating properties of phyto stem cells into our products with our **HerbCelMax** methodology.

The herbal line has been wildly successful with BioNexus patients in over 50 countries. I sincerely hope these sacred plant extracts help you and your patients as much as they did mine.

In good health,

Jodie A. Dashore PhD, OTD, BCIP, HHP, CCH, RH (AHG)
Director, BioNexus Herbals and Apothecary

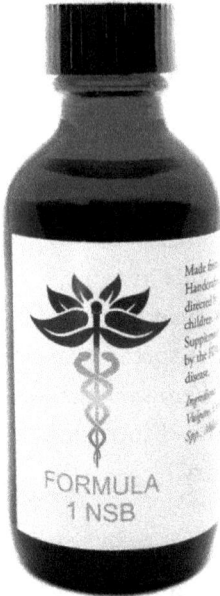

"in-vitro, a strong potential as an **alternative to current nasal spray treatment of MARCoNS** ... consistent with the requirement of the Dr. R. Shoemaker protocol for CIRS."

FORMULA
1 NSB
Nasal Spray Broad-Spectrum

A 2020 study led by Dr. Joseph D. Musto, D.A.B.B., President and Director of Laboratory Medicine at Microbiology DX in Bedford, MA, found, "32 of 33 cultures represent 97% of the cultures tested and showed very high inhibition (97.4% - 99.2%). The report concluded, "The Formula 1 NSB preparation shows in-vitro, a strong potential as an alternative to current nasal spray treatment of MARCoNS in deep nasal cultures and provides a means to eradicate nares MARCoNS consistent with the requirement of the Dr. R. Shoemaker protocol for CIRS." Additionally, "the yeast, Candida parapsilosis was also tested and showed a high level of inhibition at 97.8%."

Musto, J., Hrabec, G., & Moin, E. (2020).Report on the Effectiveness of the Antimicrobial Formula 1 NSB in Treating Multiple Antibiotic Resistant Coagulase Negative Staphylococcus (MARCoNS). Bedford, United States: MicrobiologyDX.

FORMULAS

Biotoxin Essential Oil Support

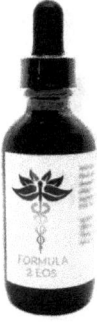

FORMULA 2 EOS

Insect Bite Tincture

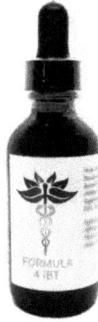

FORMULA 4 IBT

Dental Health Protocol

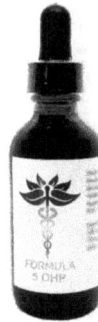

FORMULA 5 DHP

DHP - Extra Strength

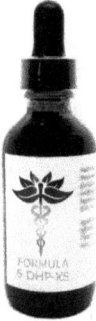

FORMULA 5 DHP-XS

Parasite Broad-Spectrum Support 1

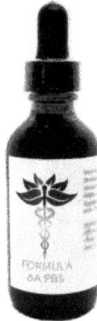

FORMULA 6A PBS

Parasite Broad-Spectrum Support 2

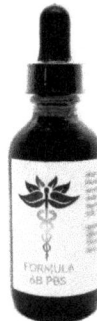

FORMULA 6B PBS

Glyphosate Detox Support

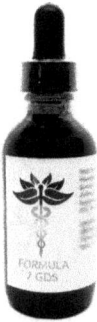

FORMULA 7 GDS

Inflammation and Joint Support

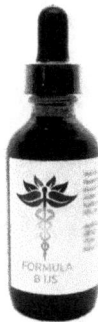

FORMULA 8 IJS

Hurt, Heartbreak and Grief

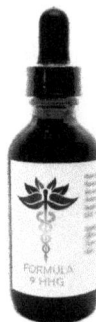

FORMULA 9 HHG

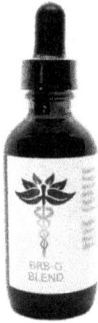

Berberine Blend G

BRB-G BLEND

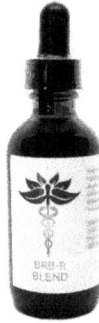

Berberine Blend R

BRB-R BLEND

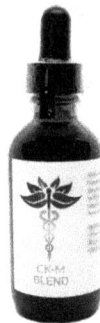

Cytokine Modulating

CK-M BLEND

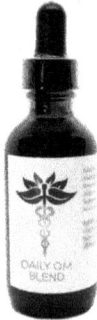

Daily Om

DAILY OM BLEND

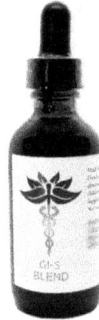

Gastrointestinal Support

GI-S BLEND

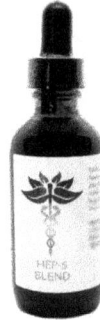

Liver/Hepatic Support

HEP-S BLEND

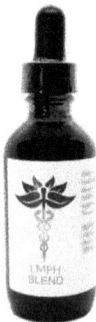

Lymphatic Support

LMPH BLEND

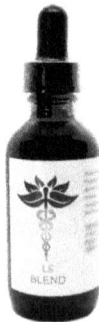

Lung Support

LS BLEND

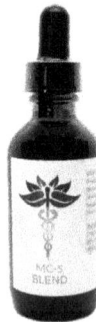

Mast Cell Support

MC-S BLEND

BLENDS

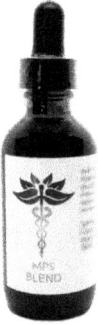

Mycoplasma Support

MPS BLEND

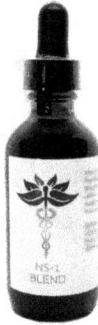

Neuro Support Level 1

NS-1 BLEND

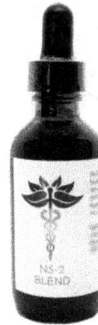

Neuro Support Level 2

NS-2 BLEND

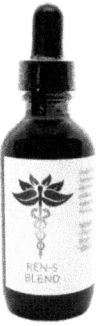

Renal/Kidney Support

REN-S BLEND

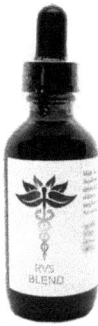

Retroviral Support

RVS BLEND

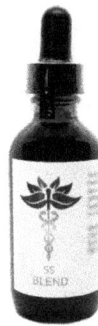

Staph and Strep

SS BLEND

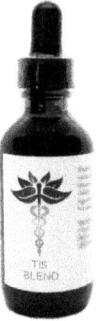

Tick-borne Infection Support

TIS BLEND

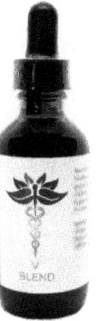

Virus

V BLEND

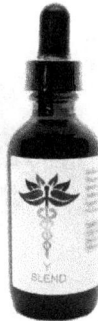

Yeast

Y BLEND

BLENDS HerbCel Max

Stem cells are the "renewal engine" of a plant known for its exceptional resilience and regenerative properties. The bioactive power of HerbCelMax enhances and supports the body's natural defenses.

Biotoxin Detox

BTXD BLEND

Immune System Boosting

IS-B BLEND

Immune System Modulating

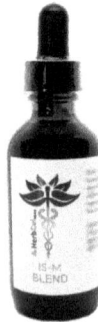

IS-M BLEND

MOLD STARTER PACK

Nasal Spray Broad-Spectrum

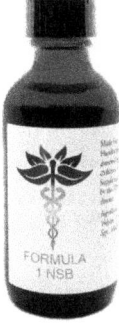

FORMULA 1 NSB

Biotoxin Essential Oil Support

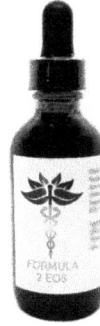

FORMULA 2 EOS

DHP - Extra Strength

FORMULA 5 DHP-XS

Biotoxin Detox

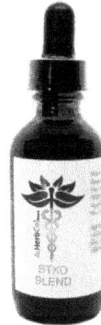

BTXD BLEND
HerbCal Max

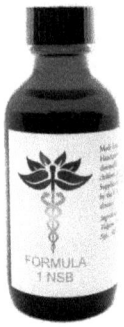

Nasal Spray Broad-Spectrum

Refrigerate on arrival travel upto 48 hours without

SHAKE WELL before each use

STORE AWAY from sunlight

GENERAL PRACTITIONER guidelines

DO NOT USE WHILE pregnant or breastfeeding

DO NOT USE WITH medical nebulizer

STORE AWAY from outlets

FORMULA 1 NSB

START	x2 per nostril per day
MAX	x2 per nostril 3x per day
SENSITIVE	Dilute 50%
	Under 5 YRS & Ultra-Sensitive:
	Dilute 75% (25% formula)
CHILD	Nostril #1 x1 wait 24 hrs
	Nostril #2 x1 wait 24 hrs
	x1 Both 2-4 days
	x1 Both 2x per day

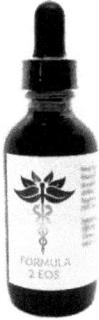

Biotoxin Essential Oil Support

FORMULA 2 EOS

Pets
Studies show that ingestion and direct skin contact with certain essential oils can be harmful to canines. Do not use essential oil sprays on or near a pet.

EXTERNAL USE ONLY
do not ingest

DO NOT USE WHILE
pregnant or breastfeeding

SHAKE WELL
before each use

STORE AWAY
from outlets

KEEP OUT OF REACH
of children

GENERAL PRACTITIONER
guidelines

Sensitive Individuals: Test on forearm before use and dilute, if needed

Diffuser: Add 5 drops per diffuser cycle, depending on diffuser and preference. Refill as needed

Room Spray: Add 40 drops to 4 oz (118 ml) distilled or purified water in a sprayer bottle. Use as an air freshener

Personal Space Spray: Add 15 drops to 2 oz (59 ml) of distilled or purified water in a sprayer bottle. Spray the immediate area around the person

External Personal Spray: Spray a mist of 2 to 3 pumps of Personal Space Spray overhead and let it cascade down on the person

Detox Bath: 5 drops into the water

Patient Recommended

Non-Toxic Cleaner: Add 5 drops into distilled water or all-natural surface cleaning solution

Floors: Add 5 drops into a full bottle of all-natural floor mopping solution

Carpets: Add 10 drops into a full fluid reservoir of a carpet cleaner or carpet streamer

Shampoo: Add 2-5 drops to 8 oz (240 ml) bottle

Laundry: Add 5-10 drops to a full load of laundry

Clothes/Drapes: Add 2-5 drops into a full fluid reservoir of a clothes steamer

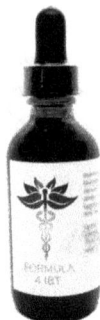

EXTERNAL USE ONLY
do not ingest

STORE AT
room temperature

KEEP AWAY FROM
heat and humidity

KEEP OUT OF REACH
of children

DO NOT USE WHILE
pregnant or breastfeeding

STORE AWAY
from outlets

GENERAL PRACTITIONER
guidelines

FORMULA 4 IBT

Suggestion for New Tick Bites: TIS Blend 10 drops 3x per day, CK-M Blend 5 drops 3x per day, and IS-M blend 10 drops 1x per day for 6 weeks

BNH BITE-SITE PROTOCOL

Transfer half Formula 4 IBT bottle to a small (travel-size) spray bottle

Day 1
1. Spray generously on the bite or sting and let dry
2. In a small bowl or glass jar, add 1/2 tsp of an organic clay powder
3. Add enough Formula 4 IBT drops to form a thick and sticky paste
4. Apply clay paste to bite or sting
5. Cover with a band-aid (optional)

Days 2-4
Mix a new batch daily
Repeat steps 1-5; 3-4x per day

Days 5-7
Mix a new batch daily
Repeat steps 1-5; 2x per day

Redness, swelling, itching, and discomfort often subside within 4 days

Removing Ticks
Correctly remove ticks from the mouthparts. Instructional videos available on lymedisease.org

Dental Health Protocol

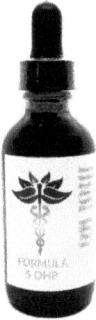

DHP - Extra Strength

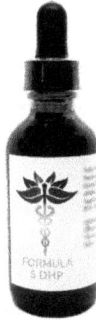

Antimicrobial to help eliminate biofilm, bacteria, mycotoxins, and MARCoNS

DO NOT USE WHILE pregnant or breastfeeding

KEEP OUT OF REACH of children

STORE AWAY from outlets

GENERAL PRACTITIONER guidelines

FORMULA 5 DHP   **FORMULA** 5 DHP-XS

	GARGLE	GUM RUB
START	2-3x per day; 10 drops in 2 oz (60 ml) filtered water	1-2 drops on gums 1x per day
MAX	3x per day; 10 drops in 2 oz (60 ml) filtered water	2 drops on gums 1x per day
SENSITIVE	2x per day; 5 drops in 2 oz (60 ml) filtered water	1 drop on gums 1x per day
CHILD	2x per day; 5 drops in 2 oz (60 ml) filtered water	1 drop on gums 1x per day

FORMULA 6A PBS	**LMPH** BLEND
FORMULA 6B PBS	**LS** BLEND
FORMULA 7 GDS	**MC-S** BLEND
FORMULA 8 IJS	**MPS** BLEND
FORMULA 9 HHG	**NS-1** BLEND
BRB-G BLEND	**NS-2** BLEND
BRB-R BLEND	**REN-S** BLEND
BTXD BLEND **Herb** Max	**RVS** BLEND
CK-M BLEND	**SS** BLEND
DAILY OM BLEND	**TIS** BLEND
GI-S BLEND	**V** BLEND
HEP-S BLEND	**Y** BLEND
IS-B BLEND **Herb** Max	
IS-M BLEND **Herb** Max	

General Practitioner Herbal Usage and Dosage Guidelines
for BioNexus Herbals formulas and blends on the previous page

Prepare herbal doses in 1-2 oz glass of distilled or purified water

DO NOT USE WHILE pregnant or breastfeeding

Wait 20 minutes after preparation to consume

KEEP OUT OF REACH of children

STORE AWAY from outlets

No food or drink 10 minutes after intake

GENERAL PRACTITIONER guidelines

START   Increase 1 drop every other day

MAX   15 drops 3x per day

SENSITIVE   **Herxheimer symptoms or die-off reactions** usually occur around 5-10 drops (sometimes sooner)

REDUCE
to 1-2 drops per day
OR
take a break for a few days

THEN RESTART with 1-2 drops per day

CHILD   1 drop per 10 lbs/ 4.5 kg of body weight divided into 2-3 doses

10 minutes after food

Report on the Effectiveness of the Antimicrobial Formula 1 NSB

In Treating Multiple Antibiotic Resistant Coagulase Negative Staphylococcus (MARCoNS)

Dr. Joseph D. Musto, D.A.B.B.
President and Director of Laboratory Medicine

George Hrabec, B.Sc., M.Sc.
Director of Microbiology

Erum Moin, B.Sc.
Clinical Technologist
Microbiology Dx, Bedford, MA

Dr. Jodie A. Dashore, PhD, OTD, BCIP, HHP, CCH, RH (AHG), Director, BioNexus Health Clinic Marlboro, NJ

February 10, 2020; Updated April 22, 2020

Introduction:

Chronic Inflammatory Response Syndrome (CIRS) describes a constellation of symptoms, associated laboratory findings and test results associated with biotoxin exposure in genetically susceptible individuals. First identified by Ritchie Shoemaker, M.D., his clinical research has resulted in a step-wise approach to patient care that has been demonstrated to treat and prevent symptoms in susceptible individuals.

In CIRS, MARCoNS have been found to colonize the deep nasal cavity in 80% of individuals with low MSH hormone. The presence of MARCoNS in the nasopharynx impairs the body to re-establish normal levels of MSH. Adequate MSH is required for recovery from biotoxin induced CIRS. MARCoNS may exist in a biofilm, which makes it more difficult to treat. A deep nasal culture is obtained and sent to Microbiology Dx, Bedford, MA. If Coagulase Negative Staphylococci are present and resistant to more than one class of antibiotics, then treatment is required.

This report shows the in-vitro evaluation of 33 patient nares cultures, 26 MARCoNS positive and 7 MARCoNS negative.

I. Objective:
To study the effectiveness of Formula 1 NSB on MARCoNS positive and MARCoNS negative bacteria in nutrient broth.

II. Materials:
    A. Formula 1 NSB Solution (2X)

    B. Organisms Tested

    1. Staphylococcus epidermidis (SE) ATCC 35984, MARCoNS positive, biofilm positive strong (3+) control.

    2. 33 Nares patient cultures, 26 MARCoNS positive and 7 Staph Coag Negative-Non MARCoNS. 25 of 26 MARCoNS cultures were biofilm positive.

III. Testing Protocol:

A. All testing was performed with a patient control.

B. A McFarland Standard (MS) of 1.0 was prepared for the MARCoNS control ATCC 35984 and for each patient culture.

C. All testing was performed in a liquid format.

D. For the MARCoNS control and each patient culture, 2 polystyrene tubes 12 x 75 mm were labeled as test and control.

E. The MS of 1.0, 100μl was pipetted into 900μl of Tryptic Soy Broth (TSB) for each patient and its control.

F. Then 1000μl of test solution for the patient test was pipetted and 1000μl of water for each patient control tubes was pipetted.

G. Both sets, 33 patients and the MARCoNS positive control were incubated for 24 hours at 37°C.

H. At 24 hours of incubation, the tubes (test and control) were removed from the incubator and a 1μl loop was taken, planted on a Blood Agar Plate (BAP) and the plate was incubated at 37°C for 24 hours. Then growth was evaluated for each patient test compared to its own control.

IV. Results:

A. The Formula 1 NSB was provided for testing in twice the concentration to take into consideration the dilution effect in the testing protocol.

B. The testing values used were such that the final concentration in-vitro was equal to the treatment nasal spray concentration.

C. There were 33 cultures, all Staph Coag Negative, 26 MARCoNS positive, 7 Staph Coag Negative-Non MARCoNS, and samples had biofilm positive strong (3+). 32 of the 33 cultures showed high level of inhibition, between 97.4% to 99.2% inhibition and 1 non-MARCoNS showed 40% inhibition. Therefore, 32 of 33 cultures represent 97% of the cultures tested and showed very high inhibition (97.4% - 99.2%).

D. Additionally, the yeast, Candida parapsilosis was also tested and showed a high level of inhibition at 97.8%.

V. Conclusion:

The Formula 1 NSB preparation shows in-vitro, a strong potential as an alternative to current nasal spray treatment of MARCoNS in deep nasal cultures and provides a means to eradicate nares MARCoNS consistent with the requirement of the Dr. R. Shoemaker protocol for CIRS.

Dr. Dashore is a clinical herbalist and an accredited registered herbalist with the American Herbalist Guild.

Formula 1 NSB is a proprietary herbal formulation created by Dr. Dashore.

PART 5

SPECIAL CIRCUMSTANCES

"Start by doing what's necessary; then do what's possible; and suddenly you are doing the impossible."

—Francis of Assisi, ~1182-1226

RISK FACTORS FOR POOR OUTCOMES

Continued biotoxin exposure
Unresolved comorbidities
Subclinical hypothyroid
Emotional trauma
Subacute cholecystitis
Gut dysbiosis
Methylation Pathways Defects
Mitochondrial Dysfunction
Biofilm
Multiple Chemical Sensitivities
Mast Cell Activation Syndrome
Porphyria
Heavy Metal Toxicity
GMOs
Other environmental neurotoxins
Retroviruses
Prescription drugs
Breast implants and associated toxins

Biotoxin illness and CIRS patients present with a variety of associated challenging conditions, including gastrointestinal and methylation issues, mast cell activation syndrome (MCAS), multiple chemical sensitivities (MCS), and poor immune health. This section covers special circumstances and poor outcome risk factors that I feel are important to highlight based on clinical experience. I urge practitioners to conduct additional research on all the considerations, including pediatric, geriatric, mast cell activation syndrome, multiple chemical sensitivities, porphyria, and breast implants.

History of GI Issues

Patients with a history of inflammatory gastrointestinal intestinal (GI) symptoms require extra precaution when transitioning to an herbal protocol. Always begin patients on a minimum or sensitive dosage. Down regulation of inflammation, and gut support and repair are usually the starting points before undertaking any antimicrobial protocol.

Methylation

A DNA epigenetic mechanism (methylation) changes the coded activity (regulation of genes). Subtle modifications to polymorphisms (genetic variations) affect gene function and predispose people to certain diseases. Studies show methylation can silence DNA transcription and is an essential part of nutrition and detoxification (Jin, Li, & Robertson, 2011). Most polymorphisms are the result of a single nucleotide change, therefore are called single nucleotide polymorphisms (SNPs). SNPs impact biochemical functions, including detoxification, metabolism, hormone balance, and vitamin D in the methylation cycle and pathway.

Biotoxin illness is a transcriptomic illness. The HLA-DR gene causes abnormal gene expression rendering the acquired immune system useless against biotoxins. Understanding and identifying SNPs help determine the most effective supplements a patient needs for health maintenance and recovery. SNPs inherited from one parent are called heterozygous (+/-). If it is from both parents, then it is homozygous (+/+). The presence of SNPs causes variable changes during methylation.

The GENIE test (See Part 3: Finding a Diagnosis) is not an SNP test. GENIE looks at differential gene activation compared to controls.

MCS, MCAS, and Porphyria

CIRS patients consistently report becoming more sensitive to pollution and lose resilience against daily life stressors. Every CIRS aware practitioner should have a working knowledge of multiple chemical sensitivities, mast cell activation syndrome, and porphyria (buildup of natural chemicals producing porphyrin). These stealth issues frequently go unnoticed, unaddressed, or misdiagnosed by physicians and practitioners. In many CIRS cases, these illnesses occur together.

Patients with MCS/MCAS require specific supplementation and very slow and gentle buildup of plant-based protocols to increase tolerance and avoid reactivity. Please refer to the Appendix section for detailed information on treatment variations required for people with MCS/MCAS.

Multiple Chemical Sensitivities (MCS)

Exposure to biotoxins and other environmental pollutants, such as solvents, volatile organic compounds (VOCs), perfumes, gasoline and diesel, smoke, household chemicals in general, pollen, house dust mites, pet fur, dander, and mold, can cause acute reactions and autoimmunities leading to chronic illness. Some physicians refer to it as "idiopathic environmental intolerance," which is more commonly known as multiple chemical sensitivities (MCS). MCS is not an allergy and affects people of all ages and all nationalities. The toxic reaction results in neurological symptoms ranging from mild to severely

Examples of Chemical Disruptors

Products enhanced with fragrance contain phthalates (perfumes, colognes, cleaning products, et cetera)

Plastics containing BPA and PVC #3 (single-use packaging, tin can lining, drinking water, toys)

Personal care products with BPA, per-fluorinated chemicals (PFCs), triclosan, parabens, and phthalates (shampoos, conditioners, lotions, nail polish, eye makeup, sunscreens, deodorant, toothpaste, shaving cream, hairspray)

The patient should carefully read the labels of products before purchase and understand any possible connection between products and symptoms. A comprehensive natural detoxification regimen should address endocrine disruptors and propose products made with safe and natural ingredients or materials.

disabling. The onset of MCS frequently occurs suddenly and is characterized by severe depression, fatigue, anorexia, chills, fever, headache, muscle pain, joint pain, nausea, vomiting, abdominal pain, and shortness of breath.

The emergence of MCS signifies a high overall toxin load. MCS presents with differing intensity and frequency of symptoms and triggers, making it is nearly impossible to describe a typical case.

Tolerance levels also change from person to person, with some people finding exposure one day knocks them out, while other days, there are no adverse effects. Many people suffering from MCS encounter severe "endocrine disruptor" reactions. Testing MCS patients typically show impaired detoxification pathways.

Endocrine Disruptors

Everyday household cleaning products, personal care products, food, cosmetics, pharmaceuticals, pesticides, plastic, water, and soil contain chemicals known as endocrine disruptors. Chemicals released into the air can spread throughout the house, creating an opportunity for inhalation or contact. Upon uptake, they can mimic a natural hormone and bind to hormone receptors that alter hormonal synthesis, transport, binding, and breakdown (U.S. Environmental Protection Agency, 2020). Stimulation or inhibition of the endocrine system causes overproduction or underproduction of hormones. In the thyroid, for example, the chemicals may cause the body to over-respond or mistime a response to a stimulus.

Mast Cell Activation Syndrome (MCAS)

Chronic exposure to environmental pathogens like toxic mold can trigger the activation of Toll-like receptors (TLRs), which activates mast cells. Without removal of the trigger, mast cells can become overactive in some individuals, leading to the development of mast cell activation syndrome (MCAS).

Bone marrow-derived mast cells play a critical role in tissue pathogen defense and chronic inflammation (Wilmott et al.,

2018). Within minutes of allergen activation, mast cells can deploy proinflammatory functions, and, potentially, immuno-regulatory mediators, including cytokines, histamine, growth factors, and leukotrienes (Amin, 2012). In biotoxin illness patients, when the body contains too many complement proteins (C4a and C3a), the innate immune system identifies it as an allergen releasing histamine. Too much histamine in the body creates excess exotoxins producing an inviting environment for quorum bacteria to produce biofilm. Mast cells also increase vascular permeability and cognitive dysfunction. The overall influx of changes can create a flurry of other autoimmune disorders, asthma, migraines, and other multisymptom illnesses.

In mast cell activation syndrome (MCAS), patients have normal or near-normal numbers of mast cells but a range of symptoms arising from the unusual activation of mast cells. Patients present with a variety of common symptoms, including food and environmental sensitivities, gut inflammation, brain fog, fatigue, skin conditions, bloating, poor digestion, motility issues, anxiety, mood disorders, and lung-related symptoms (National Organization of Rare Disorders, 2018).

Proposed Required Criteria For MCAS

1. Episodic multisystem symptoms consistent with mast cell activation.

2. An appropriate response to medications targeting mast cell activation.

3. The documented increase in validated markers of mast cell activation systemically (serum or urine) during an asymptomatic period compared with the patient's baseline values (Akin, 2017).

Identify and address each trigger for MCAS patients. Naturopathic treatment options are available in the Appendix. Each practitioner needs to create a protocol to integrate within the BioNexus Approach.

CASE STUDY - RUBY

Ruby experienced a sharp decline in health with physical pain, exhaustion, heat intolerance, cognitive decline, and an inability to care for herself or her son. For four years, she'd been on multiple high-dose antibiotics and antifungals to treat her Lyme disease, chronic fatigue syndrome, fibromyalgia, IBS, and depression. She noted the conventional protocols improved her symptoms but she relapsed soon after they moving in to a new construction townhome.

After becoming housebound and on near-constant bedrest, mold growth was found in their boiler room from a hidden slow leak. In a fragile state from the aggressive allopathic treatments, Ruby sought naturopathic options for her new symptoms, comprising of migraines, blurry vision, joint pain, hypothyroidism, and hormonal imbalances. "I seem to be allergic to life itself," the now 42-year-old Ruby said during her initial consultation when she also revealed she battled extreme fatigue and severe food sensitivities.

Ruby tested positive for CIRS, Lyme disease, Babesia, and Ehrlichia, and porphyria.

After the family moved again, Ruby started her plant-based protocol with a pinch and a drop of herbal medicines. As her tolerance grew, she began to feel better. Fourteen months into her treatment, Ruby was functioning at 60 percent, but her quality of life dramatically improved. She takes care of her son, runs errands, enjoys her marriage, and creates recipes in the kitchen.

Ruby is still a patient and focused on fully regaining her physical and mental strength. She has truly enjoyed and highly recommends two BNH recipes, which she aptly refers to as Pre-Treatment BNH Mild Soup and Post-Treatment BNH Spiced Lentil Soup (See recipes in this Part).

Porphyria

When I was deep in research trying to figure out the root causes of my son's symptoms, I stumbled upon the work on Porphyria by Professor Steven Rochlitz, PhD. After an illuminating 2-hour conversation, he mailed me his book Porphyria: The Ultimate Cause of Common, Chronic, and Environmental Illnesses - With Breakthroughs in Diet, Supplements, and Energy Balancing (2013). The book influenced my ability to understand healing possibilities, not only for my child but also for patients.

Every cell of the body makes porphyrins. Professor Rochlitz explains when iron binds with aromatic compounds (porphyrin rings), it makes heme. Porphyria is a metabolic disorder of

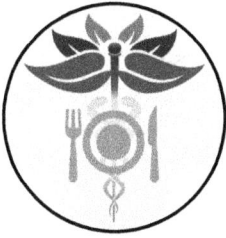

Pre-Treatment BNH Mild Soup

A mild, minimalist soup tolerable early in treatment

Ingredients (organic)

1 bunch scallions
1 small carrot
2 baby bok choy
1 tsp olive oil
1 tbsp ginger grated
4 cups water
1 tbsp medicinal mushroom powder mix
1/4 cup frozen peas
1/4 cup cooked white rice
1/2 cup shredded boiled chicken
2 tsp white miso
Salt to taste

Note: Very sensitive people may need to replace rice with magic noodles, which are devoid of starch. As starch tolerance builds, soak rice for 24 hours, and rinse until the water runs clear to help reduce starch.

Instructions

Thinly slice the scallions and carrot diagonally

Slice bok choy, keeping whites and greens separate

Heat oil in a small soup pot, sauté carrots and scallions for 1-2 minutes

Add ginger and sauté another minute

Add water and mushroom powder mix; bring to boil; reduce heat and simmer uncovered for 20 minutes

Add peas, bok choy greens, rice (or magic noodles), and chicken

In a small bowl, blend the miso with a small amount of the broth; return the miso mixture to the pot

Simmer without boiling for 5 more minutes

Post-Treatment
BNH Spiced Lentil Soup

After gut repair, try Ruby's gently spiced soup

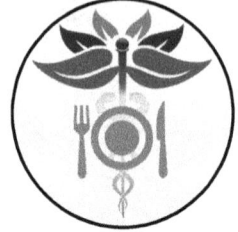

Ingredients (organic)

2 tbsp coconut oil

1 onion chopped

4 cloves garlic minced

4 or 5 carrots sliced in half-moons

3 stalks celery sliced

1 diced bell pepper

1/4 cup seaweed soup mix

2 cups red lentils

1 tsp sea salt

1 tsp ground cumin

1 tsp curry powder

1 tsp black pepper

10 cups water

5 kale leaves (ribs removed)

Instructions

In a large soup pot, sauté onions and garlic in oil

Add carrots, celery, and bell peppers; sauté for 5 more minutes

Add seaweed soup mix, red lentils, salt, and spices

Slowly stir in water; bring to a boil, then lower heat and let simmer partially covered until lentils are cooked, stir occasionally

Stir in chopped kale and cook for 5 more minutes until kale is tender, but still bright green.

Salt to taste and enjoy!

abnormal heme production. It can be a genetic or an acquired condition.

Environmental factors, alcohol, certain drugs, hormones, stress, dieting, and other illnesses can trigger porphyria. Generally, acute symptoms affect the nervous system and cutaneous, mainly affecting the skin. In addition to being a part of hemoglobin, heme is also a set of eight enzymes, including cytochrome P450 (CYP450), which aids in detoxification. However, in some people, when a substance causes CYP450 enzyme activation instead of detoxing the material, it causes excess porphyrin production and heme deficiency - elevating the body's toxicity, which affects the organs.

When materials fail to breakdown, they accumulate within the body, they can potentially act as a trigger after reaching adequate levels. A person afflicted by porphyria reach overload at much smaller concentrations causing profound fatigue, brain fog, joint pain, nausea, anxiety, irritable bowels, and more. Evidence points through proper testing methods lead to a possible explanation as to why some biotoxin illness patients cannot tolerate thyroid hormones, or respond contrary to typical results from melatonin, Benadryl, and adrenal supplementation. Porphyria could also explain patient food intolerances not revealed in lab testing for IgE and IgG.

Pediatrics

The principals and methods of treatment are the same for children as they are for adults. However, due to the delicate nature of pediatric bodies, the doses are lower. Nevertheless, younger children tend to progress relatively faster than teenagers and adults.

While using the CIRS protocol, never use Actos (pioglitazone) or Procrit (erythropoietin) on pediatric patients. VIP nasal spray may be used with careful and regular monitoring. Always follow all guidelines and instructions for pediatric prescriptions.

Dosing

Follow general pediatric guidelines for herbal dosage, unless otherwise directed. Keep in mind that herbal preparation methods and formulations change recommended herbal doses. Pediatric doses depend significantly more on the weight of the child and less on chronological age, adjust treatments accordingly.

Essential Oil Safety

Special precautions and considerations must be made before using essential oils or blends on children. Essential oils can adversely affect children's skin, immune system, and immature livers rendering them more susceptible to toxic effects.

General Age Guidelines

3-6 months: 1/20th of an adult dose

6 months to 2 years: 1/10th of an adult dose

2-5 years: 1/5th of an adult dose

5-12 years: 1/4 to 1/2 of an adult dose

12- 18 years: 1/2 to full adult dose

General Measurement Conversions

1 ml = 20 drops

5 ml = 1 teaspoon

20 ml = 1 tablespoon

75 ml = 1/2 cup

The popular rise of herbs and essential oils has led to more parents believing that natural equates to safe and harmless. A review of records by The Tennessee Poison Center (Loden, 2016) found reported toxic exposures doubled between 2011 and 2015, 80% of reports were for children.

Medicinal herbs and essential oils, when chosen according to clinical principles, can act as valuable synergists to enhance the outcomes of the patient if handled carefully. Use best practices for all pediatric patients when suggesting or prescribing essential oils and blends.

Always For Pediatrics

Keep out a reach of children
Purchase oils with child-resistant caps (when possible)
Use oils externally only
Dilute oils before adding them to bathwater
Stop use immediately if a rash or other skin reaction occurs and dilute
the area with a carrier oil, then gently wash it

Never For Pediatrics

Allow a child to ingest oils
Apply oils directly to a child's face
Put oils or blends near a child's nose
Expose children under five-years-old to strong oil vapors

When Accidents Happen

If a child accidentally ingests oils - have the child drink milk to
dilute the oils; immediately go to the emergency room

If undiluted oils get on a child's skin - immediately dilute with
a carrier oil

If essential oils get in a child's eye(s) - flush the eyes
continuously with water

Pediatric Essential Oil Dosage

Newborn to 3-Months
Do not use any form of essential oils or aromatherapy

3-Months to 2-years
Acceptable Herbs: lavender, geranium, chamomile, conifers

Do not use any form near the immunologically challenged
Only use a diffuser and keep exposure to a minimum

2-years to 5-years
Additional Acceptable Herbs: roman chamomile, orange,
bergamot, frankincense, geranium, ginger, lemon,
marjoram, tea tree, and thyme

Diffusers and diluted oil are acceptable but continue to
keep exposure to a minimum

Avoid all other oils

Geriatrics

About 10% of the BioNexus Health Clinic (BNH) patient population are senior citizens. I don't ascribe to the concept of "you're just getting older" as an explanation for declining health. I firmly believe in the body's innate ability to heal and adapt at any age. Many seniors who accompany their grandchildren to their appointments with BNH become aware of CIRS and its devastating effects. If the grandparent lives with their grandchildren, they generally become convinced that their failing health may also be biotoxin-related and ask to be tested. They are usually correct because environmental illnesses tend to affect family members living together.

Plant-based protocols resonate perfectly as a gentle, yet effective option with the relatively fragile senior physiology. Older adult patients also respond incredibly well to natural therapies. It brings me joy to see them improve and regain significant levels of vitality.

Prescriptions and Cognitive Effects

Prescription drugs can be lifesaving and essential in acute situations. With chronic illnesses, these often come with a full set of problems and adverse effects that can impede health and well-being, especially in older adults. Frequently, secondary and tertiary prescriptions or over-the-counter (OTC) medicine

CASE STUDY - VIRGINIA

Diagnosed with Lyme disease, Callie missed her sophomore year of high school, and even with intravenous antibiotics, she became bedbound. BNH diagnosed Callie with CIRS-Lyme, CIRS-WDB, and mast cell activation. Placed on a plant-based protocol, Callie steadily improved.

After, Callie's grandmother, Virginia, lost her home to Hurricane Sandy. She moved into the finished basement with Callie. Virginia described herself as a vibrant, and strong-willed senior who still had a zest for life, but recently, her health declined, sending her into depression.

She described it to her doctors as "a curtain on my mind." Her doctors reminded her that she was nearing eighty and prescribed conventional medicine for each symptom on her growing list.

When Virginia accompanied Callie to her BNH appointments, she became CIRS aware and suspected that might be her problem. She was tired of feeling like a diseased old lady, waiting to take her last breath. Virginia wanted her independent life back.

Virginia tested positive for CIRS-WDB and MARCoNS resistant to seven antibiotics, including Gentamicin. At the time, she was treated with multiple courses of Fluconazole in an attempt to manage her

IBS-like symptoms and an inflamed gut. BNH customized a slow build-up to an entirely plant-based protocol. Other than some initial die-off reactions, she responded very well.

After nine months, Virginia stopped using her walker, built a tiny house on her daughter's ranch, and now enjoys her new normal independent lifestyle. She reports that her thought process, memory, and nasal congestion have significantly improved. Her thyroid has stabilized, and her gut health feels optimal. Virginia's zest is back. She's planning to travel more and enjoys hanging out with her friends.

Virginia also mastered online navigation and, when needed, likes to connect virtually with BNH for appointments.

become necessary to combat the side effects of the initial treatment. Several common medications are anticholinergic – blocking acetylcholine. Taking a few anticholinergic drugs together can cause cognitive and neurological side effects. These side effects can go unnoticed or misdiagnosed.

Patients with CIRS, Lyme disease, and other tick-borne infections typically have dysautonomia (autonomic dysfunction) and POTS (postural orthostatic tachycardia syndrome). The autonomic nervous system in the body has two branches: sympathetic and parasympathetic. Acetylcholine is a primary neurotransmitter for the parasympathetic nervous system that helps to conserve energy, rest, digest, and heal. The body requires both branches to function correctly to maintain a state of homeostasis. An anticholinergic medication blocks the neurotransmitter acetylcholine action and can lead to an imbalance in the autonomic nervous system. An overactive sympathetic system can cause or exacerbate insomnia, anxiety, panic, and agitation symptoms. Patients may also experience dry mouth, dry eyes, blurry vision, reduced sweating, constipation, memory issues, confusion, and depression.

Studies show a significant increase in dementia risk for patients taking pharmaceutical drugs like anticholinergic antidepressants, anti-Parkinson's medications, anti-seizure drugs, bladder anti-spasmodic medications, and some antipsychotics (Molchan et al., 1992; Malaz Boustani, 2009; Alzheimer's Association, 2018). Chronic illness patients often see multiple specialists seeking relief from their numerous symptoms. When various doctors prescribe medications, the patients may take several anticholinergic drugs. Most people can tolerate a short course of treatment, but longer rounds and repeated use demands careful monitoring, especially in the older population.

Examples of Anticholinergic Medications
Cimetidine (Tagamet -antacid)
Citalopram (Celexa -antidepressant)
Dextromethorphan (cough suppressant)
Doxepin (sleep disorders, antidepressant)
Ipratropium (Atrovent -for bronchitis and COPD)
Tolterodine (Detrol -for bladder spasms)
Xanax (alprazolam)

When patients present with a multitude of symptoms and currently take several prescription medications (especially older patients), ascertain the pharmacokinetics and pharmacodynamics of each prescription.

Breast Implants

The number of female patients with breast implants diagnosed with CIRS and/or tick-borne infections at BioNexus Health Clinic has not been very high. Nevertheless, the challenges experienced in detoxification and healing are significantly notable. Other practitioners worldwide also report similar complex clinical presentations in patients with breast implants.

While not exhaustedly researched, breast implants have been associated with a long list of possible adverse reactions (U.S. Food and Drug Administration, 2019). According to the American Society of Plastic Surgery, 313,335 breast implant surgeries were performed in 2018. The National Women's Health Network (2017) reports, "within two years of having breast implants inserted, women reported experiencing signs and symptoms of connective tissue disease such as increased muscle weakness, fatigue, and muscle and joint pain. Twenty percent of patients with breast augmentations required additional surgeries after only three years due to complications. The complications included infection, loss of breast sensation, hematoma, and development of scar tissue that sometimes resulted in misshapen breasts or pain." Potential toxicity from breast implants cannot be overlooked in patients with CIRS, Lyme disease, and autism with associated immune dysfunction.

Begin at the Beginning

Laborious history taking is required. It is nearly impossible to get better unless the environment is clean, safe, and toxin-free. Consider the following questions to discover biotoxin sources.

Bio-Individualized Protocols

Every patient is unique

A small, seemingly insignificant symptom could be the missing key to unlocking biotoxin illness and CIRS

Identify The Source Building

Apply the following questions to each location: home, work, school, vehicles, recreational activities, and therapies.

Do you feel worse when leaving a location?
Do you feel better after not visiting a location for awhile?
Are there any musty smells?
Are any cardboard boxes moldy?

Exposure Building Details

Age

Building Materials

Finished or unfinished basement

Sump pump location

Flat or pitched roof

Ventilation

Insulation

Kind of cooling system

Location of cooling system

Last time filters were changed, or A/C cleaned

Kind of heating system

Location of heating system

Last time filters were changed

Duct materials used on forced hot air systems

Closed or open gutters

Attached or unattached garage

Water gathering around any area

Foundation cracks

Moss or mold growing on the outside

Windows missing flashing

Possible Leaks Or Water Intrusion

Roof

Window

Plumbing

Refrigerator

Dishwasher

Kitchen Sink

Clothes washing machine

Waterline breaks

Toilets

Bathroom sinks

Bathtub or shower

Basement

Are there any areas with water stains

Water Intrusion Repair

Did the carpet get wet or soaked

Was the carpet dried or replaced

If dried, how many days was it actively dried

Household Machines

Clothes Washing Machine

Age

Front or top loading

Clothes ever left inside overnight

Clothes left for extended periods with the lid closed

Cleaned regularly

Dishwasher

Age

Heat dry feature used

How soon after the end of a cycle is the door opened

Other Toxin Exposures

Body of water with blue-green algae

Ticks or tick-borne infections

Mycoplasma pneumoniae

Epstein Barr

Other viruses

CASE STUDY - AIDAN

BioNexus Health Clinic discharged Aidan after 16 months of treatment for CIRS. He was placed on a maintenance protocol and had been symptom-free for three months.

Aidan took the bus to school, where he maintained good grades throughout his first grading period. In December of that year, there were many days of sleet and snow. Aidan, a mold HLA-DR haplotype, developed a deep dry cough, sinusitis, low-grade fevers, and headaches. His pediatrician thought it was the common cold. As winter pressed on, his cough progressed, and his pediatrician suggested prednisone.

Aidan's mom decided it was not a lingering cold and brought him back to the clinic. He arrived pale, thin, complaining of headaches, blurry vision, indigestion, coughing, shortness of breath, difficulty sleeping, and sinus congestion. Upon request, his pediatrician ran basic labs and those for the Shoemaker panel. Aidan's TGF-beta1 was back up to 7900, C4a was normal, mycoplasma pneumoniae IgM was 2300, and IgG was 6700 (both very high), MARCoNS tested positive (small amount and resistant to three antibiotics), and he failed his VCS test.

Aidan's mom was determined to find the source of the mold exposure and traced it to the school bus. The driver told her that the window seals were compromised, and there was often condensation and water intrusion on the bus. The carpet had also been soaking wet all winter from the leaking windows and the snow on passenger's boots. The transportation department refused all requests for mycometrics testing.

Aidan missed three weeks of school, and his parents decided it was safer to drive him. It took three months for him to return to normal. Since they were unable to confirm the source, the school allowed air purifiers in each of Aidan's classrooms.

TOP LOADER WASHING MACHINE MAINTENANCE

Not a remediation solution; if there is mold, most need to purchase a new machine

Front loaders are notorious for mold infestation!

Once Per Week For Optimal Cleanliness

Select the heavy-duty cycle

Add 2 cups of vinegar directly into the inner drum (where the clothes go)

Add 1 cup of 3% hydrogen peroxide in the liquid bleach dispenser

Run the cycle

The machine feels squeaky clean when the wash completes

FLOWER & LEAF BATH

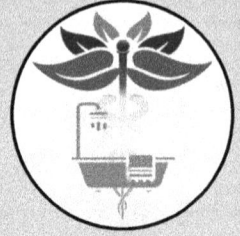

Preferences

Rose Petals & Buds: Relieves inflammation and soothes the heart

Lavender Blossoms: cleanses and induces a sense of calm

Elder Flowers: relieves inflammation and tones the skin

Rosemary Leafs: relieves fatigue and a skin cleansing tonic

Basic Bath

Combine a handful of each herb desired in a large pot

Fill the pot with water and heat to a near boil with the lid on

Remove the pot from the heat

Let the herbs infuse for at least 20 minutes

Fill the tub with filtered water

Strain the infused liquid into the tub (optional - use a muslin bag for the herbs and add it into the bath)

ECZEMA POULTICES

Herbs can be very potent; always choose the medicinal, organic version of all herbs

Chamomile
Known to soothe skin, and is also an antiseptic and antibacterial. Soak a poultice cloth in the refrigerator before using as a wash for itchy, painful, or irritated skin.

Goldenseal
A powerful all-natural herbal wash to fight bacteria and soothe the skin. Heavily dilute poultice and use externally only.

Calendula
A cooling herb that cleanses and soothes. Soak cotton balls in poultice and apply to aggravated areas.

Other Medicinal Herbs Useful for Dermatitis

Black walnut
(Juglans nigra)

Flaxseed Oil
(Linum usitatissimum)

Oregon Grape Root
(Berberis aquifolium)

Slippery Elm
(Ulmus rubra)

Uva-Ursi
(Arctostaphylos Uva-Ursi)

Borage Oil
(Borago officinalis)

Evening Primrose Oil
(Oenothera biennis)

Grapeseed Extract
(Vitis vinifera)

Patchouli
(Pogostemon cablin)

Tea Tree Oil
(Melaleuca alternifolia)

Henna
(Lawsonia inermis)

Gingko
(Ginkgo Biloba)

Daisy
(Bellis perennis)

Avocados
(Persea americana)

PART 6

THE BIONEXUS APPROACH

"I am only one; but still I am one. I cannot do everything but still I can do something. I will not refuse to do the something I can do."
                                        —Helen Keller, c. 1915

The BioNexus Approach is an all-natural, plant-based, bio-individualized program that integrates Dr. Shoemaker's treatment protocol for biotoxin illness and chronic inflammatory response syndrome (CIRS) into a functional, full 360-degree, naturopathic treatment plan. For over a decade, I developed and refined the approach. Overall, almost six years were spent on researching herbal medicine for mycotoxins and CIRS.

The idea for a holistic alternative sprung out of necessity because of my son. Brian had an extreme case of CIRS comorbid with pediatric autoimmune neuropsychiatric disorder associated with strep (PANDAS), stage three Lyme disease (neurological disseminated), Bartonellosis, Babesiosis, Rocky Mountain spotted fever, Rickettsia, chronic viruses, parasites, and yeast infections that triggered autism symptoms. Brian's myriad of early treatments included heavy doses of several powerful antibiotics, intravenous immunoglobulin (IVIG), cryosurgery, European biological therapies, and steroid nebulizers. The pharmaceutical treatments caused multiple side effects, including an immune deficiency, severe IBS, and growth delay that resulted in a failure to thrive (FTT) diagnosis.

Certain conventional treatments along with an integrative approach for Brian's Lyme disease and CIRS worked fairly well until the adverse effects of prolonged allopathic medicines outweighed the gains. Under Dr. Shoemaker's biotoxin illness treatment plan, Brian gained weight, and had significantly reduced inflammatory biomarkers. He attained astounding improvements in executive function, social cognition, reading comprehension, mathematical computation, pragmatic language, reasoning, and short-term memory. However, his gut issues and growth rate became immensely problematic. For me, it became clear that allopathic treatments could not be a long-term, life-long solution.

The majority of BioNexus Health Clinic (BNH) patients have decided that natural medicine is their preferred way to treat their conditions. A large portion of patients come from failed pharmaceutical interventions, often having spent years and thousands of dollars in trying to regain their health.

These are physically and emotionally exhausted people looking for a kinder, gentler way to heal. Then, some tolerated their pharmaceuticals, but their progress has plateaued, and they are now looking to wean off the numerous drugs they are on to a more natural regimen. Lastly, there are those looking to switch to natural plant-based treatment but want a well-rounded, holistic medicine practitioner that also understands the role of pharmaceuticals and can guide their primary care physician on a per-needed basis to enhance outcomes. At BioNexus Health Clinic, we help people of all ages while keeping their health and wellness goals and preferences in mind. Each protocol is patient-centered and custom-tailored to the individual.

The late nights and fatigued hours I spent researching, studying, collaborating, and exploring brought forth natural treatment options sensitive enough for patients like Brian, yet strong enough to eradicate MARCoNS (multiple antibiotic-resistant coagulase-negative Staphylococci). The resultant treatment template, BioNexus Approach, has improved the quality of life for BNH patients around the world.

The BioNexus Approach harnesses plant intelligence while supporting and promoting the body's natural defenses. The seven treatment steps provide an alternative plant-based treatment plan for biotoxin illness and CIRS patients. Our CIRS patients also typically have multiple chemical sensitives and other comorbid issues. This subset of patients needs a powerful yet sensitive bio-medical approach.

BioNexus Approach

The success secret to the BioNexus Approach lies within its full 360-degree approach to biochemistry, physiology, nutrition, and lifestyle. I firmly believe in the first principle of the World Health Organization's Constitution Preamble (2006) adopted in 1946, "Health is a state of complete physical, mental, and social well-being and not merely the absence of disease or infirmity." The tenet reflects upon the Age of Enlightenment's philosophical divide of rationalists and empiricists marked by Newtonian physics, which birthed modern medicine.

Evidence-based medicine, born from rationalist philosophies, provides fundamentals needed by practitioners treating chronically ill patients. Chronic illness affects the patient's life in a variety of different aspects. Formulating a complete plan of attack requires laying the foundation to address root causes by targeting underlying biochemical issues and renovating the patient's lifestyle to promote regenerative healing and maintain health. Biotoxins exist. A patient must remain diligent in preventing or limiting potential threats. As a genetic disorder,

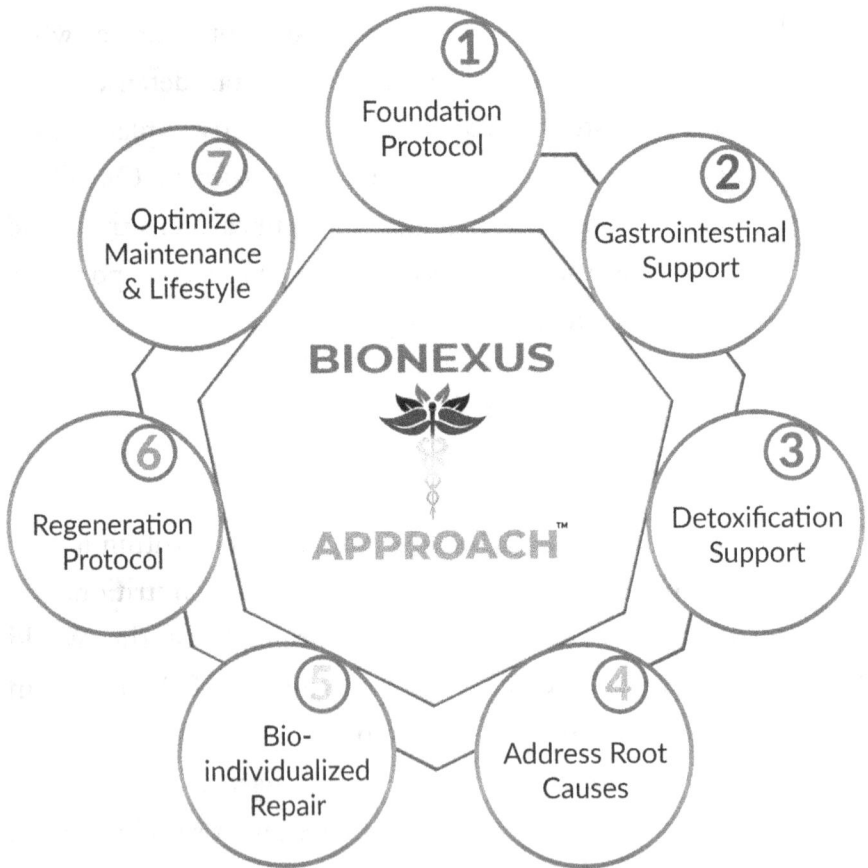

Figure 27. The BioNexus Approach: seven steps

repeated exposure to biotoxins does not dampen the effects. Re-exposure amplifies the impact and lessens the individual's time-table through the biotoxin illness stages.

Biotoxin illness patients suffer from a multitude of severe issues across multiple bodily systems. The biochemical and physiological changes require monitoring and routine testing throughout treatment. When testing is not available or an option, the patient and practitioner need to survey and monitor any improvement or deterioration. Tiers two and three in Part 3: Finding a Diagnosis contain recommended tests to track inflammatory markers, neuroendocrine abnormalities, auto-immune dysregulation, immune dysregulation, and coagulation issues.

When using plant-based protocols, the individual biology of a patient must be the predominant criterion. Each patient has their own set of symptoms, genetics, epigenetics, reactivity thresholds, and microbial and toxin load. Individualized protocols are needed to help recover and heal. There can never be a "detox in a box" approach for recovery and repair from chronic illness. Every protocol must be tailored very specifically to the individual for maximized efficacy.

Herbal medications inherently contain more active ingredients than pharmaceutical drugs. The natural ingredients synergistically function on several different biological levels and are capable of affecting a multitude of biochemical changes. These abundant factors create a protocol balancing act for the practitioner and an extended healing period for the patient. Under the guidance of a clinical herbalist, herbal medicine can be used throughout all seven steps of the BioNexus Approach without additional complications. For more information about herbal medicine, introducing herbs to patients, precautions, and preparations, please see Part 4: Prepping The Approach.

> "There is no basis in truth to the idea that repeat exposures suppress the subsequent inflammatory response. Actually, just the reverse is true. With re-exposure, "sicker, quicker."
> —Ritchie Shoemaker, MD (2011)

It is my recommendation not to attempt methylation until the inflammation is under control, unless absolutely necessary. Some sources recommend diving into methylation. At this early stage, the extent and effects of epigenetic modifying chemical compounds cannot be recognized. Attempting alterations in this fragile state, the body fails to manage the changes creating a highly unpleasant overmethylation crisis. Adverse effects can include increased inflammation, detoxification reactions, uncontrollable emotional response, headaches, body aches, and mental confusion. Therefore, it is my recommendation not to attempt methylation (see methylation sections) until after adequately addressing the patient's inflammatory crisis unless absolutely necessary as determined by scientific analysis. All genetic information, including the HLA type, methylation, and any other genetic susceptibilities, need to be considered together to obtain the big picture before introducing methylated vitamins.

The twelfth step of Dr. Shoemaker's biotoxin illness treatment protocol, vasoactive intestinal polypeptide (VIP), does not have an alternative option. VIP is a naturally occurring peptide in the body, and we have not found a substitute for this particular nasal spray. Pediatric VIP treatment is at the practitioner's discretion and only with careful monitoring of biomarkers, including lipase. A pediatric practitioner without a full understanding of the patient's status and all of their underlying issues should not prescribe VIP to pediatric patients.

The proprietary BioNexus Herbals were formulated by drawing on the wisdom of ancient eastern medicine, modern western herbalism, and the incredible power of quantum medicine. A full list of the herbal line may be found in the BioNexus Herbals section in Part 4: Prepping The Approach.

The BioNexus Approach is a broad-spectrum guide that practitioners can draw upon to enhance their skills and repair patients. It is designed for bio-individualized customization with flexibility for every practitioner's unique flair.

Patients may also learn from the BioNexus Approach; however, we recommend the guidance of a knowledgeable practitioner and consultation from their primary health care provider.

1 - Foundation Protocol

The foundation protocol addresses five corrective measures: air, water, diet, stress, and nutrition. The objective is to prepare the body for treatment, achieve the right pH balance, and provide nutrients lost to illness and pharmaceuticals. Most BioNexus Health Clinic (BNH) patients arrive after seeing several specialists and being treated with antibiotics, antifungals, antacids, mood stabilizers, and a wide variety of medications to suppress symptoms and counteract adverse effects. Candida, which can hold four times its weight in toxins, overgrowth also needs to be investigated and addressed.

Healing, detoxification, and repair consume a large amount of energy. Begin laying the foundation by addressing any nutritional deficiencies, reducing inflammatory cytokines, and providing the body with neuroendocrine support. When these three elements are combined, they ignite cellular communication and prepare the body to address the disease.

Clean Air

The home needs to be free and clear of what Dr. Shoemaker calls FAB (fungi, actinos, and bacteria) detoxification standards. FAB includes mold, mycotoxins, and microorganisms that grow in a water-damaged environment and produce endotoxins. Conduct a comprehensive review of the household to locate chemicals and mold "hot-zones" inside and out. Wearing protective gear rated for mold, inspect everything, including carpets, porous materials, windows (seals and sills), indoor plants, household products, and all areas with water access in the house like faucets, showers, tubs, under sinks, dishwasher, washing machine, et cetera. Outdoors inspect all possible water intrusion areas into the building envelope and inside the structure, including but not limited to windows, chimney, gutters, downspouts, foundation, and drainage around the property. Disturbing a mold-covered surface may release spores, dead fungi, and other toxins into the air, allowing them to travel undetected into humans. Mold can also find its way into wood, tile, wallpaper, paint, carpet, and insulation. The entire residence, depending on the findings, may require a thorough mold cleaning or, potentially, remediation.

It is of utmost importance to minimize exposure to these various toxins and microbes. Once basic remediation (if required) is completed, maintaining clean air and environmental integrity in the home can be as simple as replacing chemical-based household cleaning and personal care products with bio-friendly alternatives. White vinegar may replace most cleaning products, including cleaning, laundry, and gardening. Replace Teflon pans with stainless steel, glass, ceramic, or cast-iron. Vacuum carpets daily to pick up food crumbs, dust mites, or other potential toxins. Regularly clean porous materials: stuffed animals, pillows, mattresses, et cetera. A good HEPA vacuum is an important investment. Evacuate moldy items in a sealed plastic bag and disposed of it correctly. Continued vigilant attentiveness of the environment will help prevent relapses.

Air Filters

Furnace and air filters limit the number of spores in a given volume of air, thus limiting the reproduction capabilities of the mold. All units require a specific size for proper filtration. One micron is one-millionth of a meter or approximately 1/25,000 of an inch. A mold spore can be as small as three microns and as big as 40 microns, making them invisible to the naked eye. Air filter ratings grade the size of the particles they capture. Most filters easily remove particles larger than 10 microns. For a filter to remove mold from the air, it needs to have a rating for less than three microns.

Replace the filters within the recommended guidelines for maximum performance.

MERV Rating

Minimum Efficiency Reporting Value (MERV), an international standard, rates a filter's ability to remove macroscopic and microscopic particles from the air on a scale of 1 to 16. A high MERV rating correlates to eliminating smaller particles. Over 98% of all known bacteria are over one micron. MERV 13 filters remove over 85% of one-micron-sized particles.

3M developed the micro-particle performance rating (MPR) system to grade a filter's ability to remove airborne particles between 0.3 to 1 micron. A typical dust particle is between 0.2 and 8 microns. MERV 13 filters correspond to MPR 1500-1900 and MERV 14 filters to MPR 2800.

The home of a patient with severe biotoxin illness may need at least MERV 13 air filters. MERV 14 filters remove most respirable bacteria and harmful particles. However, due to these filters being dense, it is very important to replace them once a month. After personal well-being is achieved, a more practical solution is MERV 11 or MERV 12 filters.

Indoor Air Quality

Indoor Air Quality (IAQ) refers to a structure's air quality as it relates to the health and comfort of the occupants. According to the Environmental Protection Agency (EPA), indoor air contains two to five times more concentrations of some pollutants than outdoor air and is a top-five environmental health risk. Contaminants, such as mold, continually regenerate. It is impossible to obtain 100% removal efficiency without uncovering the source mold. Dead fungi spores break apart into 320-514 fragments and account for 99.8% of the immunogenic burden in a water-damaged building (WDB). Ultraviolet light and ozone purifiers are not sufficient for removing these fragments.

Poor IAQ accumulates gases like radon and carbon dioxide (CO_2). Radon can seep into a home through cracks, while CO_2 is emitted by exhaling humans. Modern building practices seal homes from outside air, which magnifies poor air quality in the winter. The EPA estimates the average American receives 72% of all chemical exposures in their residence.

Improving IAQ necessitates more ventilation, fresh air, reduced humidity, and routine HVAC maintenance. Those with severe biotoxin illness will benefit from consultation with a knowledgeable indoor environmental professional (IEP).

Ensure optimal interior air quality by opening the windows more often, vacuuming using a HEPA vacuum (with a window cracked open and a small fan running thats blowing towards the open window for best results), changing to high-quality air furnace filters, using the fan mode on the air conditioner for a few hours a day (at least a few times a week), adding good quality air purifiers, and maintaining household humidity to below 50%.

Add or install air purifiers and dehumidifiers in basements, bathrooms, crawl spaces, and attics with HVAC units. Remove any humidifiers attached directly to an HVAC unit. Energy recovery ventilators (ERV) are a two-fan system connected to HVAC ductwork to draw fresh air into the home and remove stale air. ERVs include air exchangers and ventilation systems. Some ERVs also remove moisture between air streams and enable thermal transfer. Highly rated ERVs recover up to 99% of the heat and contain a defrost system.

Highly Rated: Broan, LifeBreath, RenewAire, Ultimate Air

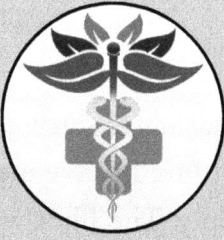

HOMEMADE POULTICE

Apply to the body to relieve soreness and inflammation

Cloth or Cotton Ball

Brew a strong cup of herbal tea using the desired herb

2 tsp of herb to 8 ounces of boiling water

Steep for 8 minutes

Soak a clean towel or cotton ball in the tea

Let it cool, if needed

Apply directly to the skin for 3-5 minutes

Directly on skin

Briefly soak herb in warm water

Lay herb gently on the skin

Cover with a clean cloth for 3-5 minutes

After determining skin reaction, more extended periods are acceptable for both applications

For dry skin, add castor oil or shea butter to application

Clean Water

Water supply regulation began in the United States during the 1970s. However, it has not been uncommon to find heavy metals or leached chemicals in the public water supply. The Flint water crisis began in 2014, led to criminal investigations and civil lawsuits. In late 2019, the EPA responded to the crisis by announcing its first significant revisions to lead and copper pipe regulations in over twenty years. A 2020 report from the Environmental Working Group (EWG) found 43 of 44 sites across 31 states and Washington D.C. had detectable levels of poly and perfluoroalkyl substances (PFAS). PFAS are the chemicals used to make Teflon, Scotchgard, and other industrial processes. The average household water filter cannot remove PFAS from water. Biotoxin illness patients should diligently refrain from drinking tap water.

Recommendation

Read *The Hidden Message in Water* by Masaru Emoto, New York Times best-selling author and Japanese scientist. His experiments document the power of consciousness and toxin-free water in the healing process.

A whole house reverse osmosis water filtration system is the best option for water purification. All the water used in the home from the kitchen sink to the bathtub needs to be appropriately filtered. When a whole house system is not possible, then place or mount countertop water filters near all faucets or use distilled and purified water in one-time-use plastic #1 or PET (polyethylene terephthalate) plastic water bottles. Shower heads also need filters; review filtration system targets listed on the packaging because most target chlorine, while others also target mold and bacteria.

Distilled and reverse osmosis water remove essential minerals. Add vital minerals back into the water by making an electrolyte drink, adding minerals and electrolyte supplements to the filtered drinking water, or adding Epsom salt to baths.

Water purified with reverse osmosis also decreases VOCs, chlorine taste and odor, microplastics, and sediment.

Use purified water for all detoxification baths and soaks. Impurities in non-purified water may absorb into the skin along with any minerals.

Grout And Caulk

Improperly maintained grout and caulk leads to cracks, leakage, and trapped moisture, which aids bathroom mold and mildew growth. Mold in the grout typically means the source mold is in the wall. Greg Weatherman, the well-known CIRS aware indoor environmental professional (IEP), advises initial installation and waterproofing are critical to avoiding bathroom mold problems. Many contractors use mastic to bond the tile directly onto moisture-resistant drywall without waterproofing — mastic and drywall fuel mold growth. Cracks in the grout and caulk expedite its visibility.

Remove the shower tile and backer board to check inside the wall cavity for mold. Waterproofing the bathroom wet area requires materials in the following order: cement board, mortar with mesh tape over the seam, coat with a waterproofing membrane, and fiber cloth over all seams and corners. Weatherman's method constructs a watertight wet area, turning the tiles, grout, and caulk into decoration.

In some milder cases, thoroughly removing the old grout and caulk, HEPA vacuuming, and cleaning the entire perimeter may solve the mold problem. The area must dry completely before applying new grout or caulk.

Clean Diet

Fatigue, illness, malaise, pain, and numerous other symptoms often contribute to a vicious cycle for CIRS patients. Exhaustion from daily life can lead patients to make poor nutrition and diet choices. These patients start feeling better with treatment and supplements, but relapse due to poor dietary choices.

Various food sensitivities, multiple chemical sensitivities, and dietary allergies are widespread in the CIRS population due to the underlying immune dysregulation. Allergies are a form of an immune system response. An immediate hypersensitivity response, anaphylactic reaction (type 1), is the most commonly recognized reaction. Within 12 minutes of exposure, the face swells, hives appear, or the throat closes.

Biotoxin illness and CIRS patients often report experiencing type 4 hypersensitivity reactions, also known as cell-mediated or delayed hypersensitivity. Within 72 hours of exposure, the immune system sends antigen-specific effector T-cells to the antigen area where they can remain for months or years. Restimulation by the antigen can cause cytokine secretion (Janeway, Travers, Walport, & Shlomchik, 2001).

The late response makes it harder to identify the sensitivity or intolerance. Prolonged exposure may lead to autoantibodies and autoimmune disease. The body can silently produce autoantibodies for up to ten years before displaying any symptoms.

Gluten is a perfect example of type 1 and type 4 hypersensitivity responses. A wheat allergy classifies as an immediate response allergy (type 1). Celiac disease, on the other hand, is an autoimmune disease where the body causes gluten sensitivity (type 4) from repeated antigen stimulation. The celiac immune system produces anti-gliadin antibodies (IgG and IgA) within 72 hours of consuming gliadin proteins in wheat, rye, barley, and oats causing mucosal inflammation, villous atrophy, and crypt hyperplasia.

ALL-PURPOSE SALVE

Ingredients

1-1 1/2 cup calendula-infused oil
(apricot kernel, lavender, sesame, or almond are best)

1 ounce beeswax pastilles or grated beeswax (vegetable wax acceptable)

10-15 drops of lavender *(Lavandula angustifolia)*, chamomile *(Matricaria recutita)*, or rose geranium *(Pelargonium roseum)* essential oil - *optional*

Directions

Make calendula-infused oil

Heat calendula-infused oil in a double boiler; add beeswax and stir until it completely dissolves

Mix in the essential oils

Test consistency: dip a spoon into the hot mix and put it in the refrigerator for a few minutes. For harder salve, add beeswax. Add calendula-infused oil to soften

Carefully pour the mixture into tins or jars

Let it cool until solid

Immune system dysregulation or impairment in CIRS-WDB and CIRS-Lyme patients may trigger a type 4 response and gliadin antibody production. When the body produces anti-gliadin, the body cannot digest gluten, setting off a volatile inflammatory response. A transglutaminase enzyme releases proinflammatory histamine, leukotrienes, prostaglandins, and cytokines resulting in gastrointestinal symptoms like constipation, cramping, and diarrhea. These responses and symptoms may also contribute to headaches, fatigue, and joint pain.

For CIRS patients, recognizing and identifying all food-related sensitivities reduces inflammation and alleviates symptoms. Since there is a delayed allergy response, following a strict diet helps narrow the potential sources. A careful elimination diet will help discover the trigger food(s). Remove gluten and sugar from the menu entirely. If there is constipation, replace cow-based dairy with goat, sheep, llama, donkey, rice, oat, almond, or coconut milk. Camel milk has a unique hypoallergenic molecular structure with potent immunoglobulin content. Reserve camel milk for medicinal purposes. Initial consumption should be under the guidance of a practitioner until reaching the optimum dosage.

Preferences: Feingold Program (KP Diet), Paleo Autoimmune Protocol (AIP), Specific Carbohydrate Diet (SCD), Wahls Protocol

The popularity of gluten-free diets have made food-like products readily available in supermarkets. Avoid all gluten-free junk food, snacks, and meal items. These products are usually made with starches, binders, gums, corn syrup, corn solids, yeast extracts, spices extractives, and other forms of hidden MSG-like substances. Organic, non-GMO, food is always the best option.

Diligently avoid food dyes, processed foods, and artificial colors and flavors.

CIRS patients who have already advanced to multiple chemical sensitivities (MCS) and/or mast cell activation syndrome (MCAS) generally should avoid all the major food allergens. In addition to personal sensitivities, gluten, sugar, and dairy, they should also avoid soy and corn. A simple home-cooked nutritious diet is the way to go. After gut repair, most patients will be able to slowly add food items back in into their diet.

Fortunately, the health impact of food sensitivities is widely recognized. There are numerous online resources and a staggering number of food choices made with clean and allergen-free ingredients that are minimally processed. It makes clean eating easily accessible with a little online research. Major retailers and membership warehouses also offer organic grocery and produce options, which helps to keep costs down. Local organic farms typically provide community supported agriculture (CSA) shares during the summer months. Most CSA options are incredibly reasonable for local, in-season, organic produce. Some farms even offer home delivery.

With a little effort, it's possible to augment a plant-based treatment protocol with a nutrition-rich diet. Proper nutrition keeps inflammation in check, can help shorten the length of treatment, and enhance overall wellness.

Diet and Medications

Turn off the television, put down the phone, and remove distractions during meals and when consuming herbal cocktails and supplements. Focus on the body's motions and reactions. Be grateful for the therapeutic benefits received from foods and herbs.

In *The Miracle of Mindfulness*, Thich Nhat Hanh explains that mindfulness or awareness of the present raises the vibrations of the items consumed. Relax, listen, and note any messages or feedback the body provides. Make a note of those responses.

Nutritional Support with Essential Micro & Macro Nutrients

Drug-induced Nutrient Deficiency

Chronic illness patients, including those with tick-borne infections, are often on long-term medications. Treatments may include antibiotics, antacids, steroids, analgesics, anti-inflammatories, diuretics to lower blood pressure, anticon-vulsants, antidepressants, and/or anxiolytics. Prolonged use of pharmaceutical medications, including many over-the-counter drugs, can cause a multi-nutrient deficiency (Harvard Health

Publishing, 2016). Frequently, patients are depleted of essential nutrients like calcium, folic acid, crucial B vitamins, and magnesium.

Symptoms of nutrient deficiency are easily confused with symptoms of the underlying disease process itself. Magnesium deficiency can present as muscle cramps, irregular heartbeat, and mood changes. Zinc depletion may exhibit as a weakened immune system, rash, hair loss, diarrhea, and taste or smell changes. A low vitamin B12 issue may present as low red blood cells, tingling, weakness, numbness, and confusion.

Proton pump inhibitors can help reduce acid reflux and heartburn. While alleviating symptoms, the body, typically, cannot absorb vitamin B12. Some blood pressure diuretics zap magnesium, potassium, and calcium. Tegretol (carbamazepine), an anticonvulsant, can reduce DHA fatty acids and vitamins B7, B9, D, and E, which may cause hair loss, depressions, skin problems, cardiovascular problems, bone and muscle weakness, and anemia. Depakote (divalproex sodium) is used to treat manic episodes and may drain carnitine, copper, DHA, selenium, zinc, and vitamins B6, B9 and E.

Potential Nutritional Deficiencies

The following lists provide a snapshot of potential drug-induced nutritional deficiencies interfering with health and wellness. A specialized diet is an easy way to replenish essential nutrients.

Antacids: calcium, melatonin, phosphate, vitamin B9 (folic acid)

Antibiotics: calcium, copper, helpful bacteria, iron, magnesium, potassium, vitamin B1 (thiamine), vitamin B2 (riboflavin), vitamin B3 (niacin), vitamin B5 (pantothenic acid), vitamin B6 (pyridoxine), vitamin B7 (biotin), vitamin B9 (folic acid), vitamin B12, vitamin D, vitamin K, zinc

Anticonvulsants: calcium, carnitine, copper, DHA fatty acid, selenium, vitamin B1 (thiamine), vitamin B7 (biotin), vitamin B9 (folic acid), vitamin B12, vitamin D, vitamin E, vitamin K, zinc

Antidepressants: coenzyme Q10, melatonin, vitamin B2 (riboflavin), vitamin B6 (pyridoxine)

Antidiabetic: coenzyme Q10, vitamin B9 (folic acid), vitamin B12

Antigout: calcium, phosphorous, potassium, sodium, vitamin A, vitamin B12

Antihistamine: calcium, chromium, iron, magnesium, melatonin, potassium, selenium, sodium, vitamin A, vitamin B5 (pantothenic acid), vitamin B9 (folic acid), vitamin B12, vitamin C, vitamin D, zinc

Anti-Parkinson: carnitine, copper, potassium, SAMe, vitamin B6 (pyridoxine), vitamin B12, zinc

Antihypertensives: calcium, coenzyme Q10, magnesium, potassium, sodium, vitamin B1 (thiamine), vitamin B6 (pyridoxine), vitamin B9 (folic acid), vitamin C, zinc

Beta Blockers: coenzyme Q10, melatonin, potassium

Cardiac Glycosides: calcium, magnesium, phosphorus, vitamin B1 (thiamine)

Cholesterol-Lowering Agents: almost any vitamin or mineral can be affected, coenzyme Q10, electrolytes, vitamin A, vitamin B12, vitamin D, vitamin E, vitamin K

Gastrointestinal System: calcium, iron, vitamin B6 (pyridoxine), vitamin B9 (folic acid), vitamin B12, zinc

Hormones: magnesium, selenium, vitamin B1 (thiamine), vitamin B2 (riboflavin), vitamin B3 (niacin), vitamin B6 (pyridoxine), vitamin B9 (folic acid), vitamin B12, vitamin C, vitamin E, zinc

Laxatives: calcium, phosphorus, potassium, vitamin A, vitamin D, vitamin E, vitamin K

Thyroid Medication: iron

Respiratory Medications: ACE inhibitors, potassium, vitamin B6 (pyridoxine), zinc

Functional Blood Analysis And Biochemistry

Understanding the entire spectrum of lab result reference ranges, and health implications when correlated with the clinical evaluation, presentation of symptoms and follow-up facilitates the practitioner's ability to create bio-unique therapeutic protocols.

The basic panels like a complete blood count, lipid panel, comprehensive metabolic panel, electrolytes, vitamins, iron, ferritin, viral titers, some bacterial markers, immunoglobulins, histamine, and urinalysis are typically covered by insurance. Specialty tests like the Shoemaker Panel (see Part 3: Finding a Diagnosis) may be beyond the scope of a primary care practitioner. BNH patients come from over 50 countries, and we have run tests in all of them.

The following lab tests are examples of tests BNH commonly run for our CIRS patients.

Thyroid

Patients reporting an unresponsive thyroid despite using several different medications. Look for underlying heavy metal toxicity because metals like mercury and aluminum act as thyroid receptor disruptors and impact the red blood cells. Run MCH, MCHC, and uric acid tests. If all three results return low normal or decreased, suspect heavy metals. Consider following up with a hair or urine metals test for specifics.

Oxidative Stress

High or high normal ranges of ferritin, bilirubin, LDL, and uric acid. Low or low normal ranges of platelets, cholesterol, lymphocytes, and albumin.

Parasites

High or high normal ranges of eosinophils (EOS), absolute eosinophils, and IgE. Low or low normal levels of serum iron and hemoglobin. Identify the parasites with a follow-up stool test.

CO_2 Levels

High to high normal levels can indicate metabolic alkalosis, low stomach acid, and adrenal dysfunction. Low levels or low normal indicate a need for thiamine and metabolic acidosis.

B6 Deficiency

Often, a B6 test may reveal low to mid ranges, but the patient presents with clinical symptoms of a B6 deficiency. It is essential to identify and address it as a B6 deficiency. Many body processes rely on B6.

AMMONIA TESTING

For accurate ammonia testing, the blood draw needs to be without a tourniquet, and the sample drawn needs to be frozen within 15 minutes.

Adrenal Insufficiency

High or high normal cholesterol, triglycerides, and potassium combined with low or low normal blood glucose levels, chloride and sodium. Follow up with a 24-hour salivary test for adrenal function.

Folate and/ or B12 Deficiency Anemia

High or high normal serum iron, LDH, RDW, MCHC, MCH, and often MCV. Low or low normal of hemoglobin, WBCs, neutrophils, and uric acid.

Metabolic Acidosis

High or high normal anion gap, chloride, and potassium, along with low CO_2.

Toxin Burden Labs

In addition to inflammation, neurotransmitter balance, microbial overgrowth, and gut health knowing a patient's toxin burden helps determine an individualized regimen.

Organic Acids Test (OAT)

Glyphosate Level

Urinary Mycotoxins: This test is not directly related to CIRS but can help practitioners overview the toxin load to determine a comprehensive detoxification program. According to Dr. Shoemaker's research, CIRS is not directly related to gut mycotoxins, nor is this test a part of the CIRS protocol. Patients often request this test because of their internet research. Once again, simply put, urinary mycotoxins are a detox item and most certainly not a CIRS diagnostic item. It is important to understand the distinction.

Read Dr. Shoemaker's robust 2019 paper, Urinary Mycotoxins: A Review of Contaminated Buildings and Food in Search of a Biomarker Separating Sick Patients from Controls.

ERMI and HERTSMI-2: Determine if the patient had exposure to a water-damaged building (WDB). If a WDB plays a role in the patient's history, even if the mycotoxins test negative, microbial amplification is a factor.

History of WDB exposure adds 30 different classes of substances that could trigger CIRS, including mycotoxins. The ERMI and HERTSMI-2 tests contain sensitive markers to determine if a building is a WDB. Analyzed dust samples from these tests rarely match mycotoxins found in urine testing.

Envirobiomics tests ERMI, HERTSMI, endotoxins, and actinos.

Other Useful Labs

Stool Test: GI Map and GPL comprehensive stool analysis to look for strep and clostridial overgrowth, often seen with an enzymatic deficiency

DNA Connexions: Tick-borne infections

DiagnosTechs Labs or Dutch Labs: Hormonal panels, including adrenal panel

GI Map: Gut-related information

Mito Swab: Mitochondrial status information

Methylation Panel: Identify SNPs

GENIE (Genomic Expression: Inflammation Explained): In-depth analysis of hypometabolism, coagulation abnormalities, the effectiveness of IV therapies in Lyme disease (especially PICC lines), VIP therapy, cytokines upregulation/dysregulation (especially TGF-beta1)

Complete a functional nutritional analysis before continuing.

Primary Nutritional Support Constituents

Some patients only need the recommended daily allowance (RDA), while others are so depleted they may need several times above the RDA. It all depends on clinical presentation and lab results, if available.

B Vitamins
BioNexus Herbals BTXD Blend
BioNexus Herbals Formula 2 EOS
BioNexus Herbals Formula 4 IBT
BioNexus Herbals LS Blend
Collagen Support
DHA/EPA

Electrolytes
Iodine
Iron Deficiency Anemia Check
Pranayama Breathing
Trace and Essential Minerals
Vitamin D, K2, A, C, and E

DOSAGE

Several factors determine prescribed doses.
Therefore, any provided dosages should be
considered recommendations and not absolutes.

Please refer to Part 4: Prepping the Approach for dosage recommendations. For patients with MCS or MCAS, always start with the smallest possible amount and build up (See Appendix).

Trace And Essential Minerals

Most people can eat a wide variety of foods to achieve the appropriate amount of trace minerals. However, chronic illness, various pathogens, and medications need more trace minerals to support numerous metabolic processes. Trace and essential minerals boost the absorption of vitamins, minerals, and other nutrients to fuel several cellular functions. Usually, starting with a tablespoon daily or the dosage indicated on the bottles is enough.

Many medicinal herbs contain minerals, and some have high mineral content. Some examples include horsetail, horseradish, stinging nettle, and dandelion. Nettle is high in calcium, chromium, cobalt, magnesium, manganese, phosphorus, protein, riboflavin, selenium, silicon, thiamine, zinc, and vitamins A and C. Fennel is well-known for its beneficial properties to aid digestive ailments but is also packed with calcium, magnesium, phosphorus, selenium, and thiamine.

Preferences: Akamai Fulvic Mineral Complex, Body Ecology Ancient Earth Liquid Minerals, Mini Minerals, Pure Himalayan Shilajit, Vital Earth Minerals

Magnesium

Many studies have looked into the importance of adequate levels of magnesium, especially with underlying pathogens, microbial, and environmental biotoxins. A study reported in the American Heart Journal (Liao, Folsom, & Brancati, 1998) followed 13,922 middle-aged adults. The research concluded that magnesium levels correlate directly with overall heart health. Another study, in the American Journal of Cardiology (Song et al., 2005), found that adequate magnesium levels were associated with normal heart rhythm.

Magnesium encourages bodily functions, including:
- healthy calcium absorption, dental health, insulin levels;
- regulating nerve and muscle function;
- aiding over 300 enzymes in blood glucose control, blood pressure regulation, and protein synthesis;
- promoting emotional well-being in premenstrual women;
- energy production and amino acid metabolism;
- structural development of bone;
- aids calcium and potassium ion transportation across cell membranes for nerve impulse conduction, muscle contraction, and normal heart rhythm.

MAGNESIUM

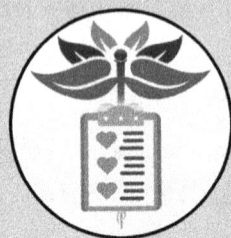

When supplementing with magnesium, look at vitamins B1, B2, and B6. A little daily boron helps improve magnesium uptake. Some patients may need added taurine and/or potassium to help with the intracellular uptake. Highly sensitive people will notice a difference in histamine levels at this early stage.

There are several different types of magnesium – malate, threonate, citrate, glycinate, orotate, oxide, aspartate, taurate, chloride, and sulfate. Clinically, people with glutamate toxicity or sensitivity cannot tolerate glycinate.

Preferences: chloride (foot soaks), citrate, malate, taurate

Clinical Notes: Most people respond best when using two to three different versions of magnesium to reach optimal results. Epsom salts are magnesium sulfate. Magnesium oxide helps with constipation and magnesium threonate is good for the brain.

Magnesium needs to be accompanied with bicarbonate, boron,

and vitamin B6 to significantly improve absorption and functional utilization at the tissue level. When using magnesium threonate, it is helpful to know threonine requires active thiamine to be broken down, and deamination is B6 dependent. Your patient can have issues taking B6 due to low intracellular thiamine, and the B6 problem can create an extreme sensitivity to glycine for some patients.

Testing: RBC Magnesium looks at the cellular magnesium level. Raise and maintain magnesium levels towards the higher end of the normal range.

Preferences: Allergy Research Group, Biogena 7-Salt Magnesium, Ecological Formulas, Klaire Labs, Mini Minerals, Nobi Nutrition, Raise Them Well Magnesium Oil with Aloe Vera (transdermal application), ReMag, Thorne

Magnesium and Vitamin D

Studies have demonstrated vitamin D deficiencies play a significant role in the development of dozens of diseases, including a variety of cancers, such as breast cancer, prostate cancer, and colon cancer, as well as diabetes, heart disease, arthritis, osteoporosis, psoriasis, and mental illness.

Most, if not all, of the enzymes that metabolize vitamin D, require magnesium. Inadequate magnesium levels impair overall vitamin D effectiveness and benefits. Magnesium assists in activating vitamin D to regulate calcium and phosphate homeostasis that influence bone growth and maintenance.

Electrolytes

Electrolytes form electrically charged particles (ions) in body fluids. These ions carry the electrical energy necessary to help regulate nerve and muscle function, hydrate the body, balance blood acidity and pressure, and help rebuild damaged tissue. A suitable electrolyte balance is vital for recovery from illness.

Preferences: homemade or BioPure matrix electrolytes

SIMPLE HOMEMADE ELECTROLYTE DRINK

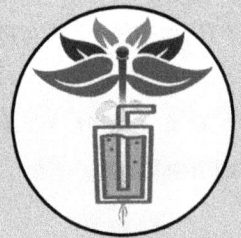

Ingredients

1/2 cup fresh orange juice
2 strawberries to taste
1/4 cup fresh lemon juice
2 cups of coconut water
1 tbsp ionic liquid magnesium
2 tbsp organic honey
(raw if preferred)
1/8 tsp Himalayan pink salt

Directions

Blend all ingredients

Store refrigerated in a glass jar

Cucumber, lemon, or ginger slices can be added to the jar for taste according to preference

Ginger is especially useful for nausea

The B Vitamins

Nutrients usually act in a coordinated manner within the body. Intestinal absorption and subsequent metabolism of a particular nutrient, to a certain extent, is dependent on the availability of other nutrients.

The B vitamins all work in synergy with one another and with other nutrients like magnesium.

For example, B2 helps B6 convert to its active form. A vitamin B2 deficiency can lead to an inadequate supply of the active form of B6, which can lead to B6 irritating tissues. It is also important to have adequate magnesium to prevent phenol and yeast-like symptoms due to enzyme suppression in the sulfation pathway.

Dosing for B vitamins varies from person to person and across B vitamins. One person may need pyridoxal 5'-phosphate (the active form of B6), while another person needs Pyridoxine (B6) because they have enough B2.

Vitamin B1 (Thiamine)

Thiamine pyrophosphate (TPP) is the active form of thiamine (B1) and is involved in several metabolic enzyme functions. A B1 deficiency affects the autonomic system and appetite. Certain foods contain anti-thiamine factors (ATFs), which oxidize thiamine rendering it inactive. Consuming moderate to large amounts of tea or coffee has been associated with thiamine

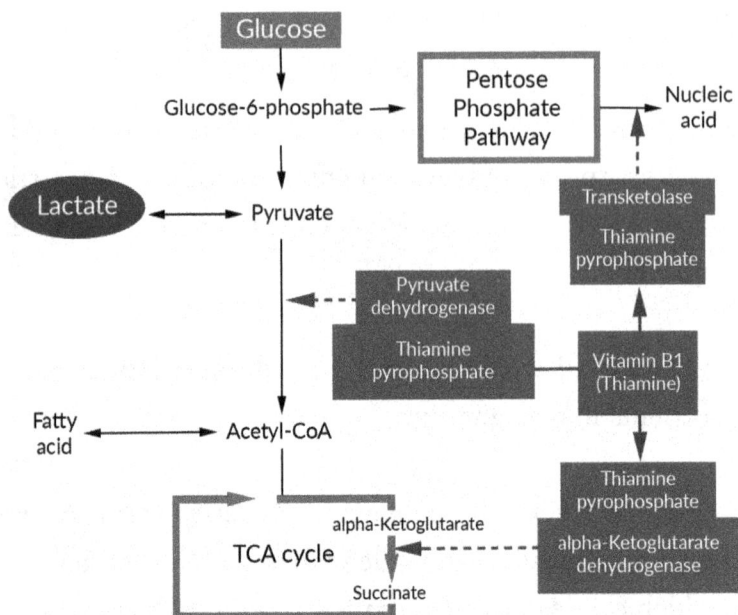

Figure 28. Thiamine (B1) serves enzymes as cofactor

deficiency due to the presence of ATFs. Mycotoxins and certain high-mold foods may have a similar effect. Also, growth spurts, Babesia, stress, chronic illness, certain viruses, and high carbohydrate diets deplete thiamine.

Vitamin B2 (Riboflavin)
Vitamin B2 is a water-soluble vitamin. It plays a role in energy production in the body and is crucial for breaking down food components, absorbing other nutrients, and maintaining tissues. It can be found in milk, meat, eggs, nuts, enriched flour, and green vegetables.

Vitamin B6 (Pyridoxine)

Vitamin B6 is involved in a wide variety of physiologic processes, including gluconeogenesis, and neurotransmitter and sphingo-lipids synthesis within the body. It also functions as a cofactor for many enzymes required for amino acid metabolism. Studies have shown B6 to be an essential factor in brain inflammation. Adequate levels of magnesium and B2 are necessary to make B6 more functional and convert to its active form, pyridoxal 5'-phosphate (P-5-P).

A subclinical deficiency can precipitate biochemical changes that become more obvious as the deficiency progresses. Hyper-homocysteinemia is a critical cardiovascular event risk factor associated with vitamin B-6 deficiency. Adequate levels of B6 are also needed for tryptophan (precursor of the neurotransmitter serotonin) metabolism, which helps keep the neurotoxin quinolinic acid levels in check. Often chronic Lyme patients are comorbid with kryptopyrrole urea (KPU). KPU causes a B6 deficiency as well.

Suggested Reading: Kynurenine Pathway Metabolites: Relevant to Vitamin B-6 Deficiency and Beyond (Ciorba, 2013)

Vitamin B7 (Biotin)

The body needs biotin, a water-soluble B vitamin, to help convert certain nutrients into energy. Vitamin B7 also promotes healthy hair, skin, and nails. Eggs, milk, and bananas contain small amounts of biotin.

Vitamin B9 (Folate) and Vitamin B12

Vitamins B9 and B12 need to be added after careful consideration of the person's methylation pathways and clinical symptoms to prevent an over methylation crisis. If lab tests are not available, cautiously start with folinic acid, then buildup to one drop of low dose methylfolate drops. With B12, adenosyl or hydroxy versions are good options.

How To Supplement

Typically start with a supplement, which does not contain any folate or B12.

The B vitamins can interfere with sleep. Use the modified B complex in the morning and other Bs in the afternoon or at least 6 hours before bedtime (Lonsdale, 2006).

Certain patients may benefit from added B1, B2, and B7. Prescribe them 4 to 6 hours after the first dose of modified B complex.

Thiamine (B1) plays a vital role in energy metabolism. Thiamine has also been useful for poor appetite and poor weight gain issues.

Preferences: allithiamine, benfotiamine, coenzymated sublingual thiamines, and thiamine HCL

After a couple of weeks, add B12 adenosyl/hydroxy at 2000 to 4000 mg per day. Add methylfolate two weeks later.

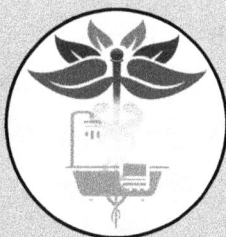

EPSOM SALT BATH
Use chlorine-free filtered water

Ingredients

2 cups of Epsom salt

1 cup of baking soda (optional)

Directions

Prepare bath with warm water to tolerance level

Add Epsom salt and baking soda when the tub is a quarter full, which gives enough time for them to melt into the bathwater

Baking soda is particularly useful to add for alkalizing, to help decrease cytokine flares, and after exposure to X-rays and other imaging procedures

Enhancing Options

<u>Essential Oils</u>
2 to 5 drops of lavender oil helps reduce stress
2 to 4 drops of ginger oil promotes detoxification sweating
2 to 5 drops of eucalyptus oil helps clear sinus and chest congestion

<u>Parsley Tea Bags</u>
Adding in 2 to 3 parsley tea bags helps with lymphatic drainage and supports the kidneys

<u>Burdock Root Tea Bags</u>
Adding in 2 to 4 burdock root tea bags helps with acne issues on the back, neck, and torso

Preferences: Holistic Heal Methyl Folate drops (depending on individual tolerance), Holistic Heal Ultimate B Complex (to slowly building up B complex), Vital Nutrients B12/Methyl Folate

Pediatrics: Hypersensitivity reactions and food intolerances prevent some kids from taking folate, only use folinic acid. Start at 1/4 capsule a day and slowly work up to a full dose.

Preferences: Biotics Research, Holistic Heal, Seeking Health, Thorne

Migraines

Patients who experience migraines report relief with daily supplementation of coenzyme Q10, magnesium, melatonin, vitamin B2, and vitamin D (Gaul, Diener, & Danesch, 2015). Another useful supplement is called Preventa. It contains butterbur, magnesium, and other useful herbs.

Magnesium, Phenol Sulfur-transferase (PST), Sulfur

A balance of amino acids, ammonia, and sulfur is important for homeostasis. Phenol metabolism is the body's only mechanism for removing excessive sulfur-containing amino acids to maintain homeostasis. Sulfation and compound detoxification of artificial food coloring and flavoring, and salicylates, require phenol metabolism.

Patients who find garlic, onions, and medications like Bactrim intolerable require additional consideration before starting any sulfur related therapies. People who have a low or no ability to convert compounds to sulfate also have problems handling environmental chemicals and some medications.

Vitamin B6 is an essential cofactor for numerous enzymes, including cystathionine beta-synthase (CBS). Using a supplement like No-Fenol enzymes can help remove certain carbohydrate groups from the phenols or at least modify their structure, allowing normal processing by the detoxification pathways. The Feingold diet (Feingold Program) can also help eliminate toxins and supply the body with available sulfate.

Some patients have seen detoxification improvements by supplementing with sulfur-containing amino acids, including cysteine and taurine, or methylsulfonylmethane (MSM).

Overall, most people obtain benefits from Epsom salts because it is already sulfate. Epsom salt baths and magnesium chloride foot soaks are two great patient recommendations.

DHA/EPA
According to Dr. Shoemaker's guidelines, the goal is at least 2.4 grams of EPA and 1.5 grams of DHA in divided daily doses.

Preferences: Dropi, Nordic Naturals, Rosita cod liver oil, Sports Research Omega 3, Cymbiotika (vegan)

Patients with MCAS have reported histamine flares with fish oil.

Other Options: Barlean's organic, Cataplex F, OmaPrem, Walkabout Emu Oil

Vitamins A, E, D, C, and K2

Vitamins A and E

Typically, a good cod liver oil supplement should provide adequate vitamins A and E. However, when there are absorption issues, supplementation is beneficial, especially with symptoms such as visual stress, floaters, snow, pain, and fatigue. Short term higher doses of vitamin A have been reported to be extremely useful during viral infections. Additionally, studies show vitamin E tocopherols plays an essential role in the suppression of inflammatory transcription factor NF-κB.

Preferences: Life Extension, OcuDyne II, Ocuvite, Pure Encapsulations, Thorne

Vitamin D

Vitamins K2 and A are beneficial in assisting with the absorption of vitamin D. Many patients self-medicate with high doses of liposomal vitamin D. It's imperative that if a patient self-medicates, they do so in moderation before seeing a health care practitioner. Studies show taking too much vitamin D can cause hypercalcemia resulting in potassium wasting and adrenal stress.

Clinical Note: 2000 IUs 1 to 2 times per day. Do not exceed 70 to 80 vitamin D levels on lab tests (Mangin, Sinha, & Fincher, 2014).

In some cases where even relatively higher doses of vitamin D3 fail to raise levels, one needs to look at underlying causes,

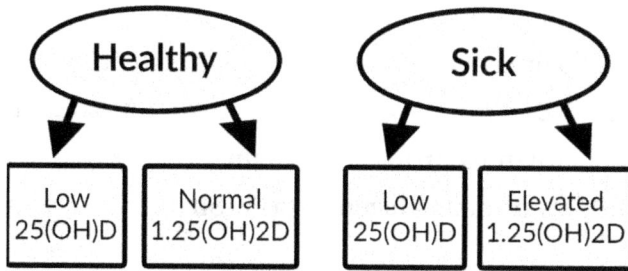

Figure 29. Assess Vitamin D Deficiency: measurement of 1,25(OH)2D via calcitriol measurement instead of low 25(OH)D, which is found in healthy and chronic inflammatory diseases

including the vitamin D receptor (VDR). Certain microbes have shown to slow innate immune defenses by down-regulating the VDR to avoid detection. When intracellular pathogens suppress the VDR, the body almost becomes resistant to calcitriol and continually needs more. Calcitriol activates the VDR. In such cases, it's advisable to test vitamin D3 and a metabolite called calcitriol (1,25-dihydroxyvitamin D). After treating identified pathogens, vitamin D supplementation provides better results. Anti-microbial therapy and vitamin D supplementation may begin simultaneously.

Preferences: Allergy Research Group vitamin D3 Complete with A and K2

Clinical Notes: Low 25(OH)D is found in both healthy persons and autoimmune or chronic inflammatory patients making interpretation of vitamin D deficiency via calcitriol measurement more difficult. Assess vitamin D status with a measurement of 1,25(OH)2D.

Vitamin C

Vitamin C is considered an essential nutrient in chronic and inflammatory conditions with well-known antioxidant potential. It has been shown to protect the brain from oxidative damage in various models of neurodegeneration (Shah, Yoon, Kim, & Kim, 2015).

Preferences: NutriGold Vitamin C Gold, organic amla powder

Co-Factors

An important point to remember is that some people may require additional co-factors (COQ-10, taurine, carnitine, L-theanine, molybdenum, inositol, iodine) for optimal nutritional balance and homeostasis.

BioNexus Herbals For Foundation Protocol

LS Blend

The BioNexus Herbals LS (lung support) Blend is a nourishing and supportive for the respiratory system. Combine the LS Blend with pranayama yogic breathing exercises.

Formula 9 HHG

BioNexus Herbals Formula 9 HHG (hurt, heartbreak, & grief) helps cultivate a calm, balanced, and uplifting mood. It also supports access to the profound healing powers of a focused mind.

Formula 2 EOS

Four years of research lead to our external use only, BioNexus Herbals Formula 2 EOS (essential oil support). Formula 2 EOS helps to keep biotoxins (mold spores, bacteria, and viruses) at bay by cleansing the air and energizing a room. BNH patients successfully use it in baths, shampoo, household cleaning products, air freshening, and much more.

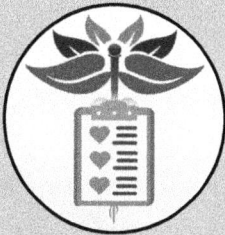

IODINE

Bio-Available Iodines: alaria, digitate dulse, kelp, kombu, nori

Thyroid imbalances are often prevalent in people with CIRS. Iodine deficiency, along with a comprehensive thyroid hormone panel, can be easily measured with basic lab testing.

David Brownstein, MD, is a leading expert on the use of iodine for endocrine health and balance. At BNH, we use transdermal, oral, or nebulizer iodine supplementation depending on the individual need.

Preferences: Biotics Research, Lugols, Nascent Iodine

MEDICINAL HERB GLYCERITE

Glycerite base to use with teas and elixirs

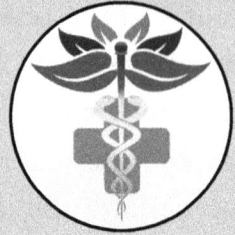

A glycerin (or honey) extraction process produces a solution with higher medicinal properties for essential oil plants

Plants high in essential oil are usually also fragrant like lemon balm, lavender, and sacred basil

Use 100% glycerin with fresh herb; if using dried herbs, dilute 3 parts distilled water to 1 part glycerin

Directions

Chiffonade fresh herbs or ground dried herbs

Add herbs to mason jar, leaving at least 1 inch at the top

Fully cover herbs with glycerin, while releasing air bubbles

Label mason jar with date and herbs

Store in dark area

Agitate mason jar daily for 4-6 weeks

Top off glycerin, if needed

Elixirs are traditionally made with a glycerin or honey base and a little bit of alcohol as a preservative

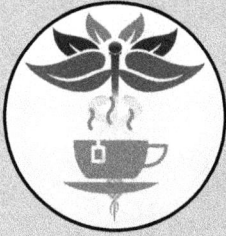

GLYCERITE TEA

See Medicinal Herb Glycerite recipe

Ingredients

Homemade Medicinal Herb Glycerite

Distilled water

Directions

In a quart glass jar, add 4-6 tbsp herb glycerite

Fill the jar to the top with boiling water

Steep with a lid on for 45 minutes

Drink 1 cup and breathe in the steamy vapors while sipping

Refrigerate excess infusion and heat it up before drinking

MAGNESIUM CHLORIDE FOOT SOAK

Remember to use filtered water

Prepare Bath

One cup of magnesium chloride flakes in a foot soaking basin with warm purified water

A few teaspoons of magnesium oil in the water may be added to help boost magnesium levels

Notes

Applying magnesium oil topically after the soak is also an option

Sometimes magnesium preparations can cause a harsh reaction on sensitive skin or skin conditions

Preference: Life Flo pure mag flakes

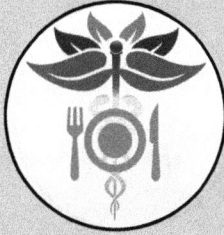

LAND & SEA STIR FRY

Serve over a bed of brown rice, garnish with thinly sliced scallions, a wedge of lime, and sprinkle roasted sesame seeds on top

Ingredients

Seaweed
Any vegetables (broccoli, cauliflower, bok choy, zucchini, onions, squash, and mushrooms) cut as desired
Any protein (chicken, cod, sprouted tofu cubes, etc.)
2 tbsp sesame oil
2 tsp roasted sesame seeds

Spice Mix: 1 tsp each -rice vinegar, gluten-free and low-sodium tamari (or coconut aminos), honey, sesame oil, and chili-garlic paste (optional)

Directions

Soak desired seaweed in warm filtered water until tender, 10 to 15 minutes, depending on the variety

Remove seaweed from soak, press down on the seaweed to remove excess liquid, drain well, and pat dry

In a small bowl, make spice mix

In a skillet, heat sesame oil and on medium-high heat; stir fry vegetables for 2 to 3 minutes

Add seaweed and spice mix; stir to coat vegetables

Add protein; cook until protein finishes

WINTER & SEA SOUP

Experiment with this recipe because it is endlessly customizable

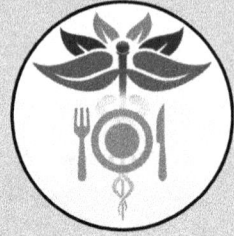

Herbs

1 sprig (about 1/4 to 3/4 tsp) each – rosemary, thyme, bay leaf, and tarragon

1 clove of garlic

Salt and black pepper

Any vegetables of choice cut (slant cut, crinkle cut, sticks, julienned, circles): celery, carrots, parsnips, shallots, butternut squash, baby potatoes, baby tomatoes, green beans, broccoli, shitake or whole baby mushrooms

My son loves 4 oz petit Copper River Sockeye salmon

Directions

Soak 1/4 cup of dried seaweed in warm water to rehydrate

I like to use Alaria and Kombu for this soup

In a medium soup pot, heat olive oil over medium heat

Add shallots and cook, stirring until softened

Add garlic and cook for 1 more minute

Add celery, carrots, and parsnips, stir for 3-4 minutes

Add chicken or vegetable stock, herb sprigs, and a dash of salt and pepper

Raise heat to medium-high and bring to a boil

Lower heat to medium-low and simmer for 10 minutes

Add potatoes, green beans, other veggies of choice, and the protein, then simmer an additional 10-15 minutes, or until vegetables are tender

Optionally, add frozen peas or kidney beans and simmer 5 minutes

Optionally, add tomatoes by hand-crushing them into the soup, including the juice

Add sea vegetables and simmer 5 more minutes, to allow flavors to blend

If the soup is too thick, add more stock

Salt and pepper to taste

Add more fresh thyme leaves, if desired

Garnish with fresh chopped parsley and a lemon wedge

Serve hot with gluten-free bread rolls or crackers

2 - Gastrointestinal Support

Step two of the BioNexus Approach, gastrointestinal support, tackles gut health and metabolic function by binding mycotoxins and reducing inflammatory cytokines.

Place a strong emphasis on reducing gut inflammation, replacing enzymes, and improving microbial balance.

HOMEMADE JOINT RELIEF REMEDY

Do not use on broken skin or on rashes; sensitive patients should test a small area before use

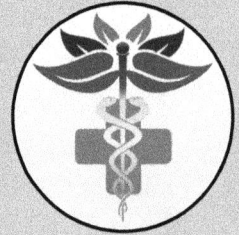

Directions

Blend one capsule of Enhansa 600 mg (or 1 tbsp of organic turmeric) with 1 tbsp of warm ghee (or sesame oil)

Add a few drops of freshly squeezed ginger juice

Apply on the inflamed joint area

Cover with gauze and wrap with a cloth bandage

Leave on overnight

Reducing inflammatory cytokines is a crucial aspect of protecting the gut and bringing down localized inflammation along with food reactivity, immune dysfunction, and neurotransmitter imbalance. Rebuild the microbiome diversity in the gastrointestinal tract by rotating probiotics. Patients need to report any constipation as it needs to be addressed before moving to the next step, detoxification.

Binders

Preferences (Rotate binders every month.): BIND, Luvos, MicroChitosan, Takesumi Supreme, Ultra Binder

BTXD Blend
Use BioNexus Herbals BTXD (biotoxin detox) Blend with each binder for gentle but faster results, even for the most sensitive of patients.

Anti-Inflammatory Therapy

Preferences: CytoQuel, Enhansa, InflammaGen Therapeutics, NRF2 activator, Thorne Meriva

Formula 8 IJS
BioNexus Herbals Formula 8 IJS (Inflammation and Joint Support) quells systemic inflammation and provides joint support. It makes a strong combination when paired with curcumin 600 mg 2x/day.

Digestive Support

Ancient Ayurvedic wisdom tells us that the wise physician (and patient) cultivates the "temperature of the field." The root of good health is the fertility of the soil (body). Foods with reliable enzymatic power provide vitality to the body, while devitalized (non-organic) foods weaken it. The temperature of the digestive system needs to be balanced - not too hot (hyperactive, inflammatory states) and not too cold (hypoactive, sluggish, damp).

Digestive Enzymes
Preferences: Digestive enzymes ultra - Digest, Digestzymes, Kidz Digest

Special Circumstances: Betaine HCL with pepsin, No-Fenol

Gut Repair
Heal and support healthy microbiomes with ghee, a traditional Ayurveda remedy. Ghee (clarified butter) is made when one removes milk solids by liquifying unsalted butter. It retains its rich source of short-chained saturated fats, including butyric acid, making it easily digestible and anti-inflammatory. Research shows unhealthy gastrointestinal tracts do not produce butyric acid that assists in aerobic energy metabolism and healing of the small and large intestines (Barcenilla et al., 2000, p. 1655). Ghee also contains antioxidants and fat-soluble vitamins A, D, E, and K.

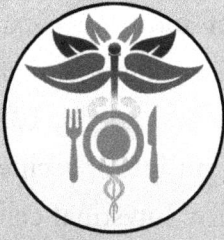

BNH GUT BUTTER

Replace the butter every two weeks

Ingredients

1 cup organic ghee (clarified butter); softened
1/2 cup organic, cold-pressed real extra virgin olive oil
3 tsp (or 4 capsules) strep-free probiotic powder
2 tsp L-glutamine (powder)*
300 mg zinc L-carnosine complex
1 tbsp organic, raw honey
1 tsp marshmallow root powder
1 tsp slippery elm powder
15 drops tulsi glycerite
1,200-1,600 mg sialic acid
2,000 mg butyric acid

*Skip, if sensitive to oxalates or glutamate

Directions

Mix ingredients in a bowl or food processor, until even

Keep refrigerated in a toxin-free storage container

Use 1-2 tbsp (14-28g) daily

Gut butter may be chased with 1 tsp digestive bitters for hypochlorhydria (low stomach acid) issues

Add to snacks, meals, soups, veggies, or stir fry like regular butter

Ayurvedic medicine uses ghee as an herb carrier and to lubricate the gastrointestinal tract. Ghee is the foundation of homemade gut butter, an alternative to butter for Crohn's and colitis, IBS, lactose intolerance, leaky gut, and CIRS. Most gut butter recipes add L-glutamine to repair intestinal permeability. Intestinal cells use glutamine for metabolic fuel.

The goal of all gut butter recipes is to promote healthy microbiomes and recover the gastrointestinal tract. The BNH gut butter recipe is specially concocted for CIRS patients.

DRIED MARSHMALLOW ROOT TEA
Drink 1-2 cups per day

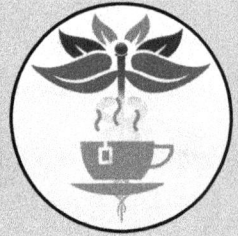

Ingredients

1 tbsp of dry marshmallow root

2-4 fresh peppermint leaves

1/2 piece of peeled ginger

Directions

Combine ingredients in a warm cup of (not boiling) water with a lid

After the infusion cools down, shake gently, and put the lid on it

Refrigerate for a few hours (or overnight)

Strain with cheesecloth (or nut milk bag) and thoroughly press mucilage (thick, gluey substance) out of the herb matter

Keep liquid refrigerated

Immune Modulation

Patients with gut challenges often benefit from custom herb blends. Use the herbal guides in Part 4: Prepping The Approach and recipes to teach them how to use and prepare beneficial herbs.

Immune modulators, nervous system trophorestoratives, and mucilaginous herbs soothe and heal the GI system. Immune modulatory herbs serve to "retrain" a hyper-reactive (or sensitive) immune response by modulating it to manageable levels.

Trophorestorative herbs nourish, restore, and balance tissues and organs. The best approach is small calculated doses over short periods.

Preferences:
BioNexus Herbals IS-M Blend (Immune Support - Modulating), a great broad-spectrum created specifically for CIRS patients

Gastrointestinal Issues - chamomile, dandelion, licorice, mint, slippery elm, yellow dock

Liver - dandelion, milk thistle, turmeric

Kidneys - nettle seed

Stomach - licorice, meadowsweet

DO NOT USE PREBIOTICS AND PROBIOTICS IN YOGURT AT THE SAME TIME.

COMBINED THEY CAN CREATE MOLD.

HOMEMADE YOGURT

A simple coconut cream recipe taught to me by a vegan chef I met at a yoga retreat

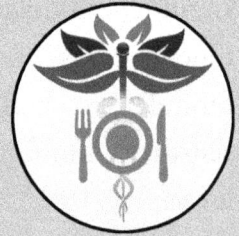

Ingredients

High-fat coconut heavy cream (canned or fresh)

2-3 strep-free probiotic capsules (opened)

Directions

Slowly mix in each probiotic capsule

Tie a cheesecloth around the jar neck (or yogurt maker); set aside overnight at room temperature

For added thickness, strain excess liquid through a cheesecloth

The yogurt will last up to two weeks in the refrigerator

Optional toppings: granola, fruit toppings, parfaits, etc

One of my favorite herbs for mucosal issues and gut repair is marshmallow root. It is very mild, nourishing, soothing, and cooling on irritated and "angry" mucosa.

Patients with poor digestive health, food allergies, autoimmune bowel disease, reflux, or gastroenteritis can use marshmallow root in a very soothing gut repair tea (see dried marshmallow root tea recipe).

Yogurt
An excellent source of probiotics is homemade, plant-based yogurt. Add the daily dose of probiotics to the recipe.

Preferences:
Gut Motility - Energetix Colon Clear, herbal enemas, senna, magnesium, Smooth Move teas

Gut Support Supplements - aloe vera juice (inner fillet), bile salts, CP-1, curcumin, digestive bitters, digestive enzymes, fulvic and humic minerals, gut butter, IBgard, L-glutamine, Life Start Pro Dairy-Free, marshmallow root, MegaSporeBiotic, Mentharil, Restore, Saccharomyces Boulardii, slippery elm

Herbal Cholagogues
Cholagogues and choleretics herbs stimulate liver and gall bladder bile production and aid flow to the small intestine. These essential therapeutic agents for detoxification and organ support contain compounds (saponins and iridoid glycosides) that help stimulate taste buds, enliven digestion, and help maintain a healthy appetite.

Most bitter herbs (arugula and dandelion) are cholagogues and choleretics that energize a sluggish digestive system. They also beneficially affect the hepatobiliary system to help ensure an active and healthy liver. Several cholagogues and choleretics provide antispasmodic action on biliary ducts.

Due to the myorelaxant and spasmolytic action on the intestines, carminative essential oils and extracts are used in gastrointestinal remedies. Carminative herbs, many are aromatic plants, also help with flatulence and the associated abdominal distension and pain.

Preferences:
Carminative - cinnamon, dill, oregano, peppermint, Russian and Persian sage

Cholagogues - dandelion, burdock, chamomile, field gentian, ginger, milk thistle, orange peel, rosemary, yarrow

Notable Choleretic Properties: black pepper, cayenne, cilantro or coriander, cumin, onion, red chili, turmeric

Advanced Metabolic Support

Alterative herbs gradually restore body functions by gently increasing metabolic waste removal through elimination pathways. They can clear a congested liver, encourage urination, support the lungs, open the skin pores, and move lymph and the bowels.

Antidyscratic agents are alteratives that have a more significant effect on the kidneys, aiding in the removing purines, uric acid, and other water-soluble wastes.

Preferences: burdock (Arctium Iaapa), calendula (Calendula officinalis), celery (Apium graveolens) seed, cleavers (Galium aparine) herb, dandelion (Taraxacum officinale) root, echinacea (Echinacea purpurea, E. pallida, E. angustifolia) root, elder (Sambucus nigra) flower, nettle (Urtica dioica) leaf

Comorbid IBS/Crohn's and Colitis

Patients with IBS/Crohn's and Colitis can use small amounts of traditional spices like bay leaves, black pepper, caraway, cardamom, chamomile, cinnamon, clove, coriander, cumin, fennel, ginger, and long pepper as tolerated.

Preferences:
Anti-inflammatory - boswellia, curcumin

Mucosal Lining Support - fennel, ginger, licorice, marshmallow root, slippery elm

Supportive - basil, dill, hyssop, lemon balm, marjoram, oregano, peppermint, rosemary, sage, savory, tarragon, thyme, tulsi

Dyspepsia and Indigestion

Preferences: anise, caraway, chamomile flowers, coriander, cumin, fennel seeds, ginger root, lemon balm, mint, peppermint leaves

Constipation

Preferences: chamomile, lavender, dandelion root, fennel, flaxseed, ginger, peppermint, psyllium, slippery elm powder, Triphala

Hydrochloric Acid Imbalances and Esophageal Reflux

Preferences: chamomile, coriander, fennel, flaxseed, geranium, goldenseal, lavender, lemon balm, licorice, marshmallow root, peppermint, Roman chamomile, slippery elm

Camel Milk Therapy

After introducing herbs to the patient (see Part 4: Prepping The Approach), if they need stronger immune modulation, it is acceptable to add camel milk therapy.

Camel milk is the nutrient-dense milk that is the closest to human milk. It contains high amounts of bioavailable vitamins, minerals, antioxidants, proteins, blood sugar-stabilizing insulin, and unique antibodies. There are more antibodies in camel milk than human milk; they are one-tenth the size, gaining the name nanobodies, and operate similarly to human antibodies.

Camel milk whey proteins carry immunoglobulins (including IVIg) and lactoferrin that are highly effective and protective of the immune system. Research shows that they also have medicinal benefits (Zibaee et al., 2015; Konuspayeva, Faye, Loiseau, & Levieux, 2007).

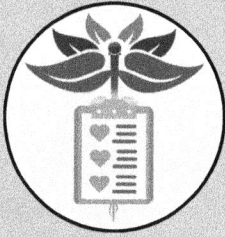

FLASH PASTEURIZED CAMEL MILK THERAPY

If the patient prefers raw camel milk, it is acceptable, but only if added later in the healing process. Diabetic CIRS patients may benefit from adding raw camel milk earlier. Sensitive people are usually unable to transition to raw camel milk.

Sensitive Start	Start	Maximum
1 drop per day and add 1 drop as tolerated until Maximum	1 tsp per day and add 1 tsp every three days until Maximum	1/2 cup 2x per day

Jarisch-Herxheimer symptoms are very common; **reduce** *to sensitive or take a break for a few days*

Lactoferrin prevents microbial growth in the gut by targeting tissues invaded by pathogens and is a systemic immune booster contributing to the non-immune host defense.

Increased serum levels of inflammatory cytokines, particularly thymus and activation-regulated chemokine (TARC or CCL17), is related to bacterial and viral infections, and asthma. Camel milk has decreased these levels (Bashir & Al-Ayadhi, 2013).

After clearing inflammation, infections, gluten, and other food sensitivities, camel milk may be used for immune modulation (regulates the activation of macrophages and neutrophils).

Ayurvedic Approach To Digestive Optimization

Understanding a body's tendencies is key to discovering the energetic constitution, or in the language of Ayurveda, dosha (see Part 4: Prepping The Approach). Adjusting diet and herbs based on an in-depth analysis of the individual's constitution can immensely benefit extreme gut sensitivities.

Vata - Dosha of Movement
Preferences: chamomile, ginger, lemon balm

Pitta - Dosha of Transformation
Preferences: dandelion, linden, rose

Kapha - Dosha of Structure And Stability
Preferences: holy basil or tulsi, peppermint, sage

NUTRITIONALLY DENSE BEET LEMON HUMMUS

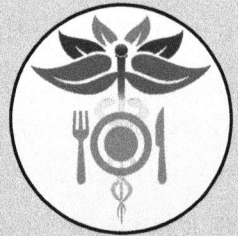

Ingredients

1/2 cup boiled beets
1 cup boiled chickpeas
1/4 cup roasted sesame seeds
1/4 cup lemon juice
1 tsp roasted, ground cumin
Sea salt

Directions

Blend beets, chickpeas, sesame seeds, and lemon juice together to a smooth, creamy paste

Stir in the cumin powder

Add salt to taste

Stress Relief

It is all in the family.

Family support, compassion, and cooperation play a critical role in the health and wellness of a CIRS patient. At BioNexus Health Clinic, we incorporate the entire family into treatment, especially when the patient tests positive for MARCoNS, parasites, streptococcal infection, mycoplasma infection, or Epstein-Barr. Any easily transmitted disease necessitates a family protocol. Joint treatment also helps the patient adjust to the new lifestyle and prevents the family (occasionally pets too) from recycling the same germs, toxins, and habits that delay or prevent healing.

Typically, once biotoxin illness becomes CIRS, it has put undue stress on the family, whether they acknowledge it or not. Chronic disease tends to bring a lot of hardship, stress, and strain into relationships. Beyond physiological health, the patient and their family probably need an emotional detox. Frequently, patients feel a sense of loneliness, abandonment, loss, and guilt.

The family dynamic is complicated to navigate, but it is essential to highlight the need for open communication to start the healing process. The parents or the partner are often overworked, overwhelmed, and exhausted. Sibling rivalry, jealousy, and acting out may also be amplified. The patient and their family need to address the factors occurring around the disease.

Low stress, fresh air, adequate water intake, and realistic self-expectations set the right tone for the body. It's reasonable for the patient to expect never to return to their old lifestyle. Graciously and with gratitude, they need to embrace their new normal. A new normal can profoundly change life for the better. They should focus on a future of better health, wellness, and longevity. Patients should begin repairing relationships and removing emotional toxins and toxic people from their life. They should also find spiritual health, daily gentle exercise, sunshine, nature, nutrition, a sleep sanctuary, and inner peace.

CASHEW MILK LATTE
Warm and comforting

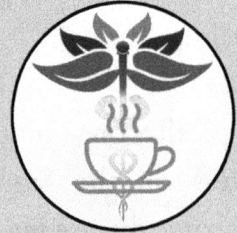

Ingredients

2 cups cashew milk
1 tsp turmeric powder
1 pinch pippali powder
2 tbsp local raw honey
1 tsp wild mushroom powder
1 tsp raw cacao powder
1 tsp crushed pistachio nuts
1 pinch cardamom powder

Directions

Mix the cacao powder, pistachios, and cardamom and keep on the side

Blend the rest of the ingredients well

Warm up to desired temperature

Use a handheld latte milk frother to stir up foam on top

Garnish with the mix

The BioNexus Approach offers renewed wellness with better health, but it cannot be achieved without also mending emotional and spiritual health.

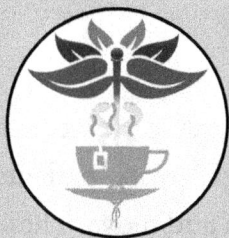

WINTER TONIC TEA

Make a batch nightly and reheat to drink the next day; several cups may be consumed throughout the day

Ingredients

2 parts nettle leaf
2 parts peppermint or spearmint leaf
1 part lemon balm leaf
1 part milky oats
1 part fresh turmeric root
1 part red clover blossom
1 part burdock root

Directions

Blend herbs together to make tea blend

Boil water

Steep 1-2 tablespoons of tea blend per cup of water for 10-15 minutes

Add honey to sweeten

A longer infusion period extracts more vitamins and minerals

3 - Detoxification Support

Step three of the BioNexus Approach, detoxification support, focuses on impeding bacterial and chemical exposure in the body and around the house. It also kickstarts the first two steps of the biotoxin illness protocol.

The Shoemaker Protocol requires patients to vacate or remediate the moldy residence before treatment. BNH treats patients globally, and it is not always possible to pick up and move. These cases must diligently detoxify their world while they create a safe living space. If the patient typically goes to a moldy area outside the residence, they need to avoid it until they reach step six of the BioNexus Approach. The practitioner's goal, for these cases, is to maintain their current state and stave off deterioration. A few patients will improve, but recovery necessitates immediate reduction with eventual elimination, and reduced exposure and re-exposure risk.

When Toxins Overflow

Patients must be diligent in toxin avoidance in vehicles and at home, work, and school. Over a lifetime, exposure occurs daily and cumulatively to a large variety and varying amounts of toxins: air fresheners, artificial "new" scents, chlorine pools, cleaning products, cooking pans, EMFs, exhaust fumes, fungicides, heavy metals, insecticides, outgassing devices, outgassing furniture, pesticides, and plastics. Unfortunately, it is a very long list of commonly used items.

If a person has MTHFR and other gene mutations that relate to detoxification, the effect of toxin accumulation is truly challenging with relentless symptoms and difficulty functioning on a day to day basis. Preexisting comorbid medical conditions may also become complicated and challenging to treat.

It is essential to understand that it is usually about more than the MTHFR genetic mutation status, whether heterozygous or homozygous. All the nutrients that support enzyme function in the methylation cycle also work hard to help the genes work correctly. CIRS patients frequently have mitochondrial dysfunction. Therefore, under these circumstances, it becomes imperative to minimize exposure to toxins.

CIRS-WDB Triggers

Exposure to mold and mycotoxins is a very potent trigger that derails the immune system and can have a devastating impact mainly on the innate immune system but also the adaptive immune system, to a certain extent. It is vital to understand that the interior environment of a water-damaged building (WDB) can contain a complex mixture of inflammagens, microbes, and toxins. There are 30 known dangerous toxins in a WDB, including VOCs, chitinases, beta-D-glucans, viruses, bacteria, and fungi (See Figure 30). Most of the trigger sources cannot be identified by spore counting. However, they are all are capable of eliciting an intense innate inflammatory response and a host cellular immune response, particularly in the HLA genetic haplotype.

When the immune system struggles and dysregulates, toxin elimination slows down, causing toxins to accumulate. Exposure also damages neuropeptide regulatory control mechanisms. When this occurs, patients typically report an explosion of inflammatory responses. This cytokine storm often results in widespread collateral damage to different organ systems in the body.

Fungi	Microbial	Others
Mycotoxins	Gram negative bacteria	Hemolysins
Bio-aerosols	Gram positive bacteria	Proteinases
Cell fragments	Mycobacteria	Chitinases
Cell wall components	Nocardia	Siderophores
Hyphal fragments	Acntiomycetes	Microbial VOC's
Spores	Protozoa	Building Material VOC's
Beta Glucans	Chlamydia	Coarse Particulates
Mannans	Endotoxins	Ultrafine particulates
	LPS - Lipopolysaccharides	Nanoparticulates
	Mycoplasma	

Figure 30. Sources of Inflammagens

Other Toxins To Consider

Before continuing, address any areas unresolved during the foundation protocol: air, water, and diet. A less than desirable kitchen environment is the most likely area to increase the chemical toxin load for an immunocompromised person. The most popular cookware has Teflon (PTFE - See Water in Foundation Protocol) coating is incredibly toxic. Many people do not know that there are temperature and use guidelines for these products. When a Teflon pan cooks too hot or the seal breaks, the chemical seeps into food and releases into the air. PTFE (and PFOA) is then consumed or inhaled by the patient. Also, avoid plastic cookware, storage containers, and utensils. Instead, everything that touches food should be stainless steel, glass, ceramic, or cast-iron.

Replace all porous cleaning supplies, including sponges, with washable cloths.

All faucets used by the patient need the appropriate filters.

Food consumed by the patient can quickly derail treatment if the diet is not toxin and trigger free. If the diet has not been overhauled or customized, the patient must change their menu. There are several diets that, when modified, fit the recommended criteria. Sensory sensitive patients typically choose a paleo, gut and psychology syndrome (GAPS) diet, autoimmune, or specific

> "Pointing at mycotoxins as the only components found in WDB that create inflammatory responses in people sickened by exposure to WDB is wrong, just dead wrong."
>
> —Ritchie Shoemaker, MD (2011)

carbohydrate diet (SCD). Recipes for all these diets are readily available and easy to follow.

<u>Preventative Tips</u>

Air Fresheners: Simple and homemade

Bath & Body: Toxin-free, replace washcloths

Car: Clean, but used vehicles to avoid the "new car" smell

Cosmetics: Paraben-free, BPA-free, toxin-free cosmetics

Filters: Change refrigerator, furnace, vacuums, car cabin filters, and window air conditioner units frequently

Dehumidifiers: Monitor hoses

Furniture: Clean, but used and aired out

Lawn & Garden: Toxin-free

Pest Control: Toxin-free

Pets: Wipe paws & bottoms before reentry

Shoes: Never wear inside

Water Filters: Test quality, install filters and change filters often in the kitchen, bathroom, and laundry

Suspected Exposure: Clean exposure areas, wash clothes and cleaning materials, shower, then wipe down shower and laundry machines

Detoxification Diet Tips

When allergens cause flare-ups and aggravate existing symptoms, review the patient's diet. Use trial and error with diets: AIP, Keto, low FODMAPS, low histamine, SCD, and Wahls.

EXCLUDE

Additional sugar	Glyphosate
Alcohol	Herbicides
Artificial colors	MSG and hidden MSG
Artificial flavors	Pesticides
Cigarettes	Processed foods
Gluten	

MSG

Food manufacturers use labeling tricks to hide MSG. Review the label for autolyzed yeast extract, extractives of food-like substances, enzyme-modified, and hydrolyzed protein. Conduct research to stay current on new methods and words used on food products.

Preferences: Allergy Research Group Acetyl-Glutathione, liposomal glutathione, Pure TheraPro Glutathione GOLD

Lung Support

Preferences: BioNexus Herbals LS Blend, fibrinolytic enzymes, InflamAway, Now N-acetyl cysteine (NAC), proteolytic enzymes, ProThera, Thorne, white willow bark extract

Clinical Notes: Now NAC, Thorne, and ProThera can clear biofilm but also can cause herxing and anxiety. Start low and slow. Do not exceed 250-300 mg per day.

There have been reports that NAC may deplete calcium and magnesium. As always, a practitioner should evaluate benefits and weigh the risks.

Herbal Detox

Toxins penetrate deep into tissues causing various symptoms of discomfort and disease. Environmental and bacterial toxins derail immune system function and can trigger autoimmune pathology.

The recipes on the following pages showcase sample remedies from beneficial herbs for various symptoms.

<u>Soft Tissue Injuries, Sprains, and Strains</u>
Herbs: ginger, Corydalis, Jamaican dogwood, lavender, meadowsweet, Solomon's seal, white willow bark

Oils: calendula, arnica, carrot seed, frankincense, ginger, helichrysum, meadowsweet, skullcap

<u>Relaxing Muscle Spasms</u>
Herbs: chamomile, kava, lavender, lemon balm, skullcap

Oils: lavender, clary sage, eucalyptus, ginger, marjoram, myrtle, pinyon pine

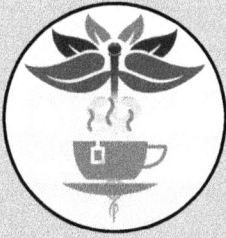

SOFT TISSUE INJURIES, SPRAINS, AND STRAINS TEA

Corydalis Tea Instructions

Prepare ginger tea
Pour 1/2 cup
Add 1/2 dropper of Corydalis
Drink 2 – 4x per day

Jamaican Dogwood Tea Instructions

Prepare ginger tea
Pour 1/2 cup
Add 1/2 dropper of Jamaican dogwood or one inch of bark
Drink 2x per day

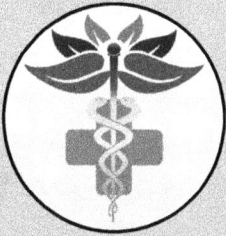

SOFT TISSUE INJURIES, SPRAINS, AND STRAINS TOPICAL RUB

Directions

Mix equal parts arnica flowers, chamomile flowers, meadowsweet, skullcap, and dry herbs

Stir 2 cups of the herb mixture into 2 cups of olive oil

Heat in a double boiler for 3-5 hours

Cool, strain, and refrigerate

Warm skin with wet compress before and after application (optional)

Apply gently over soft tissue injuries

Essential oils can be added before each application

RELAXING MUSCLE SPASMS TEA

Drink 1/2 cup; 2-4x per day

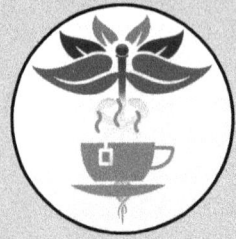

Directions

2 tbsp lemon balm (fresh herb is preferred but dried herb can be used as well) per cup of hot water

Infuse for 10-15 minutes

Add 1/2 dropper of passionflower

RELAXING MUSCLE SPASMS MASSAGE

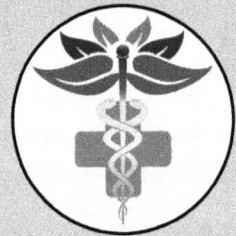

Directions

1 ounce Mahanarayan oil

Add 5 drops of each eucalyptus, myrtle and pinyon pine essential oils

Warm skin with wet compress before and after application

Massage into affected areas

Note: Test all essential oil preparations on a small area for a reaction before use

<u>Arthritic Pain</u>

Herbs: Boswellia, devil's claw, feverfew, fresh galangal root, marjoram, meadowsweet, nettles, turmeric root, white willow bark, wild yam

Oils: chamomile, conifer, eucalyptus, helichrysum, juniper, Mahanarayan, marjoram, Solomon's seal

Herbs for Autoimmune Disease

Immune Amphoterics (normalize function of an organ or a system within the body): cordyceps, licorice, maitake, reishi

Immune Regulators (reduce histamine release and allergic response): Salvia miltiorrhiza, sarsaparilla, Scutellaria, turmeric

Alteratives (increase elimination of metabolic waste via lymph, liver, kidney, lung, large intestine, or skin): Baptisia, burdock, Calendula, cleavers, dandelion, Oregon grape root, poke, red clover, violet leaf, yellow dock root

Herbs For Deeper Detoxification

For those desiring a deep cleanse, the use of the herbs below should be under the care of a knowledgeable practitioner.

Preferences: aloe vera, artichoke (Cynara scolymus), burdock (Arctium lappa), dandelion (Taraxacum officinale), chinacea (E.

ARTHRITIC PAIN TEA

Drink 1/2 cup; 2–3x per day

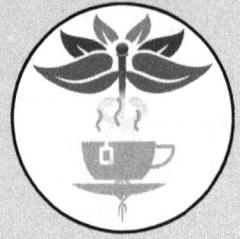

Directions

Finely chop fresh ginger root, fresh turmeric root, and fresh galangal root (dried herb may be used if fresh is not in season)

Mix equal amounts of roots, simmer 1 tsp of the mixture per cup of water for 10-15 minutes

Alternately, prepare fresh ginger root tea, then add 3-5 drops of turmeric and galangal tincture to the usual dose of ginger tea

Take 1 tablet of a guggulu preparation with the tea 2x per day

ARTHRITIC PAIN MASSAGE

Discontinue if skin irritation develops

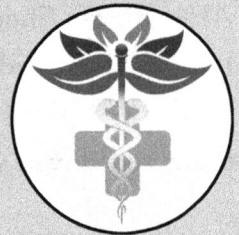

Directions

1 tbsp Mahanarayan oil, add 1 drop ginger and 1 drop black pepper

Massage into joints several times a day

Add CBD oil to the Mahanarayan oil to increase analgesic and anti-inflammatory potency

angustifolia, E. purpurea, E. pallida), figwort (Scrophularia nodosa), gentian (Gentiana lutea), goldenseal (Hydrastis canadensis), kutki (Picrorhiza kurroa), milk thistle (Silybum marianum), psyllium (Plantago ovata), red clover (Trifolium pratense), red root (Ceanothus americanus), Sarsaparilla (Smilax officinalis), Selfheal (Prunella vulgaris), senna (Cassia acutifolia), yellow dock (Rumex crispus)

Types of Binders

The liver, kidneys, lymphatic system, and adrenal glands help flush out toxins. If they poorly filter or drain, the toxins can reabsorb into the body. It is essential to keep these organs tonified and active.

Examine for swollen lymph nodes throughout detoxification. Some people respond well to lymphatic drainage massages, while others may experience a detox reaction or healing crisis similar to a herxing response from too much detoxification too fast.

<u>Binders</u>
Every binder has greater efficacy for specific toxins. Customizing binders based on individual lab results is possible. However, clinically, BNH finds the benefit of a broad-spectrum binder more economical, often outweighing the more complicated personalized approach.

Preferences:
Mycotoxins - activated charcoal, BIND, BioNexus Herbals

BTXD Blend, chlorella, Luvos, MicroChitosan, Takesumi Supreme, Ultra Binder, Welchol

Xenobiotics & Xenoestrogens - Pure Body Cleanse, Zeolite

Heavy Metals - Bioray Kids NDF Plus, chlorella, cilantro, Detox Pesto, IMD Intestinal Cleanse, Metal-Chord, MetalPul, Neuro-Chord, TRS

Vaccine Detox - CEASE therapy, BioNexus Herbals Formula 7 GDS (Glyphosate Detox Support), VAC-Chord

Organ Support

Liver - BioNexus Herbals HEP-S Blend, apo-HEPAT, Guna-Liver, milk thistle, NAC

Kidney - BioNexus Herbals REN-S Blend, Kidney-Tone, Renelix, Solidago, uva ursi

Lymphatic Drainage - BioNexus Herbals LMPH Blend, cleavers, dandelion, Itires, Lymphonest, manjistha

Adrenal - Ashwagandha, Drenatrophin PMG, Eleuthero, HPA axis daytime regulation, Loving Energy, Supren

Nebulizers - reduced glutathione, nascent iodine, magnesium chloride

Only use nebulizers with the guidance of knowledgeable practitioners. Begin diluted and very slowly build-up to the recommended dosage.

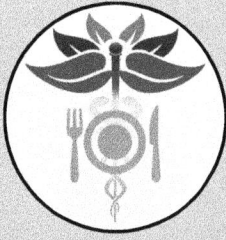

DETOX PESTO
Best when made with fresh produce

Ingredients

1 cup of cilantro leaves and stems
1/4 cup parsley leaves
1/2 cup basil leaves
1/4 cup of Holy basil (tulsi) leaves
1 garlic clove
1/4 cup fresh grated turmeric
1/4 cup fresh grated ginger
1 cup extra virgin olive oil
(sesame oil, quality water, or a combination)

According to Taste (Optional)

Spinach, dandelion, watercress, or arugula
Sprouted almonds, seeds (sunflower, pumpkin, etc.)
Honey
Lemon
Sea salt

Directions

In a blender
Add all dry ingredients (should fill about 3/4)
Add wet ingredients
Blend until smooth

Consume directly in a shot glass, use on gluten-free toast or pasta, or sprouted white or brown rice

LYME PREVENTION HERBAL COCKTAIL

1/2 - 1 tsp daily

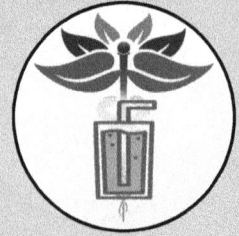

Ingredients

1 part astragalus root
1 part cat's claw
1 part neem leaf
1 part pau d'arco

Directions

Prepare in a 1:1 extract using 80 proof alcohol or organic vegetable glycerin hot water extract

Macerate for 4 weeks

Add after macerate ingredients

After Macerate Ingredients

1 tsp garlic flower essence
1 tsp tulsi
1 tsp brahmi
1/2 tsp of haritaki
(glycerite or tinctures)

In New England, Canada, England, Scotland, Ireland, Baltic States, Ukraine, and Russia, I recommend taking the Lyme Prevention Herbal Cocktail from mid-February until snowfall.

Remember, the ticks will become active any time their environment reaches 45 degrees.

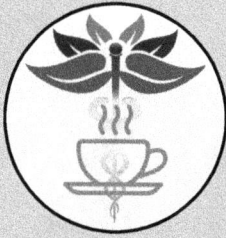

HERBAL TONIC FOR CHRONIC

If taken as directed, a 32 oz. bottle will last 32 days; avoid contamination, do not drink from the bottle

1 tbsp with breakfast and dinner

Herb Mix Ingredients

1 part turmeric root

2 parts Bidens pilosa

2 parts Japanese knotweed root

1 part wild sarsaparilla

1 part haritaki

2 parts teasel root

1 part ginger root

2 parts tulsi

1 part neem leaf

2 parts cat's claw

1/4 part white thyme leaf

1/4 part oregano leaf

Directions

Use 1 cup herb mix per gallon water

Decoct to 50%, about 64 oz

Add 3 cups raw honey

Add 1/2 cup French brandy *(optional)*

Notes

Recipe makes approx. 3 quarts
Decant HOT liquid into clean amber bottles and cap
Set aside and tighten caps in about an hour.
Average shelf life is 6 months, but always label the bottles:
"Best if used within 2 months of opening"

MASTER SAUCE

Wholesome multipurpose master sauce

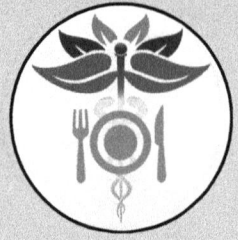

Ingredients

3 brown onions, chopped
3 stalks of celery, finely diced
4 carrots, finely diced
4 cloves garlic, crushed
1/2 inch ginger peeled and crushed

1 kg deseeded seasonal tomatoes
1/2 cup chopped red bell pepper
1/4 cup olive oil
1 tsp turmeric spice
Salt & pepper to taste

Directions

Use a heavy saucepan over low heat

Sauté the onion, carrot, celery, and olive oil for 10 minutes
Stir occasionally to prevent sticking to the bottom
Add turmeric spice in the last minute
Add a little water and simmer for another 10 minutes
(vegetables break down and turn golden)
Add the tomatoes, garlic, salt, and pepper

Simmer for 45 minutes with a lid on 3/4 of the pot, to prevent splatter

Occasionally stir, check seasoning, and thickness

Cook final 20 minutes or until the sauce becomes dense and flavorful

Add preferred protein and finishes

Serve with a side dish

Favorites: sprouted organic brown basmati rice and sprouted quinoa salad

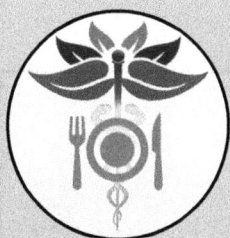

WHOLESOME DESSERT CHOCOLATE N GREEN

Ingredients

2 large frozen ripe bananas
1 large avocado
1 large handful of spinach
2 tbsp raw cacao powder
1-2 cups coconut or almond milk (or 1 tbsp coconut manna)
5 loosely chopped dates
10 organic rose petals (or 20 drops of organic rose glycerite)

Directions

In a blender, combine peeled and sliced frozen bananas, avocado, spinach, dates, rose petals, and plant-based milk of choice

Add the cacao powder and blend the contents, scraping down the sides from time to time

Blend until smooth and creamy

Taste and adjust to the preferred sweetness

Blend again

Add more plant-based milk or liquid if a thinner consistency is preferred

Serve and garnish with a chiffonade of mint leaves and crushed pistachios

A Brother's Concussion

12-year-old Mike, a CIRS patient, despite headaches, anxiety, and visual snow, had a tough time reducing the long hours of spent on his multiple devices daily. His parents struggled with Mike's defiance but also understood his compulsion with electronics.

Six months into Mike's CIRS treatment, Aaron, his 16-year-old brother, was rushed to the emergency room injured after being hit in the head with a soccer ball. The neurologist strongly cautioned against using any electronic devices for at least two weeks to allow his brain time to recover from the traumatic injury.

While Aaron and his friend hung out in the basement media room, he was convinced to play "one game." In the middle of the fast-paced video game, Aaron collapsed. Playing one high-action video game caused a seizure.

Watching Aaron convulse on the floor of the media room was traumatizing to Mike. He listened as the neurologist explained that an inflamed brain needs to remain calm, and electronics interfere with its ability to heal.

The brothers understood the importance of limiting screen time. They tried to limit use to homework and a cheat day on the weekend to help resist temptation.

EMF Vigilance

The Donegal family needed new housing after mold remediation of their house failed. They inspected seven apartment complexes before finding one that passed the mold tests. Two weeks after moving, their CIRS symptoms returned: headaches, blurry vision, light sensitivity, ice pick pain, brain fog, insomnia, poor concentration, and tingling in the arms and fingers.

They confirmed the residence was mold-free with another ERMI test. After digging deeper, they discovered their coveted corner condo had ten smart meters installed outside the master bedroom wall - the same wall as the family room. Smart power meters connect to wiring circuits creating an EMF (electromagnetic field) antenna in the walls. They open and close their electrical pulses thousands of times per second, instead of the normal sixty in the US.

The Donegals hired a building biologist to inspect EMFs and wireless radiation. He mitigated the issues in the family room and created sleeping sanctuaries in the bedrooms. Soon thereafter, the family's symptoms were alleviated.

Many CIRS patients tend to develop a high sensitivity to EMFs. There are a few websites and companies that explain EMF dangers in-depth and offer shielding devices.

EMF Awareness

Digital detox becomes more manageable when the whole household participates. While it is important to limit screen time, it is the electromagnetic effects that are a concern. Radio waves, microwaves, devices, and X-rays emit electromagnetic radiation (EMR) that drive microbial growth (Belyaev, 2011; Ahmed, Istivan, Cosic, & Pirogova, 2013). Research shows EMR fields (EMF) created by computers, Wi-Fi signals, and cellular phones increase cytokine release and impair phagocytosis capability (Oncul, Cuce, Aksu, & Inhan Garip, 2015; Lewicka et al., 2015).

In children and teens, EMFs compromise the integrity of a pediatric blood-brain barrier. Infants do not develop a viable blood-brain barrier until 18-months, which means EMFs have direct access to the brain during critical stages of development.

To limit EMFs in the home, electrically ground the house, turn off wireless routers, opt for ethernet connections, reduce overall screen time, turn off all cordless phones at night, check the SAAR rating of smartphones, and opt-out of smart electricity meters, if possible. There are several EMF protection devices based on scalar technology and Schumann frequency research that are available for purchase. A thorough online search provides a few highly-rated options.

Other Detox Considerations

Detoxification is a multipronged approach. The following are a few commonly seen concerns in my clinic and my favorite remedies or supplements.

Preferences:
Heavy Metals - Advanced TRS, BioPure MicroSilica, cilantro, Detox Pesto, detox smoothie, IMD Intestinal Cleanse

Histamine - BioNexus Herbals MC-S Blend, Allernest, BioNexus Herbals D-Hist, diamine oxidase (DAO) enzymes, Histamine Scavenger, ProAller

Glutamate - Glutamate Scavenger, magnesium, no MSG diet

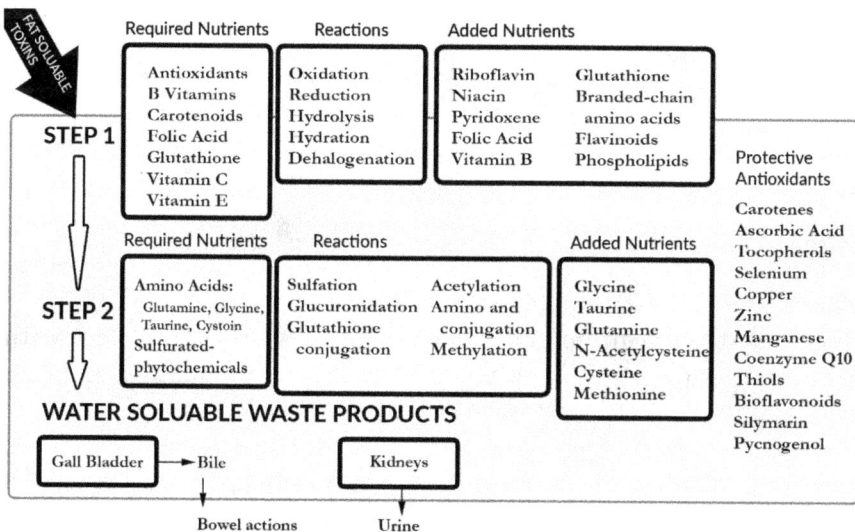

Figure 31. Detoxification pathway

Glyphosate - BioNexus Herbals Formula 7 GDS, clean living, organic diet

Zenobiotics - BioPure ZeoBind, fulvic acid, PureBody, zeolite

Detoxification and Herxheimer Support

Use a pinch of Himalayan salt in water with a squirt of lemon, Epsom salt baths, or Alka-Seltzer Gold for general detoxification and Jarisch-Herxheimer reaction.

Adrenal: Adrenal Support Tea to help the body handle the stress of detoxification and support healing

Earthing: ground yourself, house, devices, vehicle, and minimize screen time

Environmental Detox: a good air purifier, clutter-free, BioNexus Herbals Formula 2 EOS in a diffuser

Epsom Salt Baths: Alka-Seltzer Gold with a pinch of Himalayan salt in water with a squirt of fresh lemon

Foot Bath: commercially available or homemade with magnesium chloride flakes, baking soda, and apple cider vinegar

Sauna: far infrared or dry heat; three sessions: 120°f, 150°f, 180°f; hydrate before and after; mop up sweat

ADRENAL SUPPORT TEA

Make tulsi-ginger tea; cool it to room temperature

Ingredients

1 tsp turmeric powder
1 cup orange juice (freshly squeezed)
1 shot of frozen wheatgrass juice
1 tbsp of almond butter
1 tbsp flax oil
1 tsp collagen powder (optional)
2 tbsp honey

A few basil leaves for chiffonade garnish and flavor

Directions

Blend all the ingredients well in a blender. It should yield two portions

Consume one portion with breakfast for fresh energy

Prevent the mid-afternoon slump by consuming the other portion around 3 pm

For deeper adrenal rejuvenation, add 1 oz of **shilajit prep** solution per 8 oz of the adrenal blend

SHILAJIT PREP

Directions

4 oz hot water

Add a pea-sized pinch of genuine Himalayan or Kashmir Shilajit

Let sit on the countertop until it melts, then mix

It is okay to leave it overnight or to refrigerate it in a glass jar

4 - Address Root Causes

After the patient's body is supported, they are ready for the fourth step, address root causes. The patients at BNH typically have numerous coinfections per lab testing. Most have exposure to water-damaged buildings (CIRS-WDB), many have CIRS-Lyme, and there are also CIRS-WDB and CIRS-Lyme patients.

Microbial and toxin load depends on factors like immune status, the number of infections passed from the insect bites, acute versus chronic presentation, exposure to other toxins, et cetera. Below are the most common coinfections seen in the clinic.

During the treatment phase, DO NOT use immune-boosting herbs. Immune modulation is the key. BioNexus Herbals IS-M Blend is an excellent example.

Most Common Coinfections: CIRS, mycotoxins, MARCoNS, Lyme disease, tick-borne (Babesia, Brucella, Ehrlichia, Powassan virus, Rocky Mountain spotted fever, tularemia, and various species of Bartonella), coinfections (Candida, Chlamydia pneumonia, cytomegalovirus, Epstein-Barr virus, Helicobacter pylori, Mycoplasma pneumonia, parasites, parvovirus, SIBO, Streptococcus, and Toxoplasma gondii), and oral health.

Clinical Notes: Not all patients have all listed coinfections. Each patient receives a bio-individualized protocol based on laboratory testing for infections, biotoxins, and genetics. A few organism-specific treatment protocols used at BNH are listed below. These are in addition to herbs mentioned in earlier steps of the BioNexus Approach.

CIRS

Preferences:
Biotoxin Detox: BioNexus Herbals BTXD Blend and various binders previously discussed

Biofilms: bitter melon, greater celandine, NAC, Terminalia chebula

Dental Health: BioNexus Herbals Formula 5 DHP regular and extra strength

Cytokine Therapy: BioNexus Herbals CK-M Blend, GUNA low dose cytokine therapy

Multisystem Anti-Inflammatory Herbs: Ashwagandha, Bidens pilosa, BioNexus Herbals LS Blend, Chinese Senega root, Chinese skullcap, Cordyceps, curcumin, kudzu, motherwort, Pedicularis, pleurisy root, Solomon's seal, tulsi

Other: hemp oil, melatonin

MARCoNS

Eradicating MARCoNS is the priority in this step. Low MSH is a perpetual cycle due in part to MARCoNS.

BioNexus Herbals Formula 1 NSB is a proprietary herbal blend containing biodynamic Ayurvedic and western herbs that studies have shown to be effective against antibiotic-resistant organisms and biofilm. It was formulated to eradicate MARCoNS naturally. BNH and our collaborating physicians have observed excellent clinical success.

Formula 1 NSB is also used as an urgent care remedy if re-exposure is suspected, as a preventative measure, and during maintenance.

BioNexus Herbals Formula 1 NSB

Children Under 3 Years: Do not use Formula 1 NSB.

Children 3-8 Years: Begin at 25% Formula 1 NSB to 75% distilled water. Start with one spray in one nostril. Wait 24 hours. Use one spray in the other nostril. Wait 24 hours. On the third day, increase to one spray in each nostril. Do this once per day for 2-4 days or even up to 2 to 4 weeks, depending on how the child adjusts to the spray.

Decrease dilution to 50% Formula 1 NSB to 50% distilled water. Continue at the same number of sprays for 2-4 days, depending on how the child adjusts to the spray. If needed, restart the process for the 25/75 dilution. Increase to one spray in each nostril twice per day. Repeat until the child has adjusted to the sprays before increasing.

Two sprays each nostril three times per day. Do not exceed concentration beyond 50% diluted formula!

SENSITIVE	START	MAX	CHILD
Dilute 50%	x2 per nostril per day	x2 per nostril 3x per day	Nostril #1 x1 wait 24 hours
Under 5 & Ultra Sensitive Dilute 75% distilled water to 25% formula			Nostril #2 wait 24 hours
			x1 Both 2-4 days
Shake well before use. *Refrigerate on arrival.* *Travel up to 48 hours without refrigeration.*			x1 Both 2x per day

Children 8-12 Years: Begin at 50% Formula 1 NSB to 50% distilled water. Start with one spray in one nostril. Wait 24 hours. Use one spray in the other nostril. Wait 24 hours. On the third day, increase to one spray in each nostril. Do this once per day for 2-4 days or 2 to 4 weeks depending on how the child adjusts to the spray. Increase to one spray in each nostril twice per day. Repeat until the child has adapted to the sprays before increasing.

Two sprays each nostril three times per day. Do not exceed concentration beyond 50% diluted formula!

Children Over 12 and Sensitive Adults: Some people are very sensitive to change or tend to have a strong Jarisch-Herxheimer reaction. It may be necessary to dilute the spray with distilled water. Start by combining 50% Formula 1 NSB with 50% distilled water. Start with one spray in one nostril. Wait 24 hours. Use one spray in the other nostril. Wait 24 hours. On the third day, increase to one spray in each nostril. Do this once per day for 2-4 days or 2 to 4 weeks depending on how the person adjusts to the spray. Increase to one spray in each nostril twice per day. Repeat until adjusted to the sprays before increasing.

Two sprays each nostril three times per day is the goal.

Adults: Two sprays of Formula 1 NSB in each nostril four times per day.

BioNexus Herbals Formula 5 DHP and Extra-Strength

Over 65 percent of BioNexus Health Clinic patients complain about their dental health. Louis Pasteur, remembered for developing vaccines, reversed himself on his deathbed. He said, "Bernard was right. The pathogen is nothing, the terrain is everything" (as cited in Longmore, Wilkinson, Baldwin, & Wallin, 2014, p. 417).

BioNexus Herbals Formula 5 DHP and Formula 5 DHP-XS keeps the terrain in the mouth unfriendly to harmful bacteria. Use as a gargle, swish, or gum rub only.

	SENSITIVE	START	MAX	CHILD
GARGLE	2x per day 5 drops	2-3x per day 10 drops	3x per day 10 drops	2x per day 5 drops
GUM RUB	1x per day 1 drop	1x per day 1-2 drops	1x per day 2 drops	1x per day 1 drop

Use 2 oz filtered water for gargle.
Store room temperature.
No hot temperatures or humidity.

BioNexus Herbals Formula 6A PBS and Formula 6B PBS

Follow general herbal usage and dosage guidelines for BioNexus Herbals Formula 6A PBS and Formula 6B PBS, a broad-spectrum parasite medication created for treatment. It is recommended to introduce Formula 6A PBS a month before Formula 6B PBS for optimal outcomes.

Children: Take 1 drop per 10 lbs. (4.5 kg) of body weight per day divided into 2 doses 10 minutes after food; do not exceed 1/4 dropper; 2x per day

Adults: Slowly build-up to the maximum adult dose of 1/2 dropper; 3x per day; if gut sensitivity, take 15 minutes after food otherwise take on an empty stomach

THE BASIC ORIGINAL CHAI TEA

Spices can be adapted to taste

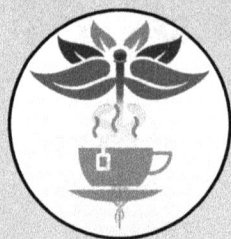

Ingredients

10-12 green cardamom pods
2 black cardamom pods (or 4 green cardamom pods)
8-10 cloves
12-15 black peppercorns
1 tbsp grated ginger
4 cups of water
2-3 tbsp Eastern black tea (Darjeeling, Assam, or Ceylon)
1 cup almond, camel, or any non-dairy milk of choice
(honey and lemon to substitute milk)
1/8 ungrated cinnamon stick

Directions

Smash cloves and black peppercorns in mortar and pestle

Smash cardamom pods twice

Bring a pot of water to boil; reduce heat

Add ginger and spices; simmer 10 minutes

Add tea; return to simmer 3–5 minutes
(stronger brew: simmer covered)

Remove from heat; add milk

Strain with a fine-mesh sieve into mugs; add cinnamon stick

Add honey to sweeten *(optional)*

Neurological Lyme Dosage

If Lyme disease is severe with multiple neurological symptoms, it is vital to prioritize frequency. Neurological disseminated Lyme disease usually takes longer to respond.

Listed below are the herbs most commonly used at BNH for tick-borne infections.

Herbs Used for Lyme and Coinfections

Lyme: Astragalus, cat's claw, cordyceps, eleuthero, haritaki, Japanese knotweed, skullcap, tulsi, and BioNexus Herbals Formula 5 DHP (XS), Formula 8 IJS and Formula 9 HHG

Bartonella: Alchornea, arjuna, Ashwagandha, Danshen, greater celandine, hawthorn, Houttuynia, Isatis, kudzu, red root, Shizandra, Sida acuta, tulsi, and BioNexus Herbals Formula 8 IJS and Formula 9 HHG

Babesia: Bidens pilosa, boneset, cordyceps, cryptolepis, fenugreek, licorice, Salvia angelica, Salvia miltiorrhiza, Sida acuta, skullcap, triphala, tulsi, and BioNexus Herbals Formula 6A and Formula 6B

Ehrlichia and Anaplasma: Danshen, Houttuynia, isatis, licorice, red root, red sage, and Sida acuta

Example Step-By-Step Treatment Plans

R stands for regular or tincture, and G stands for gentle or glycerite

Lyme Disease Tier 1: arjuna (G), cat's claw (G), Japanese knotweed (G)

Lyme Disease Tier 2: Baikal skullcap (R), Berberine (G), cat's claw (R), Japanese knotweed (R), tulsi (R)

Bartonella Tier 1: arjuna (R), Bacopa (R), Houttuynia (G), red sage (G), Sida acuta (G)

Bartonella Tier 2: arjuna (R), Centella (R), Houttuynia (R), red sage (R)

Babesia Tier 1: Artemisia annua (G), Bidens pilosa (G), Sida acuta (G)

Babesia Tier 2: cryptolepis (R), vidanga (G), neem (G), Solomon's seal (R)

Mycoplasma Pneumoniae

BioNexus Herbals MPS (mycoplasma support) Blend, BioNexus Herbals LS (lung support) Blend, nebulized (aerosol) magnesium, glutathione, and saline as needed on an individual basis.

Clinical Note: Solomon's seal and Berberine herbs may be necessary for a deep infection. With the saline, some patients need the hypertonic version.

Glutathione

Glutathione can be a beneficial complementary treatment that can reduce oxidative stress, decrease inflammation, and modulate T cell responses in the lungs. It is a tripeptide that is involved in several aspects of our metabolism. This includes the transport of gamma-glutamyl amino acids and reductive cleavage of disulfide bonds. Those with a CBS mutation or sulfur sensitivity should not do any glutathione treatments. Use sulfite strips to measure urine for sulfite sensitivity. Those who test positive for sulfites should not use glutathione.

Some patients benefit from isotonic glutathione by adding normal saline.

Retrovirus

Preferences: BioNexus Herbals RVS (Retrovirus Support) Blend

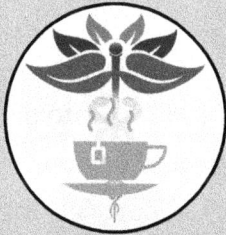

SORE THROAT TEA

Cayenne pepper soothes a sore throat and helps to open up the sinuses

Ingredients

1 part sage leaf
1/4 part cinnamon chips
1/4 part ginger root
1/2 part licorice root or slippery elm
Dash of turmeric

Optional

Add honey and lemon juice
Add a dash of cayenne pepper

5 - Bio-Individualized Repair
6 - Regeneration Protocol

Biotoxin illness genetic susceptibility markers indicate a life-long chronic illness with acute presentations during flares or re-exposures. Eliminating microorganisms facilitates the patient's ability to regain health and wellness. Repairing damage produced by the disease process and regenerating physiological health are vital steps to recovery.

Cracking the human genome at the turn of the century may have been the scientific breakthrough needed to treat the underlying cause of chronic illness. Epigenetics and transcriptomics capabilities are cutting-edge medical science. The evolution of gene testing and therapies built a solid foundation that makes a cure for biotoxin illness possible.

Until science provides a way to alter the root cause of biotoxin illness, the patient's DNA continues to authorize and stimulate volatile activity after exposure. The BioNexus Approach to biotoxin illness highlighted in this book is a great start to the patient's path to well-being. Practitioners must also complete the recovery process by implementing a repair and regeneration protocol. For biotoxin illness patients, it is advisable to address both phases together.

Introduce immune-boosting herbs based on individual needs.

Collagen support may begin during the foundation protocol, but no later than the bio-individualized repair step.

Both Lyme disease and upregulated MMP-9 with biotoxin exposure are known to affect connective tissue and soft tissue. Endocrine imbalances frequently occur in biotoxin illness cases, including tick-borne infections. The neuro-immune-endocrine connection and functional interdependence are well researched.

Neurological

Brain boosting herbs function as neural tissue protectors aiding nerve growth, increasing oxygen, as well as, improving blood flow, short-term memory, and long-term memory. Prescribe based on individual needs. Take appropriate precautions if the patient is on any neuro-psychiatric medication when using any herb that has a neurological effect.

Preferences: Bacopa, Eleutherococcus, ginkgo biloba, gotu kola, lion's mane, peppermint, rosemary, spearmint

Nootropic herbs improve spatial and long-term memory, increase learning processes, delay cognitive decline, maintain moods, sharpen social skills, stimulate concentration, and help develop self-confidence. Prescribe based on individual needs.

Preferences: Ashwagandha, Bacopa, ginkgo biloba, gotu kola, holy basil, lemon balm, peppermint, rhodiola, rosemary, saffron, spearmint

> "We can no longer assume that once a patient was a CIRS patient, one would always have susceptibility. Given that we can now correct some of T-cell synapse abnormalities it is quite possible that CIRS can actually be cured."
>
> —Ritchie Shoemaker, MD (2019)

Endocrine

Adrenal and thyroid imbalance are the most common endocrine issues in BioNexus Health Clinic's CIRS patients.

There are other concerns like sex hormonal imbalances and dysfunction. Children and teens often experience early, late, or delayed puberty, low growth rate, and irregular periods. Adult males can experience low testosterone levels, while women can experience early menopause with severe imbalances.

Balancing and regulating sex hormones requires a good endocrinologist as a part of the wellness team. If a patient presents with sex hormone imbalances or dysfunction, consider bio-identical hormonal support, hormone regulation herbs, and endocrine homeopathic dilutions as an adjunct therapy.

CIRS patients with concerns about sex hormonal imbalances and dysfunction are rightly worried. Unfortunately, this topic is too vast to explore in-depth in this book.

Adrenal Glands

The adrenal glands regulate the cortisol cycle and stress responses. Stress elevates cortisol production, which can lead to unexplained weight gain, more energy, less focus and sleep challenges. When a patient complains about being tired all day and wired at night, waking up tired with more morning inflammation and stiffness, these are symptoms of adrenal insufficiency.

Preferences: American ginseng root (a little bit goes a long way), black walnut hull, chickweed aerial parts, Eleuthero root, flaxseed, fo-ti, ginger root, licorice, Macrocarpa by Australian Bush Flower Essence (7 drops twice daily), milk thistle seed, raspberry leaf, red pepper fruit, saw palmetto berry, St. John's wort (aerial parts), third and fifth Chakra cleanse

Thyroid

Low adrenal output also causes low thyroid hormone insensitivity (TSH) thyroid output, elevated reverse triiodothyronine (rT3), and reduced cellular sensitivity.

A puffy face, dry hair and skin, weight gain, brittle nails, constipation, fatigue, muscle aches, heavy periods, fatigue, depression, and cold intolerance are symptoms of hypothyroidism.

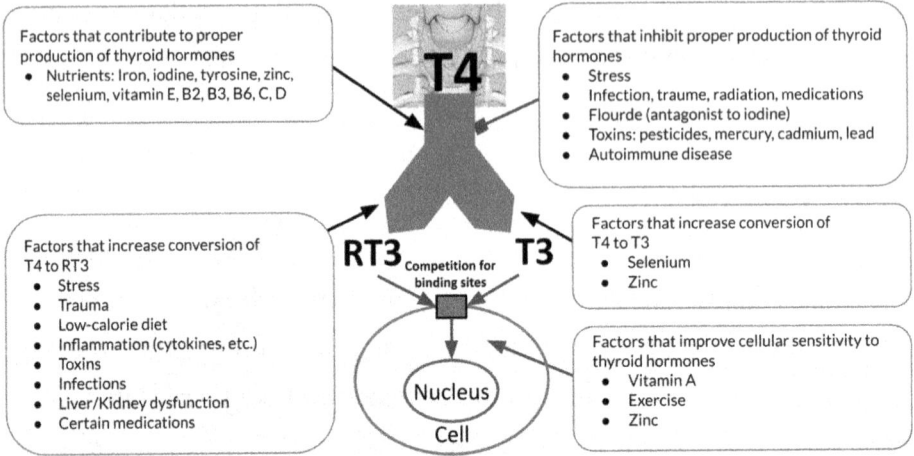

Figure 32. Thyroid factors affecting function

Avoid: teas containing lemon balm leaf and blue vervain

Preferences: American ginseng root (energetic boost), Ashwagandha root, blue flag, burdock root, chickweed aerial parts (can help with masses/lipomas), coleus (Ayurvedic herb), devil's club, elk clover, Gotu kola (Vata nervine) aerial parts, oats aerial parts, parsley aerial parts, passionflower (before bedtime), rosemary, saffron stamen (improves oxygenation), Sarsaparilla bark, schisandra, second Chakra cleanse and reset, spikenard, vitex berry, wild carrot seed, yellow dock

Immune

Preferences: BioNexus Herbals IS-M Blend, IS-B Blend, camel milk, histamine checks as needed, homemade non-cow dairy yogurt with targeted probiotics, local honey, propolis, topical nascent iodine

Gut

Natural sources of probiotics from fermented foods and drinks are preferred. Prior histamine sensitivity should show significant sensitivity reduction.

Preferences: bitter greens, green smoothies, probiotics (lactate-free and strep-free), salads, BNH Gut Butter - Modified

Lungs

Preferences: BioNexus Herbals Formula 1 NSB once a day, BioNexus Herbals LS Blend, isotonic or hypertonic saline nebulizer treatments, pranayama yogic breathing, spending time in nature

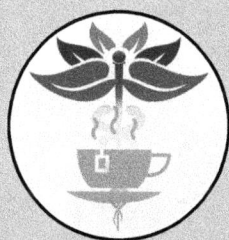

MUCOUS MELT LUNG SUPPORT TEA

The antispasmodic and expectorant properties of these herbs helps with respiratory issues

Ingredients

1 part chamomile
1 part marshmallow leaf and flower
1 part mullein leaf
1 part tulsi leaf
1 pinch long black pepper (pippali)

Optional

1 drop eucalyptus tincture
(or 5 drops glycerite)

2 drops Bidens pilosa tincture

Honey

ZESTY RAINBOW MICROGREENS SALAD

Detox-friendly

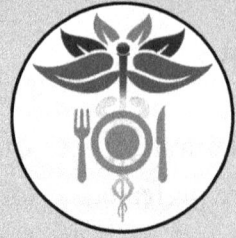

Ingredients

1 cup broccoli, beet, arugula, or microgreens
1 cup bean sprouts
1 cup heirloom cherry tomatoes
1/4 cup radicchio fine-sliced strips
4-5 shredded baby butter lettuce leaves
2 small beets (boiled) sliced into thick rounds
1/2 cup pitted Kalamata black olives
1 large lemon

Directions

Wash and prepare all the ingredients
Line a large salad bowl with the butter lettuce leaves
Toss in all the vegetables
Zest lemon on top of vegetables
Top with crushed jungle peanuts or toasted sesame seeds (optional)
Pour salad dressing according to taste

CREAMY TAHINI AVOCADO DRESSING

Blend ingredients until smooth and creamy; for lighter consistency, add 1 tsp of filtered water

1/4 cup tahini
1/4 cup tamari (optional, gluten-free and low sodium)
1 lemon, juiced
1 tbsp local raw honey

1/2 large Hass avocado
1 pinch salt (to taste)
1 pinch fresh ground cumin (optional)

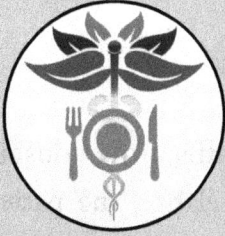

BNH GUT BUTTER - MODIFIED

Use once per day between meals; prepare fresh daily and drink immediately

At BioNexus Health Clinic, patients with a history of moderate to severe gut issues due to Lyme disease and biotoxin illness typically stay on the maintenance protocol for an additional three months, then pulse the treatment for nine months. Reassess the patient after one year.

Ingredients

4 tbsp raw camel milk
(or flash pasteurized)
1 tbsp raw local honey
1 tbsp SunButyrate
10 drops BioNexus Herbals
   GI-S Blend

Pulsing Schedule

Every day for three months

M-W-F for three months

Once a week for six months as maintenance

7 - Optimize Maintenance & Lifestyle

On a genetic level, biotoxin illness patients suffer from constant immune system dysfunction. To prevent a relapse, the patient must continuously monitor their exposure and maintain the lifestyle created in the first six steps of the BioNexus Approach. Success in step seven, Optimize Maintenance and Lifestyle, rests in the hands of the patient. Provided with the tools in the first six steps, the patient continues to bio-optimize their life from dis-ease to ease and wellness.

If reexposure occurs, the patient needs to act rapidly to prevent immune dysfunction and relapse. The patient must understand that exposure happens, and they need to be prepared for when it occurs. The BioNexus Approach factors all eventualities into a customized maintenance plan for every patient. It takes the stress out of any potential reexposures or inadvertent flare-ups.

Achieving a high quality of life is possible. BioNexus Health Clinic patients lead busy and fulfilling lifestyles. They return to work, socialize with friends, participate in school activities, and travel.

Daily Maintenance

BioNexus Health Clinic patients typically follow our daily maintenance tips for the home, first aid, dental care, and overall clean maintenance lifestyle. See the BioNexus Herbals section in Part 4: Prepping the Approach for more detailed information on the formulas.

Daily Maintenance Tips

Formula 1 NSB – one spray each nostril once a day (preferably before leaving home)

Formula 2 EOS – improve air quality

Formula 4 IBT – apply to bites sites

Formula 5 DHP (pediatric) - useful for a PANS flare related to the mouth, teething children, and before, during, and after dental visits

Formula 5 DHP-XS (adult) - used daily for maintenance and surrounding any dental procedure

Formula 6A PBS – use twice a year for maintenance and while traveling

Formula 6B PBS – use twice a year for maintenance and while traveling

Hydrogen Peroxide – a bleach replacement and general antibacterial cleaner

Borax Powder – pesticide or a bleach replacement for laundry, general cleaner, and deodorizer

Tea Tree Oil – add to household cleaning products and as an antimicrobial

Thyme Oil – add to household cleaning products and as an antimicrobial

Vinegar – general household cleaning

CIRS FLARE UP

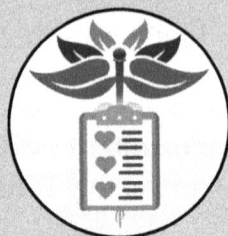

Formula 1 NSB: 2 sprays each nostril 4x/day
CK-M Blend: 10 drops 3x/day
BTXD Blend: 10 drops 3x/day
NS-1 Blend: 5 drops 3x/day
LS Blend: 5 drops 3x/day
Activated Charcoal: 560 mg 3x/day

Recommendation: pranayama yogic breathing

PRANAYAMA BREATHING

In the fresh open air for 5 minutes 2x per day, if possible

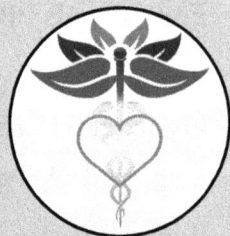

Prana, in Sanskrit, means life force or breath sustaining the body; Ayama translates as "to extend or draw out." Together, the two mean breath extension or control. There are numerous videos available online from beginners to advanced levels.

Maintenance & Lifestyle Herbs

BioNexus Health Clinic uses glycerite (G) herbs during the maintenance phase. Transition patients to regular (R) herbal tinctures based on individual patient needs.

Arjuna (R)
Artemisia annua (R)
Bacopa monnieri (G)
Baikal skullcap (G)
Baikal skullcap (R)
Berberine (G)
Berberine (R)
Bidens (G)
Bidens (R)
Cat's claw (G)
Cat's claw (R)
Chinese Senega root (G)
Cryptolepis (G)
Cryptolepis (R)
Dong quai (R)
Eleuthero (R)
Haritaki (R)

Houttuynia (G)
Houttuynia (R)
Isatis (G)
Japanese knotweed (G)
Japanese knotweed (R)
Kudzu (G)
Kudzu (R)
Lemon balm (G)
Lion's mane (G)
Motherwort (G)
Motherwort (R)
Pleurisy root (R)
Red sage (G)
Red sage (R)
Sida acuta (R)
Skullcap (R)
Tulsi (R)

During the maintenance phase, consume the prescribed herbal cocktail once a day, preferably in the morning.

After discharge from treatment, maintenance dosing continues for anywhere from six months to two years, depending on complexity. During this time, the patient should also evolve and optimize their lifestyle.

Most BioNexus Health Clinic patients enjoy the overall sense of well-being and continue on their treatment plan to minimize illness and maintain a robust immune system.

HYDROGEN PEROXIDE
Examples of potential uses

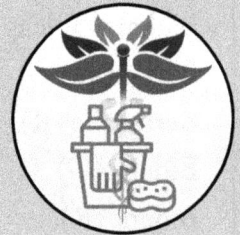

Cleaning: Daily multi-purpose cleaner, spray directly on counters, mirrors, and tables

First Aid: Use on cuts and scrapes

Kitchen: Use to sanitize cutting boards, knives, sinks, and garbage disposal

Laundry: Replace bleach to whiten clothes

Toothbrush: Daily antibacterial soak

Borax Powder Tips

Use pure borax (also known as sodium borate, sodium tetraborate, or disodium tetraborate) powder, just like hydrogen peroxide, vinegar, and baking soda, to clean around the house. A quick search online provides numerous recipes for using borax.

If mixed correctly, there should not be heavy vapors. But as a general rule, do not breathe the borax vapors.

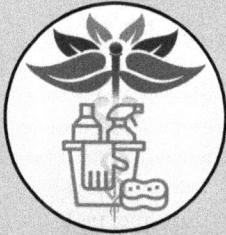

BORAX FOR MOLD

Clogged Drains: Mix 1/2 cup borax with 2 cups of boiling water. Pour it down the drain. Let it sit for 15 minutes, pour in one cup boiling water, then run the water for a few minutes.

Household Cleaner: Mix 2 tbsp borax into 2 cups of warm water. After the powder dissolves and the water cools down, transfer to a spray bottle.

Laundry: Add 1 tbsp borax powder to each load to get rid of mold and musty smells. It also helps to clean the washing machine.

Surfaces: Mix a thick paste of borax and water. Apply to moldy surface, let it dry, then rinse.

Borax Uses: A versatile household cleaner that removes mold; lifts stains; removes rust; deodorizes the refrigerator, litter box, and garbage can; and cleans the carpet, toilet bowl, sink, tub, and tiles. Borax can act as a natural pesticide and herbicide for weeds. It also unclogs drains, removes sticky residue, and helps preserve fresh-cut flowers.

Nervine Trophorestorative Herbs

Our nervous system forms one of the primary mechanisms of communication throughout the body. It is involved in direct calibration, interpretation, and assimilation of vast amounts of sensory data from the outside world to craft our automated and voluntary responses to stimuli.

Trophorestorative herbs can be powerful allies with healing and calming of a system in overdrive. They directly strengthen, tonify, and restore a depleted nervous system from long term periods of stress, lack of sleep, biotoxin exposure, chronic infections, chronic illness, and sometimes overall burnout. They can help to reset resilience to stress and indirectly assist with decreasing mast cell reactivity.

Adaptogens can also assist when taken alongside nervine trophorestorative herbals.

Preferences: Avena sativa (oat), Matricaria chamomilla (chamomile), Verbena officinalis (vervain)

Shen Tonics

Shen tonics are a group of herbs that have a beneficial effect on the spiritual heart and nervous system. They can be adaptogenic and nervines. In all cases, they ease stress and help restore balance and joy to what Traditional Chinese Medicine practitioners call the "shen," which is our energetic part that houses our spirit.

Preferences: hawthorn, holy basil (tulsi, Ocimum sanctum), mimosa (Albizia julibrissin), hawthorn (Crataegus), Rosa rugosa

Combine holy basil, nettles, and licorice for a relaxing and rejuvenating tea. Add rose and linden for a greater effect.

Disease Specific Maintenance Bundles

Below are examples of how BioNexus Health Clinic combines herbs to target specific diseases.

<u>Mold</u>
Formula 1 NSB
Formula 2 EOS
Formula 5 DHP

<u>PANS Tier 1</u>
Bacopa monnieri (G)
Baikal skullcap (G)
Cryptolepis (G)
Kudzu (G)
Motherwort (G)

VIBRANT N SPICY
GREEN CHUTNEY DIP

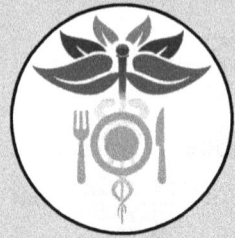

Ingredients

1 bunch/ 1 cup cilantro
1 cup mint leaves
1/2 cup spinach leaves
1/4 cup green bell pepper

1-2 diced deseeded jalapenos
2 pressed garlic cloves
1 lemon, juiced
1 lime

Directions

Wash and prep all the ingredients
Set lime aside
Blend all ingredients until smooth (vibrant green color)
Add lime juice and stir with a spoon
Zest lime on top
Adjust jalapeño and garlic level to preference

*Eat with veggies, pita, fritters, gluten-free bread, tempura, on top of
vegetarian sushi rolls, zucchini noodles, and more!*

CUCUMBER SANDWICHES

Lightly toast gluten-free bread. Add a thin layer of butter (regular raw organic or plant-based), spread green chutney dip, thin (peeled) cucumber slices, and salt and pepper to taste.

Serve as an open face sandwich for an afternoon snack.

Add a slice of toast on top to turn it into lunch. Cut the sandwich diagonally. On a toothpick, add one pitted olive, a small piece of sheep manchego cheese, and a purple heirloom cherry tomato and push into each sandwich wedge. Drink a hot cup of green tea with ginger, hot cashew latte, or decaf chai with a sprinkle of golden turmeric.

PANS Tier 2
Angelica sinensis
Berberine (G)
Chinese Senega root (G)
Dong quai (R)
Gotu kola (R)
IS-M Blend
Kudzu (R)
Tulsi (R)

Herpes
Isatis (G)
Lemon balm (G)
Tulsi (G)

Mycoplasma Tier 1
Bidens pilosa (G)
Cryptolepis (G)
Pleurisy root (G)
Sida acuta (G)

Mycoplasma Tier 2
Berberine (R)
Isatis (G)
Solomon's seal (G)

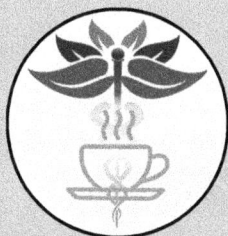

HOT HERB CHOCOLATE

Ingredients

1-2 tbsp cocoa
1/2 tsp kudzu glycerite or powder
1/2 tsp licorice powder
1 tsp chicory powder
1 tsp reishi powder
1 tsp vanilla extract
1 tsp turmeric powder
1 pinch black pepper
6-8 oz almond or camel milk

Directions

Simmer for 5 minutes, covered

Sweeten with local raw honey and a sprinkle of cinnamon powder

Add a pinch of cayenne (extra hot option) for chronic post nasal drips and lung congestion

ADAPTOGENIC MASALA CHAI BLEND

Supports the immune system and adrenals during cold and flu season; drink up to 3-4 cups throughout the day

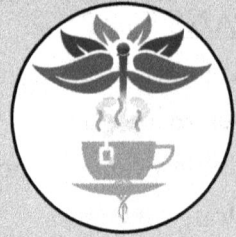

Ingredients

1 tbsp medicinal mushroom powder blend
1 tbsp eleuthero or ashwagandha root
1 tbsp burdock root
1 tsp tulsi leaves
1 tsp mint leaves
2 cups of water
1 tsp cinnamon chips
2 tsp dried ginger (or 7 slices fresh ginger)
5 cardamom pods
1/4 teaspoon cloves
1 cup non-dairy milk (camel milk is okay)

Directions

Combine mushrooms, eleuthero, burdock, tulsi, mint, and water in a pot; bring to a gentle simmer for 15-20 minutes

Gently smash cardamom pods

Add remaining herbs and milk, return to simmer for 10-15 minutes

Add a small pinch of Himalayan shilajit for an extra "perk" *(optional)*

Strain with a fine-mesh sieve into a mug

Sweeten with a small amount of local raw wild honey or Ayurvedic rose petals jam

Refrigerate unused portion unsweetened and reheat later
Only sweeten when ready to drink

APPENDIX

"The art of healing comes from nature, not from the physician. Therefore the physician must start from nature, with an open mind."
— Paracelsus (as cited in Lewis, 2013)

Some patients need additional consideration before beginning treatment. The following sections offer some clinical wisdom, more information, and developing theories to help practitioners further understand the complexity of biotoxin illness and CIRS cases.

Biofilm

Current research has identified a four-step process to biofilm formation: adherence, accumulation, maturation, and detachment.

Adherence, in the case of MARCoNS, occurs in the nasal mucous membranes. When sensing a quorum, the participating microbes trigger the production of an autoinducer molecule. The primary mechanism is a series of enzyme reactions, including the LuxS enzyme and the synthesis of autoinducer (AI)-2, a class of pheromones (Berndtson, 2013). Microbial surface components recognize adhesive matrix molecules' (MSCRAMMs) binding serum proteins (Clarke & Foster, 2006). S. epidermidis' binding proteins include MSCRAMM fibrinogen-binding protein SdrG and bifunctional adhesins/autolysins (Pei & Flock, 2001; Heilmann, Hussain, Peters, & Gotz, 1997; Heilmann et al., 2003). These proteins also release extracellular DNA (eDNA), which has been proven to be an essential adherence/aggression factor in both S. epidermidis and S. aureus biofilm formation (Qin et al., 2007; Rice et al., 2007). The known antibiotic resistance mechanisms do not apply to bacterial protection within the biofilm (Berndtson, 2013).

The accumulation phase is the most understood mechanism of biofilm formation because the synthesis of polysaccharide intercellular adhesion (PIA) is the most studied. PIA increases the persistence of infections and aids in the decreased efficacy of antibiotic-induced bactericidal activity. S. epidermidis strains expressing PIA increase the architecture of maturing biofilm. When proteinaceous factors substitute PIA negative isolates during biofilm formation, the resulting biofilm is not as well-formed (Rohde et al., 2007; Qin et al., 2007). Additionally, the deacetylation of PIA in PIA attachment on the cell surface aids in immune system evasion (Fey & Olson, 2010). Quorum sensing induces highly effective and efficient cellular cooperation with each bacteria taking on a specific task. The bacteria successfully creates a harmonious and cooperative community.

The maturation stage is defined as having a variety of adhesive molecules, including eDNA, PIA, proteinaceous factors (Bhp, Aap, and Embp), and teichoic acids (Fey & Olson, 2010). Studies demonstrated the average S. epidermidis and S. aureus growing in biofilm shift their physiology towards anaerobic or microaerobic metabolism, and downregulate protein, cell wall and DNA synthesis (Beenken et al., 2004; Resch, Rosenstein, Nerz, & Gotz, 2005; Stewart & Franklin, 2008). The biofilm matrix protects the bacteria by preventing antibiotics from penetrating the barrier (Shoemaker et al., 2005). Approximately 80% of people who have low melanocyte-stimulating hormone (MSH) and suffer from biotoxin illness, chronic inflammatory response syndrome (CIRS), or chronic fatigue and immune dysfunction syndrome (CFIDS) are found to have MARCoNS (Shoemaker & Katz, 2013).

CIRS and PANS

Mold is an established trigger for PANS. Dr. Scott McMahon led a research group that found 100% (33/33) of children with clinically diagnosed PANS (pediatric acute-onset neuro-psychiatric syndrome) or PANDAS (pediatric autoimmune neuropsychiatric disorder associated with Strep infection) had CIRS biomarkers.

After treatment for CIRS, 94% of the children had CIRS symptom improvement, and more than 80% had a reduction in PANS/ PANDAS symptoms and demonstrated a decrease or cessation in their neuropsychiatric medicines.

The basal ganglia and cerebellum modify body movement every nanosecond. Exposure to water-damaged buildings and mold affects the basal ganglia, which then affects the cerebral cortex feedback loop. Smooth, coordinated actions require a balance between the systems.

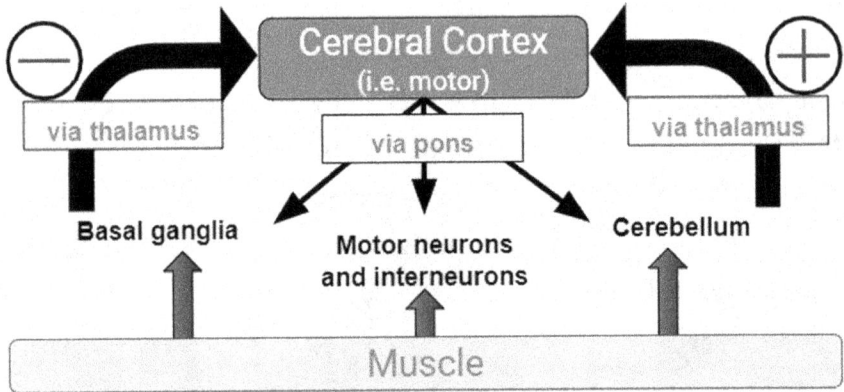

Figure 33. CIRS and PANS connection: basal ganglia and cerebellum modify movement on a minute-to-minute basis. Motor cortex sends information to both, the output of the cerebellum to cortex is excitatory, while the basal ganglia are inhibitory. Disturbance in either system will show up as movement disorders.

Enhancing Therapies

Autonomic Balance

Patients who need to calm their nervous system need to enhance the parasympathetic (rest and digest) response and dampen the sympathetic (flight or fight) response. For these patients, consider adding programs like the Tomatis method, amygdala retraining program, yogic breathing exercises, or a neural retraining program. BioNexus Health Clinic patients report varying degrees of success with various tapping protocols.

Thought Field Therapy (TFT) combined with similar techniques like the Emotional Freedom Technique (EFT), Iridology, and eye movement therapy has proven helpful in some patients.

Patients with emotional and sensory triggers have reported success with sound therapy and sound healing. Sound can cause positive effects on the person's physical, emotional, and spiritual being — from balancing the brain and nervous system to aiding homeostasis and autonomic balance.

Auto Iso Nosode Therapy and basic auto-nosode therapy are systematic homeopathic serial dilutions of the offending substance with biocompatible frequency infusion. It is a highly specialized method of helping people overcome their sensitivities and modulating the immune system.

Camel Milk

Certain herbs and essential oils are synergistic with camel milk, especially for children diagnosed with autism.

Fat: low-fat concentrations (2%), consisting mainly of polyunsaturated fatty acids (PUFAs) present as microcells, in natural homogenate

Lactose: easily absorbed lactose (4.8%), even by those suffering from lactose intolerance

Vitamins: camel milk contains calcium, iron, and vitamin C in high concentrations

Proteins: do not contain allergens (ruminant-like beta-casein or beta-lactoglobulin), but do contain insulin, lysozyme, immunoglobulins, and lactoferrin

Non-Immune Host Defense: lactoperoxidase

For more resources, visit camelmedforum.com.

Melatonin

Melatonin is a natural scavenger that helps to detox the liver (Meki, Abdel-Ghaffar, & El-Gibaly, 2001).

The liver detoxes several molecules. Excess toxic reactive oxygen species (ROS) cause oxidative damage to hepatocytes compromising liver function. A variety of antioxidants protect the liver from free radical-mediated damage; melatonin is one of the best. Clinical studies have confirmed melatonin is also a precursor tryptophan (Chojnacki, Walecka-Kapica, Romanowski, Chojnacki, & Klupinska, 2014).

Biotoxin illness patients typically have low MSH, which is related to melatonin synthesis in the hypothalamus. Low MSH affects melatonin and cortisol levels.

Decreased REM sleep is also associated with certain classes of

Melatonin - Not Just For Sleep

Amphiphilic easily crosses cell membranes and acts as a direct scavenger for oxygen radicals

Binds to MT1 & MT2 receptors expressed by immunocompetent cells acting as an anti-inflammatory

Decreases leptin secretion at night

Effects feedback to nuclei in the hypothalamus

Enhances cell and nuclear membrane integrity

Essential vitamin B6 cofactor

Improves daytime alertness and function

Lipophilic antioxidant easily crosses cell membranes and acts as a direct scavenger for oxygen radical

medications like SSRIs, tricyclic antidepressants, and benzodiazepines. Studies show melatonin can increase REM sleep (ScienceDirect, 2020). Vivid dreaming or nightmares can be related to melatonin supplementation and REM sleep deprivation. If so, lower the dose, or in some cases, adding magnesium can bring relief from the REM rebound effect.

Melatonin supplement tolerance varies significantly in patients. Taken an hour before dinner, start the patient at 1 mg of melatonin, but do not exceed 20 mg. Higher doses may be needed in certain patients if the tolerance levels observed have been good.

Female Hormone Therapy

Hormone replacement therapy is a hotly debated topic that seeks to balance the estrogen and progesterone fluctuations in women. Improving these hormone levels helps lessen adverse effects on neurotransmitters that lead to over one hundred symptoms of perimenopause and premenstrual syndrome (PMS). Many patients with biotoxin illness experience highly irregular hormonal and life transitions, often find bioidentical hormone replacement therapy to be a useful adjunct.

Lifestyle changes may help to alleviate symptoms. Excessive adipose (fat) tissue produces surplus estrogen. By maintaining a healthy weight, patients can decrease this pseudo-endocrine fat. Broccoli, bok choy, Brussels sprouts, cabbage, cauliflower, and kohlrabi metabolize to produce diindolylmethane (DIM) that helps modulate estrogen. Bean sprouts, flax seeds, sunflower seeds, and peas balance hormones with phytoestrogens. Brew a tea with an herb below to reduce the correlating symptom.

Preferences:
PMS - alfalfa, black cohosh, dandelion root, fennel, nettles, raspberry leaves, skullcap, vervain, wild yam

Dysmenorrhea - California poppy, cramp bark, damiana, Jamaican dogwood, motherwort, yarrow

Menopausal Symptoms - Ashwagandha, black cohosh, rosemary, sage, Shatavari, valerian, vitex

Therapies to Enhance Herbal Regimen

Biochemic tissue salts

Gemmo Therapy

Restorative Oligotherapy

EFT: Emotional Freedom Technique

TFT: Thought Field Therapy

Tapping

Family Constellation Therapy

Mindful Living

Conscious Fitness

Diligently avoiding glyphosate exposure

Future of GENIE

"We can no longer assume that once a patient was a CIRS patient, one would always have susceptibility. Given that we can now correct some of the T-cell synapse abnormalities, it is quite possible that CIRS can actually be cured," Ritchie Shoemaker (2019).

CIRS is a transcriptomic illness, a failure of regular gene expression that renders the acquired immune system useless against biotoxins. The potentiality of GENIE testing and epigenetic research brings hope that we can soon discover and activate the master control gene to turn off HLA-DR effects permanently.

The next phase for GENIE is finding the marker for defective apoptosis that causes a pathological release of intracultural particles upon cell lysis. Apoptosis is one of the least studied and most important factors for CIRS treatment.

MCAS

Mast cell activation syndrome refers to a group of disorders with diverse causes presenting with episodic multisystem symptoms as the result of mast cell mediator release.

Validated MCAS Markers
Tryptase: Typically increased in hypotensive mast cell activation episodes. Measure within four hours of an episode and compare it to a baseline. The most specific marker.

Urinary Histamine Metabolites: Diet or bacterial contamination may influence results, but is rather specific for mast cell activation.

Urinary Prostaglandin D2 or Metabolites: Do not use as a single marker, usually increased in MCAS patients.

Urinary Leukotriene E4: Frequently elevated in patients with mast cell activation. May indicate a need for leukotriene-targeting therapy.

MCS, MCAS, and Porphyria

Options Before Foundation Protocol

MCS and MCAS patients may need a gentle introduction to the foundation protocol. For these patients, consider European biological treatments, including biochemic tissue salts, gemmotherapy, homotoxicology, and oligotherapy.

Biochemic Tissue Salts

Adding trace minerals and electrolytes to the foundation protocol for advanced MCS and MCAS patients can provoke reactivity, which presents a problematic clinical challenge. German physician Dr. Wilhelm Heinrich Schuessler identified a system of twelve inorganic tissue salts essential for healthy bodily function and maintaining homeostasis. Consider starting advanced MCS and MCAS patients with homeopathic tissue salts to introduce their systems to the foundation protocol.

Twelve Biochemic Tissue Salts

Calcarea Fluor (calcium fluoride)
Calcarea Phos (calcium phosphate)
Calcarea Sulf (calcium sulfate
Ferrum Phos (ferrum phosphate) [powerful oxygenator]
Kali Mur (potassium chloride)
Kali Phos (potassium phosphate)
Kali Sulf (potassium sulfate)
Mag Phos (magnesium phosphate)
Natrum Mur (sodium chloride)
Natrum Phos (sodium phosphate)
Natrum Sulf (sodium sulfate)
Silicea (silica)

The biochemic tissue salts provide support throughout the body, including membrane stability, cytoplasmic homeostasis, oxygenation, and detoxification. They act as subtle cellular building blocks and a biochemical support system to rebuild on a cellular level, then on a systemic level. Most homeopathic pharmacies carry a potency 6X needed for MCS and MCAS patients.

Preferences: UNDA Melange Combination Schuessler Tissue Salts is usually my remedy of choice that helps a patient maintain general mineral metabolism. Depending on the individual blood chemistry analysis, the recommended dose ranges. The patient should allow them to dissolve under the tongue.

Gemmotherapy - Advanced Cellular Homeopathy

A gentle but direct-acting extract remedy made from the fresh, new growth of young buds, shoots, and embryonic tissue of various trees and shrubs. Supports the immune system's ability to respond to pathogens and inflammation by draining toxins from intracellular spaces, enhancing cellular illumination, and harmonizes electromagnetic communication.

Only use pure materials and biodynamically grown or wildcrafted herbs to capture a complete set of highly-concentrated active constituents.

Preferences:
OCD and Infection-Oriented Anxiety Symptoms - Ficus carica

Stress Relief and Sleep Difficulties - Tilia tomentosa

Viral Infections, Cold Sores, and Canker Sores - Acer campestre

Homotoxicology

Dr. Hans-Heinrich Reckeweg combined classical homeopathy with modern medical science in the 1950s. Homotoxins act as a molecular sieve in lymph vessels, capillary system, and cells, causing inflammation by blocking nutrients and waste removal. Homotoxicology gently unblocks the extracellular matrix to stimulate the immune system in highly sensitive patients.

Preferences: Pekana, Pleo Sanum, Nestmann, Soluna

Digestion Herbs

MCAS requires a focus on improving digestion and stimulating digestive enzyme production.

Clinical Note: Limit high histamine-containing foods, retrain the system, and use botanical support (bitters) to increase digestive enzymes.

Tincture alcohol can sometimes act as an MCAS trigger for sensitive and histamine intolerant patients. Many sensitive patients are introduced to medicinal herbs with weak teas then are very slowly transitioned to tinctures.

Preferences: glycerites, teas, capsules, diet changes

Clinical Note: Foster a positive attitude toward food because patients can become afraid to eat.

Sodium cromoglycate (cromolyn sodium) intranasal format OTC is most effective when used before antigen exposure. A prescription version of the same is orally administered and can be a good option to consider.

Histamine Intolerance Herbs

Patients with histamine intolerance may need additional targeted herbal remedies with antihistaminic and anti-inflammatory properties.

Preferences: BioNexus Herbals MC-S Blend, Moringa oleifera (Moringa), Nigella sativa (black cumin), Urtica dioica (nettles)

NETI POT

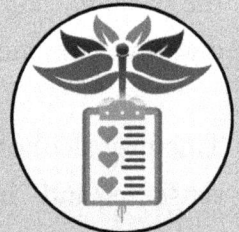

BioNexus Herbals Formula 1 NSB-SF (Silver-Free) in a neti pot is a good option to consider for some sensitive patients in the beginning. The papaya extract helps open biofilm and release mucus.

Foundation Protocol Herbs

Consider adding the following to the foundation protocol based on individual needs. Clinically, it may sometimes be important to address inflammation, cytokines, and toxins well before the body can be ready for antimicrobial intervention.

BioNexus Herbals:
MC-S Blend, CK-M Blend, and Formula 7 GDS

AIP diet	Low Histamine Diet
Allernest	NasalCrom
Bacillus Coagulans	No-Fenol
Bromelain	Ox Bile
Butterbur	ProAller
Cromolyn Sodium	Proteolytic Enzymes
D-Hist	Quercetin
DAO Enzymes	Stinging nettle
Histamine Scavenger	

MCAS Immune Modulating Herbs

Mast cell stabilizers settle the membrane preventing mediator release. MCAS patients regularly benefit from potent immune modulators, nervous system trophorestorative, and mucilaginous herbs that soothe and heal the GI system. Immune modulatory herbs "retrain" hyper-reactive immune responses and help anti-allergic actions.

Preferences: BioNexus Herbals MC-S Blend, CK-M Blend, IS-M Blend, Boswellia serrata (frankincense), Curcuma longa (turmeric), Scutellaria baicalensis (skullcap)

MCAS Gastrointestinal System Herbs

Several MCAS patients find strong reactivity to a variety of foods. Healing the GI system becomes a clinical challenge because dietary intake requires support to calm mucosa.

Preferences: Althaea officinalis (marshmallow), Ulmus rubra (slippery elm)

Nervous System Trophorestorative Herbs

Nervous System Trophorestorative herbs decrease mast cell reactivity by assisting the overtaxed system in recalibrating a resilience to stress.

Preferences: Avena sativa (oat), Matricaria chamomilla (chamomile), Verbena officinalis (vervain)

FENNEL TEA

Drink 1/2 - 1 cup warm with 1 tsp local wild honey (according to preference)
2-3x per day between meals

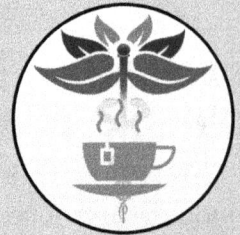

Ingredients

1 tsp fennel per cup of hot water

1/4 tsp licorice root powder

1/4 tsp marshmallow root powder
(or slippery elm powder)

Directions

Infuse fennel with hot water

Add licorice root powder and marshmallow root powder before consuming

Regenerative Oligotherapy

A unique method to add bio-available essential trace minerals that are indispensable cofactors for cellular enzymatic reactions. "Oligo" derives from Greek for a very tiny quantity. Oligotherapy precisely measures one or several oligo-elements to prevent deficiency and create a complementary therapeutic effect, typically with gemmotherapy.

Regenerative oligotherapy applications help restore functions diminished by antibiotics.

Examples:
Tetracyclines Support - calcium, chelated magnesium, copper, iron, manganese, nickel, zinc

Pediatric Rhinopharyngitis (subacute or chronic) - consider alternating manganese and copper with calcium, copper, and zinc. If adenitis, otitis, or sinusitis also present, then focus on copper, gold, and silver or copper, magnesium, manganese, and zinc.

Clinical Note: It is important to monitor the copper and zinc balance in these patients. When using copper, signs of nervousness or insomnia indicate toxicity.

Methylation

DNA methylation is the most broadly understood epigenetic change. As a general rule, it is vital to understand tests may show genetic mutations or SNPs; however, it does not mean SNPs are expressing. Clinically, sometimes, it becomes clear that the patient has severe detoxification challenges and neurotransmitter imbalances. Under these circumstances, it is critical to look at methylation polymorphisms closely and help with rebalancing the detoxification pathways. Gradually progress patients from non-methylated B vitamins and cofactors (see Part 5: The BioNexus Approach) to methylation Bs with careful monitoring. A slow approach helps to reduce detoxification reactions, which can include a temporary increase in inflammatory cytokines.

Studies found an upwards of 90% of autism spectrum disorder children with methylation deficiencies had a mutation of the methylenetetrahydrofolate reductase (MTHFR) gene (Sener, Oztop, & Ozkul, 2014). The single nucleotide polymorphisms (SNP) issues are less critical than real-life expression.

Recent studies show that high-dose niacin supplementation causes unfavorable changes in liver health and methyl donor levels (Scoffone et al., 2013; Adiels et al., 2018). If niacin treatment is not resolving, try the Yasko approach as an alternative.

Pediatric patients need riboflavin in higher doses to assist the pentose phosphate pathway (PPP), which aids the adrenals and liver. When the PPP slows, the body stops producing B1, reduces glutathione, and develops red blood cell issues. Children with behavioral or detox challenges need riboflavin for their neurotransmitters.

In patients with neurodegenerative diseases and CIRS, look at the role of and ensure adequate levels of alpha-lipoic acid (ALA) and methylation profile. Alpha-lipoic acid has antioxidant and anti-inflammatory properties. The effects modulate NF-kB. It also helps modulate inflammatory cytokines, including IL-1b and IL-6, in different tissues and cell types (Dinicola, Proietti, Cucina, Bizzarri, & Fuso, 2017).

Clinical Note: Take strong precautions and work closely with a knowledgeable practitioner when addressing methylation in Epstein-Barr positive patients.

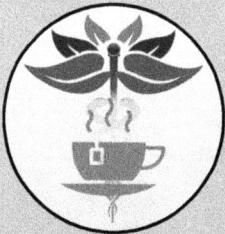

BRONCHIAL RELAXER TEA

Valerian root relaxes deep spastic coughs and helps restful sleep

Ingredients

1 part licorice root
1 part valerian root
1/4 part cinnamon chips
1/4 part ginger root

Optional

5 drops max. CBD hemp oil

Resources

Become a free member of BioNexusHealth.com for more general information, including simple tips, recipes, and more.

Crawl Spaces

Renowned CIRS-literate indoor environmental consultants, Vince Neil and John Banta advise that it is challenging to seal a crawl space without toxins and VOCs permeating into other areas.

Killing mold and bacteria does not remove the pathogen-associated molecular pattern molecules (PAMPs) and damage-associated molecular patterns (DAMPs).

If there is contamination in the crawl space, remove it. Eliminate ongoing moisture ingress, then clean and replace the underside of the flooring.

Depending on the sensitivity of the individual, any remaining low-level exposure may still produce an inflammatory impact.

New dust needs to settle before a post-remediation ERMI. Wait 4-6 weeks after remediation to test.

EMFs

The JRS Eco 100 router automatically switches to Full Eco mode, completely radiation-free, when WiFi devices are not connected. The router only sends a connection request when WiFi is turned on, or the listed devices become available.

Although the router reduces radiation during standby mode and partly during operation, it does not lessen any radiation from wireless devices. WiFi is two-way traffic, for each piece of data sent from the WiFi router, a confirmation is sent back by the device.

WiFi radiation from devices is powerful, and we frequently keep them very close to the body. Data-intensive applications like video apps intensify radiation. Using hardwired internet (i.e., ethernet) can minimize exposure to electromagnetic radiation. Hardwired adaptors are available for tablets and mobile phones. Purchase low radiation devices and accessories, including baby monitors whenever possible.

There is a serious concern with 5G technology that began rolling out in select cities in 2018. According to GSMA Intelligence (2019), the United States, South Korea, Japan, China, Mexico, India, Brazil, Mexico, and Europe are expected to lead 5G coverage.

More than 180 scientists and doctors from 36 countries made an appeal to the European Union about the danger of 5G, which will lead to a massive increase in involuntary exposure to electromagnetic radiation (5gappeal.eu).

Communities around the globe, including Australia, Bangladesh, Brussels, France, Ireland, Italy, Switzerland, the UK, and the USA began banning or limiting 5G networks in 2019 over health concerns.

Home Hunting

Credit goes to Vince Neil, IEP, CIRS Literate and Dr. Scott McMahon.

Looking for a mold-free home can be overwhelming and taxing for biotoxin illness patients. The following tips help to navigate the unknown environments of while looking for a home - rental or purchase.

VCS Test: Upon entry into the home, conduct a hand-held VCS test. After at least 60 minutes inside with the windows closed, retest in the same spot.

Windows: Look for condensation mold. Check aluminum for indented scrub marks. Obvious scour marks may indicate mold cleaning.

Windows, Doors, and Nearby Walls: Examine the skirting boards for swelling. Look at seals for discoloration or deterioration.

Walls Near Wet Rooms: If the adjoining walls have timber bases, look for discoloration as a sign of a water leak. Check all carpet near bathrooms and kitchens for stains on the carpet gripper with a small pair of long nose pliers - lift the carpet about 5mm. Tuck the carpet back in place.

Sink Cabinets: Inspect cabinets under all the sinks. Look for swelling, bloating cracks, visible watermarks, and discoloration. Using the fingertips, feel for abnormalities on panels that touch the floor.

Built-ins and Cabinets: Poke the head into all built-ins and cupboards for 20 seconds and access physiological reactions. Observe the behind walls (interior and exterior) for yellow, brown, or orange spots. Discoloration indicates condensation molds and a moisture vapor issue. Turn all drawers upside down to inspect the back for moisture-related evidence.

Ceilings: Look for discoloration and cellulosic browning. Mold without cellulosic marks indicates condensation-related growth.

Floor: If possible, examine the subfloor for any evidence of moisture.

A quality moisture meter and EMF measuring device are handy tools to have when touring homes.

It is best to proceed towards moving in, only if all of the above points pass your initial personal inspection.

32 Simple Tips

Additional tips that have proven clinically useful over the years.

1. Keep the lymphatic system in good condition by jumping on a trampoline or dry brushing.

2. Keep the colon moving with periodic cleanses.

3. Get massages.

4. Decrease stress and listen to pleasant or spiritual music.

5. Get quality sleep.

6. Be cautious of new clothing, much of it contains bromides, heavy metals, and toxic treatments.

7. Only use natural and minimally processed lotions, make-up, creams (coconut oil, shea butter, etc.), shampoo, soap, and deodorant with pronounceable ingredients. Avoid parabens and phthalates.

8. Avoid vaccines that contain a plethora of toxic ingredients.

9. Avoid pharmaceuticals or minimize use.

10. Never get a root canal. Visit a biomimetic dentist and have a biologic dentist remove any mercury amalgam fillings.

11. Avoid adding glyphosate and other toxic products to the yard and plants.

12. Avoid artificially scented products, including candles, perfumes, and air fresheners.

13. Use natural cleaners for laundry, dishes, and home cleaning.

14. Filter all drinking water (reverse osmosis or very high-quality filtering).

15. Use naturally grown whole and organic products; chew every bite thoroughly to pre-digest the food.

16. Add magnesium through food, supplements, Epsom salts, and magnesium oil.

17. Increase vegetable and fruit intake by adding a variety to meals; making fresh multi-produce juice (carrots, celery, beets, ginger, apple, etc.); blending superfood smoothies (flax seeds, chia seeds, whole lemon, hemp seeds, matcha green tea, spinach leaf, fruits, etc.). Eat the rainbow everyday!

18. Throw away all Teflon non-stick cookware, aluminum cookware, and aluminum foil.

19. Try intermittent fasting.

20. Never heat food in a microwave.

21. Eliminate plastic: utensils, dishware, food storage (baggies, containers, etc.), one-use products, and drinkware (glasses, pitchers, etc.).

22. Never consume high fructose corn syrup, trans fat (hydrogenated oils or partially hydrogenated oils), sodium nitrate, and monosodium glutamate (MSG), and processed meats (pepperoni, bacon, salami, jerky, deli meat, or hot dogs). Learn all the new words used on labels to hide MSG in food products.

23. Avoid food preservatives (BHT, BHA, benzoate, and sulfites); colorings (FD&C Yellow #5 and #6, and Red #5); artificial sweeteners (sucralose and aspartame); white flour; white salt; unprocessed sea salt; white sugar products; and soy products (hydrolyzed protein, soy oil).

24. Use aluminum-free baking powder and don't buy products with baking powder unless it's aluminum-free.

25. Avoid most conventional restaurants. They may use aluminum pots and pans, and hidden food ingredients. If restaurant food is necessary, only eat food served hot, avoiding uncooked food: raw salads, juices, and sushi.

26. Vegan "meat" is full of processed soy and other proteins to mimic the taste of meat.

27. Environmental Working Group posts regular updates on the recent versions of "Dirty Dozen" (foods that are high in pesticide residues) and the "Clean 15" (foods that are typically low in pesticide residues) on their website (ewg.org/foodscores).

28. Get out in nature, enjoy more sunshine, and exercise to tolerance.

29. Cherish the ones you love.

30. Live and express thankfulness and gratitude.

31. Take more time for relaxing and rejuvenating activities.

32. Reduce EMF exposure.

Cancer

A patient with a cancer diagnosis needs to take all clean tips to an extreme level and begin aggressive natural treatments immediately. It is very important to rule out underlying chronic infections and inflammation, along with the root causes of the same.

Many patients and practitioners have reported good experiences focusing on targeted nutrition and adding Rick Simpson oil, Gerson therapy, Essiac tea, hyperbaric oxygen therapy, baking soda protocol, 35% food grade peroxide protocol, IV Vitamin C, and B17 to treatment.

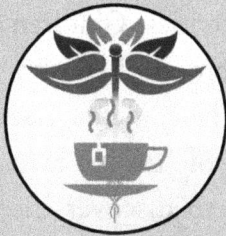

NO NAUSEA TEA
For nausea, upset stomach, and indigestion

Ingredients

1 part lemon balm
1 part chamomile
1 part peppermint leaf
1/4 part dill leaf and seed
1/4 part fresh grated ginger
1/2 part fennel

Directions

Add splash of apple cider vinegar in cold tea before drinking

Add 1 tsp honey to taste (optional)

Cold steeped tea - seltzer (optional)

Triggered Autism

Immune system dysregulation is recognized as an inherent feature of autism spectrum disorders (ASD). MARCoNS (multiple antibiotic-resistant coagulase-negative Staphylococci) is antibiotic-resistant staph that resides deep in the nasal passage of 80% of people suffering from biotoxin illness, and its advanced stage known as chronic inflammatory response syndrome (CIRS). The bacterial exotoxins produced by MARCoNS can cross the blood-brain barrier and cause structural brain changes, especially in those that carry one of the six CIRS related HLA-DR genetic haplotypes.

Neural inflammation and dysregulation of the innate immune responses lead to decreased endocrine and inflammatory regulation in the gastrointestinal tract initiating malabsorption, mast cell activation, and multiple chemical sensitivities. Children with ASD are not typically tested for altered blood chemistry biomarkers nor toxic environmental exposures. The epidemic rise in ASD diagnoses requires an investigation of the known symptoms, genetic links, and biological testing to discover the underlying cause or causes of ASD and ASD-like conditions.

The growth in the ASD patient population at BioNexus Health Clinic drove the discovery of a subset of pediatric patients whose diagnosis was misled by Lyme disease, biotoxin illness, CIRS-WDB, and/or MARCoNS. All patients treated for mycotoxins and MARCoNS eradication with biodynamic herbal formulas and bio-individualized integrative protocol, resulted in decreased (often dramatically) ASD and comorbid symptoms.

Women (Pregnancy and Breastfeeding)

Always consult a practitioner when using herbs while pregnant or breastfeeding.

Preferences:
Promote Milk - Ashwagandha, fennel, milk thistle, nettles, Shatavari

Decrease Milk - peppermint, sage

Avoid: black cohosh, garlic, gentian, ginkgo, goldenseal, licorice, lobelia, kava, Oregon grape root, osha, rhubarb (Essiac), St. John's wort, vitex, white willow bark, wormwood, yellow dock

REFERENCES

Abrhaley, A., & Leta, S. (2017). Medicinal value of camel milk and meat. Journal of Applied Animal Research, 46(1), 552–558. https://doi.org/10.1080/09712119.2017.1357562

Achilly, N. P. (2016). Properties Of Vip+ Synapses In The Suprachiasmatic Nucleus Highlight Their Role In Circadian Rhythm. Journal of Neurophysiology, 115(6), 2701–2704. https://doi.org/10.1152/jn.00393.2015

Adiels, M., Chapman, M. J., Robillard, P., Krempf, M., Laville, M., & Borén, J. (2018). Niacin action in the atherogenic mixed dyslipidemia of metabolic syndrome: Insights from metabolic biomarker profiling and network analysis. Journal of Clinical Lipidology, 12(3), 810-821.e1. https://doi.org/10.1016/j.jacl.2018.03.083

Ahmad, I., & Beg, A. Z. (2001). Antimicrobial And Phytochemical Studies On 45 Indian Medicinal Plants Against Multi-Drug Resistant Human Pathogens. Journal of Ethnopharmacology, 74, 113–123. Retrieved from http://citeseerx.ist.psu.edu/viewdoc/download?doi=10.1.1.459.3169&rep=rep1&type=pdf

Ahmed, I., Istivan, T., Cosic, I., & Pirogova, E. (2013). Evaluation of the effects of Extremely Low Frequency (ELF) Pulsed Electromagnetic Fields (PEMF) on survival of the bacterium Staphylococcus aureus. EPJ Nonlinear Biomedical Physics, 1(1). https://doi.org/10.1140/epjnbp12

Ahuja, A. (2014, December). Living Medicine Stephen Harrod Buhner On Plant Intelligence, Natural Healing, And The Trouble With Pharmaceuticals. Retrieved from https://www.thesunmagazine.org/issues/468/living-medicine

Akin, C. (2017). Mast cell activation syndromes. Journal of Allergy and Clinical Immunology, 140(2), 349–355. https://doi.org/10.1016/j.jaci.2017.06.007

Alberts, B., Johnson, A., Lewis, J., Raff, M., Roberts, K., & Walter, P. (2002). Molecular Biology of the Cell (4th ed.). New York, United States of America: Garland Science.

Albrecht, E., Kirkham, K. R., Liu, S. S., & Brull, R. (2012). Peri-operative intravenous administration of magnesium sulphate and postoperative pain: a meta-analysis. Anaesthesia, 68(1), 79–90. https://doi.org/10.1111/j.1365-2044.2012.07335.x

Ali, O., & Donohoue, P. A. (2016). Nelson Textbook of Pediatrics, 2-Volume Set. In R. M. Kliegman, B. F. Stanton, J. W. St. Geme, N. F. Schor, & R. E. Behrman (Eds.), Hypofunction of the testes (20th ed., pp. 2735–2740). Philadelphia, USA: Elsevier Health Sciences.

Alzheimer's Association. (2018). 2018 Alzheimer's disease facts and figures. Alzheimer's & Dementia, 14(3), 367–429. https://doi.org/10.1016/j.jalz.2018.02.001

American Museum of Natural History. (2013, November). Bacteria Evolving: Tracing the Origins of a MRSA Epidemic [Video]. Retrieved November 2018, from https://www.amnh.org/learn-teach/curriculum-collections/bacteria-evolving-tracing-the-origins-of-a-mrsa-epidemic

American Psychiatric Association. (1980). Diagnostic and Statistical Manual of Mental Disorders: DSM-III (3rd ed.). Washington, D.C., USA: American Psychiatric Assoc.

American Psychiatric Association. (1987). Diagnostic and Statistical Manual of Mental Disorders: DSM-III-R (Rev. ed.). Washington, D.C.: American Psychiatric Assoc.

American Psychiatric Association. (2000). Diagnostic and Statistical Manual of Mental Disorders: DSM-IV (4th ed.). Washington D.C., USA: American Psychiatric Publishing.

American Psychiatric Association. (2013). Diagnostic and Statistical Manual of Mental Disorders: DSM-V (5th ed.). Washington D.C., USA: American Psychiatric Publishing.

American Society for Plastic Surgery. (2018). 2018 Plastic Surgery Statistics Report. Retrieved from https://www.plasticsurgery.org/documents/News/Statistics/2018/plastic-surgery-statistics-full-report-2018.pdf

Amin, K. (2012). The role of mast cells in allergic inflammation. Respiratory Medicine, 106(1), 9–14. https://doi.org/10.1016/j.rmed.2011.09.007

Anderson, O. S., Sant, K. E., & Dolinoy, D. C. (2012). Nutrition and epigenetics: an interplay of dietary methyl donors, one-carbon metabolism and DNA methylation. The Journal of Nutritional Biochemistry, 23(8), 853–859. https://doi.org/10.1016/j.jnutbio.2012.03.003

Archer, G. (1978, September). Antimicrobial Susceptibility and Selection of Resistance Among Staphylococcus epidermidis Isolates Recovered from Patients with Infections of Indwelling Foreign Devices. Retrieved from https://www.ncbi.nlm.nih.gov/pmc/articles/PMC352464/

Archer, G., & Climo, M. (1994, October). Antimicrobial Susceptibility Of Coagulase-Negative Staphylococci. Retrieved from https://www.ncbi.nlm.nih.gov/pmc/articles/PMC284723/

Argou-Cardozo, I., & Zeidán-Chuliá, F. (2018). Clostridium Bacteria and Autism Spectrum Conditions: A Systematic Review and Hypothetical Contribution of Environmental Glyphosate Levels. Medical Sciences, 6(2), 29. https://doi.org/10.3390/medsci6020029

Autism Speaks. (2018, April 26). Cdc Increases Estimate Of Autism's Prevalence By 15 Percent, To 1 In 59 Children. Retrieved from https://www.autismspeaks.org/science-news/cdc-increases-estimate-autisms-prevalence-15-percent-1-59-children

Bachir, R. G., & Benali, M. (2012). Antibacterial activity of the essential oils from the leaves of Eucalyptus globulus against Escherichia coli and Staphylococcus aureus. Asian Pacific Journal of Tropical Biomedicine, 2(9), 739–742. https://doi.org/10.1016/S2221-1691(12)60220-2

Bag, A., Bhattacharyya, S.K., Pal, N.K., & Chattopadhyay, R.R. (2009). The Kill Kinetics of Phenolics of Chebulic Myrobalan (Fruit of Terminalia chebula Retz .) against Methicillin-Resistant Staphylococcus aureus and Trimethoprim-Sulphamethoxazole-Resistant Uropathogenic Escherichia coli.

Bag, A., Bhattacharyya, S. K., & Chattopadhyay, R. R. (2013). The development of Terminalia chebula Retz. (Combretaceae) in clinical research. Asian Pacific Journal of Tropical Biomedicine, 3(3), 244–252. https://doi.org/10.1016/S2221-1691(13)60059-3

Baio, J., Wiggins, L., Christensen, D. L., Maenner, M. J., Daniels, J., Warren, Z., ... Dowling, N. F. (2018). Prevalence of Autism Spectrum Disorder Among Children Aged 8 Years — Autism and Developmental Disabilities Monitoring Network, 11 Sites, United States, 2014. MMWR. Surveillance Summaries, 67(6), 1–23. https://doi.org/10.15585/mmwr.ss6706a1

Baker, C. M., Ferrari, M. J., & Shea, K. (2018a, December 4). Beyond dose: Pulsed antibiotic treatment schedules can maintain individual benefit while reducing resistance. Retrieved from https://www.nature.com/articles/s41598-018-24006-w

Baker, C. M., Ferrari, M. J., & Shea, K. (2018b). Beyond dose: Pulsed antibiotic treatment schedules can maintain individual benefit while reducing resistance. Scientific Reports, 8(1). https://doi.org/10.1038/s41598-018-24006-w

Balakrishnan, P., & Ashwini, M. (2014). Conceptual Analysis of Physiology of Vision In Ayurveda. Journal of Ayurveda and Integrative Medicine, 5(3), 190. https://doi.org/10.4103/0975-9476.140486

Balas E.A., Boren S.A. (2000). Managing Clinical Knowledge For Health Care Improvement. In: Bemmel J, McCray AT, editors. Yearbook of Medical Informatics 2000: Patient-Centered Systems. Stuttgart, Germany: Schattauer Verlagsgesellschaft mbH; 2000:65-70.

Baluška, F., & Mancuso, S. (2009). Deep evolutionary origins of neurobiology: Turning the essence of 'neural' upside-down. Commun Integr Biol, 2(1), 60–65. Retrieved from https://www.ncbi.nlm.nih.gov/pmc/articles/PMC2649305/

Baluška, F., & Mancuso, S. (2009). Plant neurobiology. Plant Signaling & Behavior, 4(6), 475–476. https://doi.org/10.4161/psb.4.6.8870

Baluška, František, Volkmann, D., & Menzel, D. (2005). Plant synapses: actin-based domains for cell-to-cell communication. Trends in Plant Science, 10(3), 106–111. https://doi.org/10.1016/j.tplants.2005.01.002

Barcenilla, A., Pryde, S. E., Martin, J. C., Duncan, S. H., Stewart, C. S., Henderson, C., & Flint, H. J. (2000). Phylogenetic Relationships of Butyrate-Producing Bacteria from the Human Gut. Applied and Environmental Microbiology, 66(4), 1654–1661. https://doi.org/10.1128/aem.66.4.1654-1661.2000

Bartlett, J. G., Gilbert, D. N., & Spellberg, B. (2013). Seven Ways to Preserve the Miracle of Antibiotics. Clinical Infectious Diseases, 56(10), 1445–1450. https://doi.org/10.1093/cid/cit070

Bashir, S., & Al-Ayadhi, L. Y. (2013). Effect of camel milk on thymus and activation-regulated chemokine in autistic children: double-blind study. Pediatric Research, 75(4), 559–563. https://doi.org/10.1038/pr.2013.248

Beck, K., & Schachtrup, C. (2011). Vascular damage in the central nervous system: a multifaceted role for vascular-derived TGF-β. Cell and Tissue Research, 347(1), 187–201. Retrieved from https://link.springer.com/article/10.1007/s00441-011-1228-0

Becker, K., Heilmann, C., & Peters, G. (2014). Coagulase-Negative Staphylococci. Clinical Microbiology Reviews, 27(4), 870–926. Retrieved from https://cmr.asm.org/content/27/4/870

Beenken, K. E., Dunman, P. M., McAleese, F., Macapagal, D., Murphy, E., Projan, S. J., . . . Smeltzer, M. S. (2004). Global Gene Expression in Staphylococcus aureus Biofilms. Journal of Bacteriology, 186(14), 4665–4684. https://doi.org/10.1128/jb.186.14.4665-4684.2004

Bell, J. S., Bell, M., Gottfried, K., & Veltman, M. (2001). John S. Bell on the Foundations of Quantum Mechanics. Singapore: World Scientific.

Belmonte, G., Cescatti, L., Ferrari, B., Nicolussi, T., Ropele, M., & Menestrina, G. (1987). Pore formation by Staphylococcus aureus alpha-toxin in lipid bilayers. Dependence upon temperature and toxin concentration. - PubMed - NCBI. Retrieved from https://www.ncbi.nlm.nih.gov/pubmed/2439323

Belyaev, I. (2011). Toxicity and SOS-response to ELF magnetic fields and nalidixic acid in E. coli cells. Mutation Research/Genetic Toxicology and Environmental Mutagenesis, 722(1), 56–61. https://doi.org/10.1016/j.mrgentox.2011.03.012

Benarroch, E. E., Westmoreland, B., Daube, J., Reagan, T., & Sandok, B. (1999). Medical Neurosciences: An Approach to Anatomy, Pathology, and Physiology by Systems and Levels (3rd ed.). Philadelphia: Lippincott Williams & Wilkins.

Bent, S. (2008). Herbal Medicine in the United States: Review of Efficacy, Safety, and Regulation. Journal of General Internal Medicine, 23(6), 854–859. https://doi.org/10.1007/s11606-008-0632-y

Berberoğlu, M. (2009). Precocious Puberty and Normal Variant Puberty: Definition, etiology, diagnosis and current management - Review. Journal of Clinical Research in Pediatric Endocrinology, 1(4), 164–174. Retrieved from https://www.ncbi.nlm.nih.gov/pmc/articles/PMC3005651/

Berndtson, K. (2013). Review of evidence for immune evasion and persistent infection in Lyme disease. International Journal of General Medicine, , 291. https://doi.org/10.2147/ijgm.s44114

Berndtson, K., McMahon, S. W., Ackerley, M., Rapaport, S., Gupta, S., & Ritchie C. Shoemaker Center for Research on Biotoxin Associated Illness. (2016, January 19). Medically sound investigation and remediation of water-damaged buildings in cases of chronic inflammatory response syndrome. | Dr. Ritchie Shoemaker. Retrieved January 15, 2019, from https://www.survivingmold.com/docs/MEDICAL_CONSENSUS_1_19_2016_INDOOR_AIR_KB_FINAL.pdf

Berry, Y. (2014). A Physician's Guide to Understanding & Treating Biotoxin Illness [PDF]. Retrieved from https://www.survivingmold.com/legal-resources/works-citing-dr.-shoemaker/a-physicians-guide-to-biotoxin-illness

Bertin, M. (2016, July 6). Understanding Behavioral Therapy for Autism. Retrieved from https://www.psychologytoday.com/us/blog/child-development-central/201607/understanding-behavioral-therapy-autism

Biello, D. (2007, April 13). When It Comes to Photosynthesis, Plants Perform Quantum Computation. Retrieved from https://www.scientificamerican.com/article/when-it-comes-to-photosynthesis-plants-perform-quantum-computation/

Bilbey, D. L., & Prabhakaran, V. M. (1996). Muscle cramps and magnesium deficiency: case reports. Canadian family physician Medecin de famille canadien, 42, 1348–1351.

Biontology Arizona. (n.d.). Dr. Popp Biophoton Theory. Retrieved from https://www.biontologyarizona.com/dr-fritz-albert-popp/

Biswas, M., Voltz, K., Smith, J. C., & Langowski, J. (2011). Role of Histone Tails in Structural Stability of the Nucleosome. PLoS Computational Biology, 7(12). https://doi.org/10.1371/journal.pcbi.1002279

Blendon, R. J., DesRoches, C. M., Benson, J. M., Brodie, M., & Altman, D. E. (2001). Americans' Views on the Use and Regulation of Dietary Supplements. Archives of Internal Medicine, 161(6), 805. https://doi.org/10.1001/archinte.161.6.805

Böhm, M., Luger, T. A., Tobin, D. J., & García-Borrón, J. C. (2006). Melanocortin Receptor Ligands: New Horizons for Skin Biology and Clinical Dermatology. Journal of Investigative Dermatology, 126(9), 1966–1975. https://doi.org/10.1038/sj.jid.5700421

Boles, B., & Horswill, A. (2008, April). agr-Mediated Dispersal of Staphylococcus aureus Biofilms. Retrieved from https://www.ncbi.nlm.nih.gov/pmc/articles/PMC2329812/

Bommarito, P. A., & Fry, R. C. (2019). The Role of DNA Methylation in Gene Regulation. Toxicoepigenetics, 127–151. https://doi.org/10.1016/B978-0-12-812433-8.00005-8

Bose, J. (1926). The Nervous Mechanism of Plants. Retrieved from https://archive.org/details/in.ernet.dli.2015.163904/page/n3

Bove, M. (2001). An Encyclopedia of Natural Healing for Children and Infants (2nd ed.). McGraw-Hill Education.

Boundless Psychology. (2017, June). Introduction to Consciousness. Retrieved from https://courses.lumenlearning.com/boundless-psychology/chapter/introduction-to-consciousness/

Bove, M., & Costarella, L. (1997). Herbs for Women's Health: Herbal Help for the Female Cycle from PMS to Menopause (Good Herb Guide Series) (1st ed.). Keats Pub.

Bray, D. (1995). Protein molecules as computational elements in living cells. Nature, 376(6538), 307–312. https://doi.org/10.1038/376307a0

Brown, C., Redd, S., Damon, S., Division of Environmental Hazards and Health Effects, & National Center for Environmental Health. (2004, March 12). Acute Idiopathic Pulmonary Hemorrhage Among Infants: Recommendations from the Working Group for Investigation and Surveillance. Retrieved April 3, 2019, from https://www.cdc.gov/mmwr/preview/mmwrhtml/rr5302a1.htm

Bryant, M. G. (1978). Vasoactive intestinal peptide (VIP). Journal of Clinical Pathology, s1-8(1), 63–67. https://doi.org/10.1136/jcp.s1-8.1.63

Buhl, R., Meyer, A., & Vogelmeier, C. (1996). Oxidant-Protease Interaction in the Lung. Chest, 110(6), 267S-272S. https://doi.org/10.1378/chest.110.6_supplement.267s

Buhner, S. H. (2012). Herbal Antibiotics, 2nd Edition: Natural Alternatives for Treating Drug-resistant Bacteria. North Adams, United States of America: Storey Publishing, LLC.

Buhner, S. H. (2014). Plant Intelligence and the Imaginal Realm: Beyond the Doors of Perception into the Dreaming of Earth. Rochester, United States of America: Inner Traditions/Bear.

Buhner, S. H. (2017, January 6). Plant Intelligence: The Evidence That Plants are Conscious. Retrieved from https://www.consciouslifestylemag.com/plant-consciousness-intelligence-feeling/

Burroughes, D. (2013, February 14). WHAT FOODS ARE HIGH IN BIOPHOTONS? Retrieved from http://www.dianeburroughes.com/blog---listen-up-listen-in/what-foods-are-high-in-biophotons

C., S. (2009, February 17). Bio-photons detect food quality. Retrieved from http://www.teatronaturale.com/technical-area/science-news/124-biophotons-detect-food-quality.htm

Cai, D., & Liu, T. (2011). Hypothalamic inflammation: a double-edged sword to nutritional diseases. Annals of the New York Academy of Sciences, 1243(1), 1–39. Retrieved from https://www.ncbi.nlm.nih.gov/pmc/articles/PMC4389774/

Caraka., Kaviratna, A.C. (1913). Charaka-samhita: translated into English. Calcutta: Printed by G.C. Chakravarti [etc.].

Carrel, M., & Bitterman, P. (2015). Personal Belief Exemptions to Vaccination in California: A Spatial Analysis. Retrieved from https://pediatrics.aappublications.org/content/136/1/80.long

Carson, C. F., Hammer, K. A., & Riley, T. V. (2006). Melaleuca alternifolia (Tea Tree) Oil: a Review of Antimicrobial and Other Medicinal Properties. Clinical Microbiology Reviews, 19(1), 50–62. https://doi.org/10.1128/CMR.19.1.50-62.2006

Casey, J., & Euclid. (2007). Project Gutenberg's First Six Books of the Elements of Euclid [PDF] (3rd ed.). Retrieved from http://www.gutenberg.org/files/21076/21076-pdf.pdf

Centers for Disease Control and Prevention. (n.d.). CDC - Mold - General Information: Facts about Stachybotrys chartarum and Other Molds. Retrieved April 3, 2019, from https://www.cdc.gov/mold/stachy.htm

Centers for Disease Control and Prevention. (2006). Mold Prevention Strategies and Possible Health Effects in the Aftermath of Hurricanes and Major Floods. MMWR, 55(RR-8). Retrieved from https://www.cdc.gov/mmwr/PDF/rr/rr5508.pdf

Centers for Disease Control and Prevention. (2013). Antibiotic Resistance Threats in the United States. Retrieved from https://www.cdc.gov/drugresistance/pdf/ar-threats-2013-508.pdf

Centers for Disease Control and Prevention. (2018, September 27). Antifungal Resistance. Retrieved from https://www.cdc.gov/fungal/antifungal-resistance.html

Centers for Disease Control and Prevention. (2019, May 7). The biggest antibiotic-resistant threats in the U.S. Retrieved from https://www.cdc.gov/drugresistance/biggest_threats.html

Centers for Disease Control and Prevention. (2019, July 12). Candida auris. Retrieved from https://www.cdc.gov/fungal/candida-auris/index.html

Cerca, N., Martins, S., Cerca, F., Jefferson, K., Pier, G., Oliveira, R., & Azeredo, J. (2005, August). Comparative assessment of antibiotic susceptibility of coagulase-negative staphylococci in biofilm versus planktonic culture as assessed by bacterial enumeration or rapid XTT colorimetry. Retrieved from https://www.ncbi.nlm.nih.gov/pmc/articles/PMC1317301/

Chaitow, L. (2008). Naturopathic Physical Medicine: Theory and Practice for Manual Therapists and Naturopaths. London, UK: Elsevier Health Sciences.

Chen, T. (2011). Mechanistic and Functional Links Between Histone Methylation and DNA Methylation. Progress in Molecular Biology and Translational Science, 335–348. https://doi.org/10.1016/B978-0-12-387685-0.00010-X

Chen, Y., Harapanahalli, A. K., Busscher, H. J., Norde, W., & van der Mei, H. C. (2014). Nanoscale Cell Wall Deformation Impacts Long-Range Bacterial Adhesion Forces on Surfaces. Applied and environmental microbiology, 80(2), 637-643. https://doi.org/10.1128/AEM.02745-13

Chen, Z., & O'Shea, J. J. (2008). Th17 cells: a new fate for differentiating helper T cells. Immunologic Research, 41(2), 87–102. https://doi.org/10.1007/s12026-007-8014-9

Cheney, P. (2018, March 21). Oxygen Toxicity as a Locus of Control for Chronic Fatigue Syndrome - Source: Presentation at 15th International Symposium of Functional Medicine, May 22, 2008. Retrieved from https://www.prohealth.com/library/oxygen-toxicity-as-a-locus-of-control-for-chronic-fatigue-syndrome-source-presentation-at-15th-international-symposium-of-functional-medicine-may-22-2008-28469

Chojnacki, C., Walecka-Kapica, E., Romanowski, M., Chojnacki, J., & Klupinska, G. (2014). Protective Role of Melatonin in Liver Damage. Current Pharmaceutical Design, 20(30), 4828–4833. https://doi.org/10.2174/1381612819666131119102155

Cimanga, K., De Bruyne, T., Lasure, A., Van Poel, B., Pieters, L., Claeys, M., ... Vlietinck, A. (1996). In VitroBiological Activities of Alkaloids fromCryptolepis sanguinolenta. Planta Medica, 62(01), 22–27. https://doi.org/10.1055/s-2006-957789

Cimanga, K., De Bruyne, T., Pieters, L., Totte, J., Tona, L., Kambu, K., ... Vlietinck, A. J. (1998). Antibacterial and antifungal activities of neocryptolepine, biscryptolepine and cryptoquindoline, alkaloids isolated from Cryptolepis sanguinolenta. Phytomedicine, 5(3), 209–214. https://doi.org/10.1016/S0944-7113(98)80030-5

Ciorba, M. A. (2013). Kynurenine pathway metabolites: relevant to vitamin B-6 deficiency and beyond. The American Journal of Clinical Nutrition, 98(4), 863–864. https://doi.org/10.3945/ajcn.113.072025

Clarke, S. R., & Foster, S. J. (2006). Surface Adhesins of Staphylococcus aureus. Advances in Microbial Physiology Volume 51, 187–224. https://doi.org/10.1016/s0065-2911(06)51004-5

Cohen, H., Amerine-Dickens, M., & Smith, T. (2006). Early Intensive Behavioral Treatment: Replication of the UCLA Model in a Community Setting. Journal of Developmental & Behavioral Pediatrics, 27(2). Retrieved from https://journals.lww.com/jrnldbp/pages/articleviewer.aspx?year=2006&issue=04002&article=00013&type=abstract

Condrau, F., & Kirk, R. G. (2011). Negotiating hospital infections: the debate between ecological balance and eradication strategies in British hospitals 1947-1969. Dynamis (Granada, Spain), 31(2), 385–405.

Connelly, D. (2014). A history of aspirin. Clinical Pharmacist. https://doi.org/10.1211/CP.2014.20066661

Cook, K. (2019). Glyphosate in Beer and Wine. Retrieved from https://uspirg.org/sites/pirg/files/reports/WEB_CAP_Glyphosate-pesticide-beer-and-wine_REPORT_022619.pdf

Cookson, B. (2011). Five decades of MRSA: controversy and uncertainty continues. The Lancet, 378(9799), 1291–1292. https://doi.org/10.1016/S0140-6736(11)61566-3

Coppola, M., Cascone, P., Madonna, V., Di Lelio, I., Esposito, F., Avitabile, C., ... Corrado, G. (2017). Plant-to-plant communication triggered by systemin primes anti-herbivore resistance in tomato. Scientific Reports, 7(1). https://doi.org/10.1038/s41598-017-15481-8

Cossins, J. (2018, June 12). Plant Talk. Retrieved from https://www.the-scientist.com/features/plant-talk-38209

Costerton, J. W. (1999). Bacterial Biofilms: A Common Cause of Persistent Infections. Science, 284(5418), 1318–1322. Retrieved from http://web.biosci.utexas.edu/psaxena/bio226r/articles/Biofilm.pdf

Costerton, J. W., Geesey, G. G., & Cheng, K. (1978). How Bacteria Stick. Scientific American, 238(1), 86–95. https://doi.org/10.1038/scientificamerican0178-86

Costerton, J. W., Cheng, K. J., Geesey, G. G., Ladd, T. I., Nickel, J. C., Dasgupta, M., & Marrie, T. J. (1987). Bacterial Biofilms in Nature and Disease. Annual Review of Microbiology, 41(1), 435–464. https://doi.org/10.1146/annurev.mi.41.100187.002251

Cousens, G. (2009). Spiritual Nutrition: Six Foundations for Spiritual Life and the Awakening of Kundalini. Berkeley, United States: North Atlantic Books.

Crosby, V., Wilcock, A., Mrcp, D., & Corcoran, R. (2000). The Safety and Efficacy of a Single Dose (500 mg or 1 g) of Intravenous Magnesium Sulfate in Neuropathic Pain Poorly Responsive to Strong Opioid Analgesics in Patients with Cancer. Journal of Pain and Symptom Management, 19(1), 35–39. https://doi.org/10.1016/s0885-3924(99)00135-9

Crow, D. (2013). Plants That Heal: Essays On Botanical Medicine. Floracopeia.

Daly, M. J. (2008). Association between Microdeletion and Microduplication at 16p11.2 and Autism. New England Journal of Medicine, 358(7), 667–675. https://doi.org/10.1056/NEJMoa075974

Daniel, E. E., & Fox-Threlkeld, J. E. T. (1997). Vasoactive Intestinal Polypeptide. Molecular and Cellular Endocrinology, 517–530. https://doi.org/10.1016/S1569-2582(97)80169-9

Dashore, J. A. (2018a, May 25). Mold/Biotoxin illness and Autism: Focus on Multinuclear atrophy of Cortical Grey Matter, Stem Cells and Language, Behavioral and Neurological recovery. [Video]. Retrieved from https://www.youtube.com/watch?v=bpZx3DxBiQU

Dashore, J. A. (2018b, May 31). Mold/Biotoxin illness and Autism:Focus on Multinuclear atrophy of Cortical Grey Matter, Stem Cells and Language, Behavioral and Neurological Recovery [Video]. Retrieved from https://www.youtube.com/watch?v=bpZx3DxBiQU

Dashore, J. A., & BioNexus Health. (2019a, April 25). Formula 1 NSB Recommended Use [PDF].

Dashore, J. A. (2019b, May 28). Pediatric All-Natural Treatment Options for Brain and Digestive Health Utilizing Herbs, Ayurveda, Camel Milk, and Essential Oils [Video]. Retrieved from https://www.youtube.com/watch?v=90CxtrcoTg0

Dashore, J. A. (2019c, June 3). Biotoxin Illness From The Ground Up: Step by Step Approach to Natural Treatment Options for CIRS-WDB and CIRS-Lyme [Video]. Retrieved from https://www.youtube.com/watch?v=AdV4ADwlcKA

Davies, J., & Davies, D. (2010). Origins and Evolution of Antibiotic Resistance. Microbiology and Molecular Biology Reviews, 74(3), 417–433. https://doi.org/10.1128/MMBR.00016-10

De Allori, M. C. G., Jure, M. Á., Romero, C., & De Castillo, M. E. C. (2006). Antimicrobial Resistance and Production of Biofilms in Clinical Isolates of Coagulase-Negative Staphylococcus Strains. Biological & Pharmaceutical Bulletin, 29(8), 1592–1596. Retrieved from https://www.jstage.jst.go.jp/article/bpb/29/8/29_8_1592/_pdf/-char/en

Deer, B. (2011). How the case against the MMR vaccine was fixed. BMJ, 342(jan05 1). https://doi.org/10.1136/bmj.c5347

Delgado, M. (2004). The Significance of Vasoactive Intestinal Peptide in Immunomodulation. Pharmacological Reviews, 56(2), 249–290. https://doi.org/10.1124/pr.56.2.7

Dinges, M., Orwin, P., & Schlievert, P. (2000, January). Exotoxins of Staphylococcus aureus. Retrieved from https://www.ncbi.nlm.nih.gov/pmc/articles/PMC88931/

Dinicola, S., Proietti, S., Cucina, A., Bizzarri, M., & Fuso, A. (2017). Alpha-Lipoic Acid Downregulates IL-1β and IL-6 by DNA Hypermethylation in SK-N-BE Neuroblastoma Cells. Antioxidants, 6(4), 74. https://doi.org/10.3390/antiox6040074

Donlan, R., & Costerton, J. (2002, April). Biofilms: Survival Mechanisms of Clinically Relevant Microorganisms. Retrieved from https://www.ncbi.nlm.nih.gov/pmc/articles/PMC118068/

Drouin, P. (2017, December 5). What is Pro-Consciousness Medicine? Retrieved from https://drpauldrouin.com/what-is-pro-consciousness-medicine/

Du, G., Chen, X., Sun, F., Ma, L., Wang, J., & Qin, H. (2011). In vitro evaluation on the antioxidant capacity of triethylchebulate, an aglycone from Terminalia chebula Retz fruit. Indian Journal of Pharmacology, 43(3), 320. https://doi.org/10.4103/0253-7613.81508

Duvernelle, C., Freund, V., & Frossard, N. (2003). Transforming growth factor-β and its role in asthma. Pulmonary Pharmacology & Therapeutics, 16(4), 181–196. https://doi.org/10.1016/S1094-5539(03)00051-8

Ebell, M. H., Siwek, J., Weiss, B. D., Woolf, S. H., Susman, J., Ewigman, B., & Bowman, M. (2004, February 1). Strength of Recommendation Taxonomy (SORT): A Patient-Centered Approach to Grading Evidence in the Medical Literature. Retrieved June , from https://www.aafp.org/afp/2004/0201/p548.html

Eddy, D. M. (1990). Practice Policies: Where Do They Come From? JAMA: The Journal of the American Medical Association, 263(9), 1265. https://doi.org/10.1001/jama.1990.03440090103036

Edwards-Jones, V., Buck, R., Shawcross, S. G., Dawson, M. M., & Dunn, K. (2004). The effect of essential oils on methicillin-resistant Staphylococcus aureus using a dressing model. Burns, 30(8), 772–777. https://doi.org/10.1016/j.burns.2004.06.006

Eikeseth, S., Smith, T., Jahr, E., & Eldevik, S. (2007). Outcome for Children with Autism who Began Intensive Behavioral Treatment Between Ages 4 and 7. Behavior Modification, 31(3), 264–278. https://doi.org/10.1177/0145445506291396

Eisenberg, D. M., Kessler, R. C., Foster, C., Norlock, F. E., Calkins, D. R., & Delbanco, T. L. (1993). Unconventional Medicine in the United States -- Prevalence, Costs, and Patterns of Use. New England Journal of Medicine, 328(4), 246–252. https://doi.org/10.1056/NEJM199301283280406

Ekor, M. (2014). The growing use of herbal medicines: issues relating to adverse reactions and challenges in monitoring safety. Frontiers in Pharmacology, 4. https://doi.org/10.3389/fphar.2013.00177

Engel, G. S. (2011). Quantum coherence in photosynthesis. Procedia Chemistry, 3(1), 222–231. https://doi.org/10.1016/j.proche.2011.08.029

Environmental Working Group. (2020, January 22). PFAS Contamination of Drinking Water Far More Prevalent Than Previously Reported. Retrieved from https://www.ewg.org/research/national-pfas-testing/

Espinell-Ingroff, A. V. (2013). Medical Mycology in the United States: A Historical Analysis (1894–1996). Netherlands: Springer.

European Medicines Agency, & Committee on Herbal Medicinal Products. (2015). European Union herbal monograph on Melaleuca alternifolia (Maiden and Betch) Cheel, M. linariifolia Smith, M. dissitiflora F. Mueller and/or other species of Melaleuca, aetheroleum. Retrieved from https://www.ema.europa.eu/en/documents/herbal-monograph/final-european-union-herbal-monograph-melaleuca-alternifolia-maiden-betch-cheel-m-linariifolia-smith/other-species-melaleuca-aetheroleum_en.pdf

Faculty of Science - University of Copenhagen. (2018, September 25). Infectious bacteria hibernate to evade antibiotics. ScienceDaily. Retrieved June 26, 2019 from www.sciencedaily.com/releases/ 2018/09/180925110025.htm

Fahrenkrug, J. (2001). Gut/brain peptides in the genital tract: VIP and PACAP. Scandinavian Journal of Clinical and Laboratory Investigation, 61(234), 35–39. https://doi.org/ 10.1080/003655101317095392

Feng, G., Cheng, Y., Wang, S.-Y., Borca-Tasciuc, D. A., Worobo, R. W., & Moraru, C. I. (2015). Bacterial attachment and biofilm formation on surfaces are reduced by small-diameter nanoscale pores: how small is small enough? Npj Biofilms and Microbiomes, 1(1). https://doi.org/10.1038/ npjbiofilms.2015.22

Fey, P. D., & Olson, M. E. (2010). Current concepts in biofilm formation ofStaphylococcus epidermidis. Future Microbiology, 5(6), 917–933. https://doi.org/10.2217/fmb.10.56

Fields, D. R. (2010, July 2). Left-sided Cancer: Blame your bed and TV? Retrieved from https:// blogs.scientificamerican.com/guest-blog/left-sided-cancer-blame-your-bed-and-tv/

Fleming, A. (2001). On the antibacterial action of cultures of a penicillium, with special reference to their use in the isolation of B. influenzae. 1929. Bulletin of the World Health Organization, 79(8), 780–790. Retrieved from https://www.ncbi.nlm.nih.gov/pmc/articles/PMC2566493/pdf/ 11545337.pdf

Flemming, A. (2018, June). The Nobel Prize in Physiology or Medicine 1945. Retrieved from https://www.nobelprize.org/prizes/medicine/1945/fleming/lecture

Follmann W, Ali N, Blaszkewicz M. (2016). Biomonitoring of Mycotoxins in Urine: Pilot study in Mill Workers. J Toxicol Environ Health, 79: 1015-1025.

Folstein, S., & Rutter, M. (1977). Infantile Autism: A Genetic Study Of 21 Twin Pairs. Journal of Child Psychology and Psychiatry, 18(4), 297–321. https://doi.org/10.1111/j. 1469-7610.1977.tb00443.x

Folstein, S. E., & Rosen-Sheidley, B. (2001). Genetics of austim: complex aetiology for a heterogeneous disorder. Nature Reviews Genetics, 2(12), 943–955. https://doi.org/10.1038/35103559

Franck, J., & Teller, E. (1938). Migration and Photochemical Action of Excitation Energy in Crystals. The Journal of Chemical Physics, 6(12), 861–872. https://doi.org/10.1063/1.1750182

Freris, L. (2013). Mind and matter. Communicative & Integrative Biology, 6(6), e26658. https:// doi.org/10.4161/cib.26658

Fux, C., Stoodley, P., Hall-Stoodley, L., & Costerton, J. (2003, December). Bacterial biofilms: a diagnostic and therapeutic challenge. - PubMed - NCBI. Retrieved from https:// pdfs.semanticscholar.org/40b3/5bc778c0c18a06d425564884339a8c453187.pdf

Gaby, A. (2011). Nutritional Medicine. New Hampshire, USA: Fritz Perlberg Publishing.

Gardiner, R. M. (2002). The Human Genome Project: the next decade. Archives of Disease in Childhood, 86(6), 389–391. Retrieved from https://adc.bmj.com/content/86/6/389

Garzón F. C. (2007). The quest for cognition in plant neurobiology. Plant signaling & behavior, 2(4), 208–211. doi:10.4161/psb.2.4.4470

Gaul, C., Diener, H.-C., & Danesch, U. (2015). Improvement of migraine symptoms with a proprietary supplement containing riboflavin, magnesium and Q10: a randomized, placebo-controlled, double-blind, multicenter trial. The Journal of Headache and Pain, 16(1). https://doi.org/10.1186/s10194-015-0516-6

Gay-Jordi, G., Guash, E., Benito, B., Brugada, J., Nattel, S., Mont, L., & Serrano-Mollar, A. (2013). Losartan Prevents Heart Fibrosis Induced by Long-Term Intensive Exercise in an Animal Model. PLoS ONE, 8(2), e55427. https://doi.org/10.1371/journal.pone.0055427

Gerhart, J., Kirschner, M., & Moderbacher, E. S. (1997). Cells, Embryos and Evolution (4th ed.). New York City, United States of America: Wiley.

Gladstar, R., & Hirsch, P. (2000). Planting the Future: Saving Our Medicinal Herbs. Rochester, United States of America: Healing Arts Press.

Gläscher, J., & Adolphs, R. (2003, November 12). Processing of the Arousal of Subliminal and Supraliminal Emotional Stimuli by the Human Amygdala. Retrieved March 4, 2019, from http://www.jneurosci.org/content/23/32/10274

Global Market Insights. (2019, May 8). Glyphosate Market Share will Touch US$ 8 Billion by 2024 [Press release]. Retrieved from https://www.marketwatch.com/press-release/glyphosate-market-share-will-touch-us-8-billion-by-2024-2019-05-08

Goldberg, D. R. (2019, April 18). Aspirin: Turn-of-the-Century Miracle Drug. Retrieved from https://www.sciencehistory.org/distillations/aspirin-turn-of-the-century-miracle-drug

Gottlieb, S. (2018). Remarks by Scott Gottlieb, M.D., Commissioner of Food and Drugs. Presented at the FDA's Strategic Approach for Combating Antimicrobial Resistance, Washington, DC, USA. Retrieved from https://www.fda.gov/news-events/speeches-fda-officials/fdas-strategic-approach-combating-antimicrobial-resistance-09142018

Gough, S., & Simmonds, M. (2007). The HLA Region and Autoimmune Disease: Associations and Mechanisms of Action. Current Genomics, 8(7), 453–465. https://doi.org/10.2174/138920207783591690

Gradmann, C. (2016). Re-Inventing Infectious Disease: Antibiotic Resistance and Drug Development at the Bayer Company 1945–80. Medical History, 60(2), 155–180. https://doi.org/10.1017/mdh.2016.2

Grahn, J. A., Parkinson, J. A., & Owen, A. M. (2008). The cognitive functions of the caudate nucleus. Progress in Neurobiology, 86(3), 141–155. https://doi.org/10.1016/j.pneurobio.2008.09.004

Gray, G., & Kehoe, M. (1984, November). Primary sequence of the alpha-toxin gene from Staphylococcus aureus wood 46.. Retrieved from https://iai.asm.org/content/iai/46/2/615.full.pdf

Grayson, D. R., & Guidotti, A. (2016). Merging data from genetic and epigenetic approaches to better understand autistic spectrum disorder. Epigenomics, 8(1), 85–104. https://doi.org/10.2217/epi.15.92

Green, H. F., & Nolan, Y. M. (2014). Inflammation and the developing brain: Consequences for hippocampal neurogenesis and behavior. Neuroscience & Biobehavioral Reviews, 40, 20–34. Retrieved from https://www.sciencedirect.com/science/article/pii/S0149763414000074?via%3Dihub

Grover, N. (2010). Echinocandins: A ray of hope in antifungal drug therapy. Indian Journal of Pharmacology, 42(1), 9. https://doi.org/10.4103/0253-7613.62396

Gumbiner, B. (2001). Obesity. Philadelphia, United States of America: American College of Physcians.

Guzman, P., Fernandez, V., Gracia, J., Cabral, V., Kayali, N., Khayet, M., & Gil, L. (2014). Chemical and structural analysis of Eucalyptus globulus and E. camaldulensis leaf cuticles: a lipidized cell wall region. Frontiers in Plant Science, 5. https://doi.org/10.3389/fpls.2014.00481

Hamilton, C. (1997). The Self-Aware Universe - An Interview with Amit Goswami. Retrieved from https://www.bibliotecapleyades.net/ciencia/ciencia_consciousuniverse08.htm

Hammer, K. A., Dry, L., Johnson, M., Michalak, E. M., Carson, C. F., & Riley, T. V. (2003). Susceptibility of oral bacteria to Melaleuca alternifolia (tea tree) oil in vitro. Oral Microbiology and Immunology, 18(6), 389–392. https://doi.org/10.1046/j.0902-0055.2003.00105.x

Hamza, M., Halayem, S., Mrad, R., Bourgou, S., Charfi, F., & Belhadj, A. (2017). Implication de l'épigénétique dans les troubles du spectre autistique : revue de la littérature. L'Encéphale, 43(4), 374–381. https://doi.org/10.1016/j.encep.2016.07.007

Hansen, E. S., Hasselbalch, S., Law, I., & Bolwig, T. G. (2002). The caudate nucleus in obsessive–compulsive disorder. Reduced metabolism following treatment with paroxetine: a PET study. The International Journal of Neuropsychopharmacology, 5(01). https://doi.org/10.1017/s1461145701002681

Harapanahalli, A. K., Younes, J. A., Allan, E., van der Mei, H. C., & Busscher, H. J. (2015). Chemical Signals and Mechanosensing in Bacterial Responses to Their Environment. PLOS Pathogens, 11(8), e1005057. https://doi.org/10.1371/journal.ppat.1005057

Hardee, J. E., Thompson, J. C., & Puce, A. (2008). The left amygdala knows fear: laterality in the amygdala response to fearful eyes. Social Cognitive and Affective Neuroscience, 3(1), 47–54. Retrieved from https://academic.oup.com/scan/article/3/1/47/1612007

Hartigan-O'Connor, D. J., Hirao, L. A., McCune, J. M., & Dandekar, S. (2011). Th17 cells and regulatory T cells in elite control over HIV and SIV. Current Opinion in HIV and AIDS, 6(3), 221–227. https://doi.org/10.1097/COH.0b013e32834577b3

Harvard Health Publishing. (2016, August 11). Are your medications causing nutrient deficiency? Retrieved from https://www.health.harvard.edu/staying-healthy/are-your-medications-causing-nutrient-deficiency

Hashimoto, T., Perlot, T., Rehman, A., Trichereau, J., Ishiguro, H., Paolino, M., ... Penninger, J. M. (2012). ACE2 links amino acid malnutrition to microbial ecology and intestinal inflammation. Nature, 487(7408), 477–481. https://doi.org/10.1038/nature11228

Heilmann, C., Hussain, M., Peters, G., & Gotz, F. (1997). Evidence for autolysin-mediated primary attachment of Staphylococcus epidermidis to a polystyrene surface. Molecular Microbiology, 24(5), 1013–1024. https://doi.org/10.1046/j.1365-2958.1997.4101774.x

Heilmann, C. (2003). Identification and characterization of a novel autolysin (Aae) with adhesive properties from Staphylococcus epidermidis. Microbiology, 149(10), 2769–2778. https://doi.org/10.1099/mic.0.26527-0

Helmy, K. Y., Patel, S. A., Silverio, K., Pliner, L., & Rameshwar, P. (2010). Stem cells and regenerative medicine: accomplishments to date and future promise. Therapeutic Delivery, 1(5), 693–705. https://doi.org/10.4155/tde.10.57

Henning, R. (2001). Vasoactive intestinal peptide: cardiovascular effects. Cardiovascular Research, 49(1), 27–37. https://doi.org/10.1016/s0008-6363(00)00229-7

Henning, R. J. (2013). VIP. Handbook of Biologically Active Peptides, 1443–1449. https://doi.org/10.1016/B978-0-12-385095-9.00196-2

Henry, R. (2005, July 7). The Mental Universe. Nature, 436(29). Retrieved from http://henry.pha.jhu.edu/The.mental.universe.pdf

The Herbarium. (2009, February 1). Tinctures & Fluid Extracts. Retrieved from https://theherbarium.wordpress.com/2009/02/01/tinctures-fluid-extracts/

Hideg, È. (1993). On the spontaneous ultraweak light emission of plants. Journal of Photochemistry and Photobiology B: Biology, 18(2–3), 239–244. https://doi.org/10.1016/1011-1344(93)80070-p

Hill, J. (2007). Vasoactive Intestinal Peptide in Neurodevelopmental Disorders:Therapeutic Potential. Current Pharmaceutical Design, 13(11), 1079–1089. https://doi.org/10.2174/138161207780618975

Hoffman, D. D., & Prakash, C. (2014). Objects of consciousness. Frontiers in Psychology, 5. https://doi.org/10.3389/fpsyg.2014.00577

Hope, J. (2013). A Review of the Mechanism of Injury and Treatment Approaches for Illness Resulting from Exposure to Water-Damaged Buildings, Mold, and Mycotoxins. The Scientific World Journal, 2013, 1–20. https://doi.org/10.1155/2013/767482

Horton, P. (2012). Optimization of light harvesting and photoprotection: molecular mechanisms and physiological consequences. Philosophical Transactions of the Royal Society B: Biological Sciences, 367(1608), 3455–3465. https://doi.org/10.1098/rstb.2012.0069

Huang, J. (2017, July). Brain Dysfunction by Location. Retrieved March 7, 2019, from https://www.msdmanuals.com/home/brain,-spinal-cord,-and-nerve-disorders/brain-dysfunction/brain-dysfunction-by-location

Hudnell, H. K. (2005). Chronic biotoxin-associated illness: Multiple-system symptoms, a vision deficit, and effective treatment. Neurotoxicology and Teratology, 27(5), 733–743. https://doi.org/10.1016/j.ntt.2005.06.010

Hudnell, H. K., & Shoemaker, R. C. (2002). Correspondence: Visual Contrast Sensitivity as a Diagnostic Tool & Response. Environmental Health Perspectives, 110(3), A 121-A 123. Retrieved from https://ehp.niehs.nih.gov/doi/pdf/10.1289/ehp.110-a120

Hu-Lince, D., Craig, D. W., Huentelman, M. J., & Stephan, D. A. (2005). The Autism Genome Project. American Journal of PharmacoGenomics, 5(4), 233–246. https://doi.org/10.2165/00129785-200505040-00004

Huseby, M. J., Kruse, A. C., Digre, J., Kohler, P. L., Vocke, J. A., Mann, E. E., . . . Earhart, C. A. (2010). Beta toxin catalyzes formation of nucleoprotein matrix in staphylococcal biofilms. Proceedings of the National Academy of Sciences, 107(32), 14407–14412. Retrieved from https://www.researchgate.net/profile/Ethan_Mann/publication/45366356_Beta_toxin_catalyzes_formation_of_nucleoprotein_matrix_in_staphylococcal_biofilms/links/552692480cf2628d5afeefc2/Beta-toxin-catalyzes-formation-of-nucleoprotein-matrix-in-staphylococcal-biofilms.pdf

ifarm LLC. (2016, July 22). Making Herbal Tinctures and Infused Oils with Herbalist Margi Flint - July 24 [Slides]. Ifarm LLC. https://ifarmboxford.com/event/making-herbal-tinctures-and-infused-oils-with-herbalist-margi-flint-july-24/

Indoor Science. (2018, March 29). Mold Testing and Inspections. Retrieved April 5, 2019, from https://indoorscience.com/mold-testing/

Institute of Medicine. (2004). Damp Indoor Spaces and Health. Retrieved from https://www.ncbi.nlm.nih.gov/books/NBK215643/

Institute of Medicine (US) Immunization Safety Review Committee. (2004). Immunization Safety Review: Vaccines and Autism. Washington D.C., USA: National Academies Press.

Isenberg, D. A., Morrow, W. J., & Snaith, M. L. (1982). Methyl prednisolone pulse therapy in the treatment of systemic lupus erythematosus. Annals of the Rheumatic Diseases, 41(4), 347–351. https://doi.org/10.1136/ard.41.4.347

Jabr, F. (2012, January 30). Redefining Autism: Will New DSM-5 Criteria for ASD Exclude Some People? Retrieved from https://www.scientificamerican.com/article/autism-new-criteria/

Janeway, C., Travers, P., Walport, M., & Shlomchik, M. (2001). Immunobiology (5th ed.). New York, USA: Garland Science.

Jernberg, C., Lofmark, S., Edlund, C., & Jansson, J. K. (2010). Long-term impacts of antibiotic exposure on the human intestinal microbiota. Microbiology, 156(11), 3216–3223. https://doi.org/10.1099/mic.0.040618-0

Ji, H., & Khurana Hershey, G. K. (2012). Genetic and epigenetic influence on the response to environmental particulate matter. Journal of Allergy and Clinical Immunology, 129(1), 33–41. https://doi.org/10.1016/j.jaci.2011.11.008

Jiménez Barbosa, I. S., Boon, M. Y., & Khuu, S. K. (2015). Exposure to Organic Solvents Used in Dry Cleaning Reduces Low and High Level Visual Function. PLOS ONE, 10(5). https://doi.org/10.1371/journal.pone.0121422

Jin, B., Li, Y., & Robertson, K. D. (2011a). DNA Methylation: Superior or Subordinate in the Epigenetic Hierarchy? Genes & Cancer, 2(6), 607–617. https://doi.org/10.1177/1947601910393957

Jirtle, R. L., & Skinner, M. K. (2007). Environmental epigenomics and disease susceptibility. Nature Reviews Genetics, 8(4), 253–262. https://doi.org/10.1038/nrg2045

John, J., & Harvin, A. (2007, December). History and evolution of antibiotic resistance in coagulase-negative staphylococci: Susceptibility profiles of new anti-staphylococcal agents. Retrieved from https://www.ncbi.nlm.nih.gov/pmc/articles/PMC2387300/

Johnson, L. B., & Kauffman, C. A. (2003). Voriconazole: A New Triazole Antifungal Agent. Clinical Infectious Diseases, 36(5), 630–637. https://doi.org/10.1086/367933

Jolanta Wasilewska, J., & Klukowski, M. (2015). Gastrointestinal symptoms and autism spectrum disorder: links and risks – a possible new overlap syndrome. Pediatric Health, Medicine and Therapeutics, 153. https://doi.org/10.2147/PHMT.S85717

Joshi, K. (2012). Insights into Ayurvedic biology-A conversation with Professor M.S. Valiathan. Journal of Ayurveda and Integrative Medicine, 3(4), 226. https://doi.org/10.4103/0975-9476.104450

Joshi, K., & Bhonde, R. (2014). Insights from Ayurveda for translational stem cell research. Journal of Ayurveda and Integrative Medicine, 5(1), 4. https://doi.org/10.4103/0975-9476.128846

Juang, L.-J., Sheu, S.-J., & Lin, T.-C. (2004). Determination of hydrolyzable tannins in the fruit ofTerminalia chebula Retz. by high-performance liquid chromatography and capillary electrophoresis. Journal of Separation Science, 27(9), 718–724. https://doi.org/10.1002/jssc.200401741

Judson, H. F. (1996). The Eighth Day of Creation: Makers of the Revolution in Biology (3rd ed.). Cold Spring Harbor, United States of America: Cold Spring Harbor Laboratory Press.

Jukema, J. W., & van der Hoorn, J. W. (2004). Amlodipine and atorvastatin in atherosclerosis: a review of the potential of combination therapy. Expert Opinion on Pharmacotherapy, 5(2), 459–468. https://doi.org/10.1517/14656566.5.2.459

Kaku, M. (2015). The Future of the Mind: The Scientific Quest to Understand, Enhance, and Empower the Mind. New York, United States of America: Anchor Books, a division of Random House LLC.

Kali, A. (2015). Antibiotics and bioactive natural products in treatment of methicillin resistant Staphylococcus aureus: A brief review. Pharmacognosy Reviews, 9(17), 29. https://doi.org/10.4103/0973-7847.156329

Kandel, E. R., Schwartz, J. H., & Jessell, T. M. (1991). Principles of Neural Science (3rd ed.). Retrieved from http://citeseerx.ist.psu.edu/viewdoc/download?doi=10.1.1.470.551&rep=rep1&type=pdf

Kanherkar, R. R., Bhatia-Dey, N., & Csoka, A. B. (2014). Epigenetics across the human lifespan. Frontiers in Cell and Developmental Biology, 2. https://doi.org/10.3389/fcell.2014.00049

Kanner, L. (1943). Autistic disturbances of affective contact. Nervous Child, 2, 217–250. Retrieved from http://neurodiversity.com/library_kanner_1943.pdf

Kansra, A. R., & Donohoue, P. A. (2016). Nelson Textbook of Pediatrics, 2-Volume Set. In R. M. Kliegman, B. F. Stanton, J. W. St. Geme, N. F. Schor, & R. E. Behrman (Eds.), Hypofunction of the ovaries (20th ed., pp. 2743–2748). Philadelphia, USA: Elsevier Health Sciences.

Keys, T., & Hewitt, W. (1973, August 1). Endocarditis Due to Micrococci and Staphylococcus epidermidis. Retrieved from https://jamanetwork.com/journals/jamainternalmedicine/article-abstract/581642

Khalsa, K. P. (2019, August 22–25). Herbal Update: The Newest Techniques, Developments and Remedies [Presentation]. NorthWest Herb Symposium, Coupeville, WA, USA.

Khan, T., & Gurav, P. (2018). PhytoNanotechnology: Enhancing Delivery of Plant Based Anti-cancer Drugs. Frontiers in Pharmacology, 8. https://doi.org/10.3389/fphar.2017.01002

Kimera, D. (1977, September). Acquisition of a motor skill after left-hemisphere damage. - PubMed - NCBI. Retrieved March 7, 2019, from https://www.ncbi.nlm.nih.gov/pubmed/589430

King, M., & Bearman, P. (2009). Diagnostic change and the increased prevalence of autism. International Journal of Epidemiology, 38(5), 1224–1234. https://doi.org/10.1093/ije/dyp261

Kingsbury, M. A. (2015). New perspectives on vasoactive intestinal polypeptide as a widespread modulator of social behavior. Current Opinion in Behavioral Sciences, 6, 139–147. https://doi.org/10.1016/j.cobeha.2015.11.003

Klepeis, N. E., Nelson, W. C., Ott, W. R., Robinson, J. P., Tsang, A. M., Switzer, P., … Engelmann, W. H. (2001). The National Human Activity Pattern Survey (NHAPS): a resource for assessing exposure to environmental pollutants. Journal of Exposure Science & Environmental Epidemiology, 11(3), 231–252. https://doi.org/10.1038/sj.jea.7500165

Klin, A., McPartland, J., & Volkmar, F. (2005). Asperger syndrome. In F. Volkmar et al. (Eds.), Handbook of Autism and Pervasive Developmental Disorders (pp.88-125). Hoboken, NJ: John Wiley & Sons. (pg.99)

Kloos, W., & Bannerman, T. (1994, January). Update on clinical significance of coagulase-negative staphylococci.. Retrieved from https://www.ncbi.nlm.nih.gov/pmc/articles/PMC358308/

Kloos, W., & George, C. (1991). Identification of Staphylococcus Species and Subspecies with the MicroScan Pos ID and Rapid Pos ID Panel Systems. Journal of Clinical Microbiology, 29(4), 738–744. Retrieved from https://pdfs.semanticscholar.org/e3e2/cc732646f6314b7082b97b3b7f846271bf06.pdf

Kloos, W., & Jorgensen, J. (1985). Manual of Clinical Microbiology. In E. H. Lennette, & ORG. American Society for Microbiology (Eds.), Staphylococci (4th ed., pp. 145–147). Washington D.C., United States of America: American Society for Microbiology.

Kloos, W., & Schleifer, K. (1975, January). Simplified scheme for routine identification of human Staphylococcus species.. Retrieved from https://www.ncbi.nlm.nih.gov/pmc/articles/PMC274946/

Knapton, S. (2019, March 14). Harvard University uncovers DNA switch that controls genes for whole-body regeneration. Retrieved from https://sg.news.yahoo.com/harvard-university-uncovers-dna-switch-180000109.html

Knierim, J. (1997). Chapter 4: Basal Ganglia. In Department of Neurobiology and Anatomy, McGovern Medical School at UTHealth (Ed.), Neuroscience Electronic Textbook (pp. 35–35). Retrieved from https://nba.uth.tmc.edu/neuroscience/m/s3/chapter04.html

Koehler, B. (2007, April 16). Integration instead of separation the a little different access to the healing. Retrieved from http://www.infrafit.ro/wp-content/uploads/Bodo_Koehler_Samen_Genezen.pdf

Koehler, B. (2007). Life Supporting Medicine & BIT (Bio-physical Information Therapy) [Video]. Retrieved from http://lifesupportingmedicine.com/about_chapters.html

Koehler, B. (2020). Textbook for the UNITED life supporting MEDICINE: Volume 2. Norderstedt, Germany: Books on Demand.

Koinig, H., Wallner, T., Marhofer, P., Andel, H., Horauf, K., & Mayer, N. (1998). Magnesium Sulfate Reduces Intra- and Postoperative Analgesic Requirements. Anesthesia & Analgesia, 87(1), 206–210. https://doi.org/10.1097/00000539-199807000-00042

Kong, D.-X., Li, X.-J., & Zhang, H.-Y. (2009). Where is the hope for drug discovery? Let history tell the future. Drug Discovery Today, 14(3–4), 115–119. https://doi.org/10.1016/j.drudis.2008.07.002

Kontoyiannis, D. P., & Lewis, R. E. (2014). Treatment Principles for the Management of Mold Infections. Cold Spring Harbor Perspectives in Medicine, 5(4), a019737. https://doi.org/10.1101/cshperspect.a019737

Konuspayeva, G., Faye, B., Loiseau, G., & Levieux, D. (2007). Lactoferrin and Immunoglobulin Contents in Camel's Milk (Camelus bactrianus, Camelus dromedarius, and Hybrids) from Kazakhstan. Journal of Dairy Science, 90(1), 38–46. https://doi.org/10.3168/jds.S0022-0302(07)72606-1

Koob, G. F., Moal, M. L., & Thompson, R. F. (2010). Encyclopedia of Behavioral Neuroscience. San Diego, USA: Elsevier Science.

Kotchoubey, B. (2018). Human Consciousness: Where Is It From and What Is It for. Frontiers in Psychology, 9. https://doi.org/10.3389/fpsyg.2018.00567

Kottow, M. H. (1980). A medical definition of disease. Medical Hypotheses, 6(2), 209–213. https://doi.org/10.1016/0306-9877(80)90085-7

Kulik, E., Lenkeit, K., & Meyer, J. (2000). Antimicrobial effects of tea tree oil (Melaleuca alternifolia) on oral microorganisms. Schweiz Monatsschr Zahnmed, 110(11), 125–130. Retrieved from https://www.ncbi.nlm.nih.gov/pubmed/11374358

Kwieciński, J., Eick, S., & Wójcik, K. (2009). Effects of tea tree (Melaleuca alternifolia) oil on Staphylococcus aureus in biofilms and stationary growth phase. International Journal of Antimicrobial Agents, 33(4), 343–347. https://doi.org/10.1016/j.ijantimicag.2008.08.028

Lad, V. (2002). Textbook of Ayurveda. Albuquerque, USA: Amsterdam University Press.

Lafyatis, R. (2014). Transforming growth factor β—at the centre of systemic sclerosis. Nature Reviews Rheumatology, 10(12), 706–719. https://doi.org/10.1038/nrrheum.2014.137

Lam, F. F., Seto, S. W., Kwan, Y. W., Yeung, J. H. K., & Chan, P. (2006). Activation of the iberiotoxin-sensitive BKCa channels by salvianolic acid B of the porcine coronary artery smooth muscle cells. European Journal of Pharmacology, 546(1–3), 28–35. https://doi.org/10.1016/j.ejphar.2006.07.038

Larsson, E., & Wright, S. (2011). O. Ivar Lovaas (1927–2010). Retrieved from https://www.ncbi.nlm.nih.gov/pmc/articles/PMC3089401/

Ledon-Rettig, C. C., Richards, C. L., & Martin, L. B. (2012). Epigenetics for behavioral ecologists. Behavioral Ecology, 24(2), 311–324. https://doi.org/10.1093/beheco/ars145

Leonard, S. S., Cutler, D., Ding, M., Vallyathan, V., Castranova, V., & Shi, X. (2002). Antioxidant Properties of Fruit and Vegetable Juices: More to the Story than Ascorbic Acid. Annals of Clinical & Laboratory Science, 32(2), 193–200. Retrieved from http://www.annclinlabsci.org/content/32/2/193.long

Le Thuc, O., Stobbe, K., Cansell, C., Nahon, J., Blondeau, N., & Rovère, C. (2017). Hypothalamic Inflammation and Energy Balance Disruptions: Spotlight on Chemokines. Frontiers in Endocrinology, 8. Retrieved from https://www.frontiersin.org/articles/10.3389/fendo.2017.00197/full

Lett, D. (2007). Vaccine autism link discounted, but effect of "study" is unknown. Canadian Medical Association Journal, 177(8), 841–841. https://doi.org/10.1503/cmaj.071199

Letterio, J. J., & Roberts, A. B. (1998). REGULATION OF IMMUNE RESPONSES BY TGF-β. Annual Review of Immunology, 16(1), 137–161. https://doi.org/10.1146/annurev.immunol.16.1.137

Leuchte, H. H., Prechtl, C., Callegari, J., Meis, T., Haziraj, S., Bevec, D., & Behr, J. (2015). Augmentation of the effects of vasoactive intestinal peptide aerosol on pulmonary hypertension via coapplication of a neutral endopeptidase 24.11 inhibitor. American Journal of Physiology-Lung Cellular and Molecular Physiology, 308(6), L563–L568. https://doi.org/10.1152/ajplung.00317.2014

Levy, A., Steiner, L., & Yagil, R. (2013). Camel Milk: Disease Control and Dietary Laws. Journal of Health Science, (1), 48–53. Retrieved from https://pdfs.semanticscholar.org/09ab/1563ccc942dc8dde23c895d9ba46294754d4.pdf

Lewicka, M., Henrykowska, G. A., Pacholski, K., Śmigielski, J., Rutkowski, M., Dziedziczak-Buczyńska, M., & Buczyński, A. (2015). The effect of electromagnetic radiation emitted by display screens on cell oxygen metabolism – in vitro studies. Archives of Medical Science, 6, 1330–1339. https://doi.org/10.5114/aoms.2015.56362

Lewis, R. (2013). Paracelsus. Retrieved from https://5482ff13812fff93b4b0-f30566d4c910ec79e48ff03c503d3718.ssl.cf5.rackcdn.com/03_rmlewis.pdf

Lewis, S., Dove, A., Robbins, T., Barker, R., & Owen, A. (2004, February). Striatal contributions to working memory: a functional magnetic resonance imaging study in humans. - PubMed - NCBI. Retrieved April 4, 2019, from https://www.ncbi.nlm.nih.gov/pubmed/14984425

Liao, F., Folsom, A. R., & Brancati, F. L. (1998). Is low magnesium concentration a risk factor for coronary heart disease? The Atherosclerosis Risk in Communities (ARIC) Study. American Heart Journal, 136(3), 480–490. https://doi.org/10.1016/s0002-8703(98)70224-8

Littman, D. R., & Pamer, E. G. (2011). Role of the Commensal Microbiota in Normal and Pathogenic Host Immune Responses. Cell Host & Microbe, 10(4), 311–323. https://doi.org/10.1016/j.chom.2011.10.004

Liu, Y., Li, S., & Wu, Y. (2003). Advances in the study of Eucalyptus globulus Labill. Zhong Yao Cai, 26(6), 461–463.

Lloyd, S. (2011). Quantum coherence in biological systems. Journal of Physics: Conference Series, 302, 012037. https://doi.org/10.1088/1742-6596/302/1/012037

Loden, J. (2016, May 13). Tennessee Poison Center at Vanderbilt sees rise in children ingesting essential oils. Retrieved from http://news.vumc.org/2016/05/10/tennessee-poison-center-at-vanderbilt-sees-rise-in-children-ingesting-essential-oils/

Longmore, M., Wilkinson, I., Baldwin, A., & Wallin, E. (2014). Oxford Handbook of Clinical Medicine. OUP Oxford.

Lonsdale, D. (2006). A Review of the Biochemistry, Metabolism and Clinical Benefits of Thiamin(e) and Its Derivatives. Evidence-Based Complementary and Alternative Medicine, 3(1), 49–59. https://doi.org/10.1093/ecam/nek009

Lovaas, O. I. (1987). Behavioral treatment and normal educational and intellectual functioning in young autistic children. Journal of Consulting and Clinical Psychology, 55(1), 3–9. Retrieved from https://www.beca-aba.com/articles-and-forms/lovaas-1987.pdf

Loza-Correa M, Ayala JA, Perelman I, Hubbard K, Kalab M, Yi Q-L, et al. (2019) The peptidoglycan and biofilm matrix of Staphylococcus epidermidis undergo structural changes when exposed to human platelets. PLoS ONE 14(1): e0211132. https://doi.org/10.1371/journal.pone.0211132

Lu, J. F., & Nightingale, C. H. (2000). Magnesium Sulfate in Eclampsia and Pre-Eclampsia. Clinical Pharmacokinetics, 38(4), 305–314. https://doi.org/10.2165/00003088-200038040-00002

Maertens, J. A. (2004). History of the development of azole derivatives. Clinical Microbiology and Infection, 1–10. Retrieved from https://www.ncbi.nlm.nih.gov/pubmed/14748798

Mahaki, H., Tanzadehpanah, H., Jabarivasal, N., Sardanian, K., & Zamani, A. (2018). A review on the effects of extremely low frequency electromagnetic field (ELF-EMF) on cytokines of innate and adaptive immunity. Electromagnetic Biology and Medicine, 38(1), 84–95. https://doi.org/10.1080/15368378.2018.1545668

Malaz Boustani, M. (2009). The cognitive impact of anticholinergics: A clinical review. Clinical Interventions in Aging, 225. https://doi.org/10.2147/cia.s5358

Mangin, M., Sinha, R., & Fincher, K. (2014). Inflammation and vitamin D: the infection connection. Inflammation Research, 63(10), 803–819. https://doi.org/10.1007/s00011-014-0755-z

Marais, A., Adams, B., Ringsmuth, A. K., Ferretti, M., Gruber, J. M., Hendrikx, R., ... van Grondelle, R. (2018). The future of quantum biology. Journal of The Royal Society Interface, 15(148), 20180640. https://doi.org/10.1098/rsif.2018.0640

Margaret McCarthy, M. M., & Nugent, B. (2015). Epigenetic influences on the developing brain: effects of hormones and nutrition. Advances in Genomics and Genetics, 215. https://doi.org/10.2147/agg.s58625

Marzec, N. S., Nelson, C., Waldron, P. R., Blackburn, B. G., Hosain, S., Greenhow, T., Green, G. M., Lomen-Hoerth, C., Golden, M., & Mead, P. S. (2017). Serious Bacterial Infections Acquired During Treatment of Patients Given a Diagnosis of Chronic Lyme Disease — United States. MMWR. Morbidity and Mortality Weekly Report, 66(23), 607–609. https://doi.org/10.15585/mmwr.mm6623a3

Margulis, L. (2006). The Conscious Cell. Annals of the New York Academy of Sciences, 929(1), 55–70. https://doi.org/10.1111/j.1749-6632.2001.tb05707.x

Massé, D., Saady, N., & Gilbert, Y. (2014). Potential of Biological Processes to Eliminate Antibiotics in Livestock Manure: An Overview. Animals, 4(2), 146–163. https://doi.org/10.3390/ani4020146

Massey, R. C., Horsburgh, M. J., Lina, G., Höök, M., & Recker, M. (2006). The evolution and maintenance of virulence in Staphylococcus aureus: a role for host-to-host transmission? Nature Reviews Microbiology, 4(12), 953–958. https://doi.org/10.1038/nrmicro1551

Matson, J. L., & Williams, L. W. (2013). Differential diagnosis and comorbidity: distinguishing autism from other mental health issues. Neuropsychiatry, 3(2), 233–243. https://doi.org/10.2217/NPY.13.1

May, J., Chan, C., King, A., Williams, L., & French, G. L. (2000). Time-kill studies of tea tree oils on clinical isolates. Journal of Antimicrobial Chemotherapy, 45(5), 639–643. https://doi.org/10.1093/jac/45.5.639

McMahon, S. (2013). Dr. Shoemaker's 11 Step Treatment Protocol. Retrieved from https://www.survivingmold.com/docs/McMahon_11_Step_Biotoxin_Elimination_Pathway_Essay.pdf

McMillin, M. A., Frampton, G. A., Seiwell, A. P., Patel, N. S., Jacobs, A. N., & DeMorrow, S. (2015). TGFβ1 exacerbates blood–brain barrier permeability in a mouse model of hepatic encephalopathy via upregulation of MMP9 and downregulation of claudin-5. Laboratory Investigation, 95(8), 903–913. https://doi.org/10.1038/labinvest.2015.70

McTaggart, L. (2008). The Field Updated Ed: The Quest for the Secret Force of the Universe. New York, United States of America: HarperCollins.

Mehta, N. D., Haroon, E., Xu, X., Woolwine, B. J., Li, Z., & Felger, J. C. (2018). Inflammation negatively correlates with amygdala-ventromedial prefrontal functional connectivity in association with anxiety in patients with depression: Preliminary results. Brain, Behavior, and Immunity, 73, 725–730. Retrieved from https://www.ncbi.nlm.nih.gov/pubmed/30076980

Meki, A. R., Abdel-Ghaffar, S. K., & El-Gibaly, I. (2001). Aflatoxin B1 induces apoptosis in rat liver: protective effect of melatonin. Neuro Endocrinology Letters, 22(6), 417–426. Retrieved from https://www.ncbi.nlm.nih.gov/pubmed/11781538/

Mellor, I. R., Thomas, D. H., & Sansom, M. S. (1988). Properties of ion channels formed by Staphylococcus aureus δ-toxin. Biochimica et Biophysica Acta (BBA) - Biomembranes, 942(2), 280–294. https://doi.org/10.1016/0005-2736(88)90030-2

Menestrina, G., Bashford, C., & Pasternak, C. (1990). Pore-forming toxins: Experiments with S. aureus α-toxin, C. perfringens θ-toxin and E. coli haemolysin in lipid bilayers, liposomes and intact cells. Toxicon, 28(5), 477–491. https://doi.org/10.1016/0041-0101(90)90292-f

Merin, U., Bernstein, S., Bloch-Damti, A., Yagil, R., van Creveld, C., Lindner, P., & Gollop, N. (2001). A comparative study of milk serum proteins in camel (Camelus dromedarius) and bovine colostrum. Livestock Production Science, 67(3), 297–301. https://doi.org/10.1016/S0301-6226(00)00198-6

Michigan Medicine - University of Michigan. (2019, April 14). 'Superbugs' found on many hospital patients' hands and what they touch most often. ScienceDaily. Retrieved from www.sciencedaily.com/releases/2019/04/190414111500.htm

Miller, G. T. (2006). Living in the Environment: Principles, Connections, and Solutions. Belmont, United States of America: Cengage Learning.

Millington, G., Tung, Y., Hewson, A., O'Rahilly, S., & Dickson, S. (2001). Differential effects of α-, β- and γ2-melanocyte-stimulating hormones on hypothalamic neuronal activation and feeding in the fasted rat. Neuroscience, 108(3), 437–445. https://doi.org/10.1016/s0306-4522(01)00428-6

Mills-Robertson, F. C., Tay, S. C. K., Duker-Eshun, G., Walana, W., & Badu, K. (2012). In vitro antimicrobial activity of ethanolic fractions of Cryptolepis sanguinolenta. Annals of Clinical Microbiology and Antimicrobials, 11(1), 16. https://doi.org/10.1186/1476-0711-11-16

Molchan, S. E., Martinez, R. A., Hill, J. L., Weingartner, H. J., Thompson, K., Vitiello, B., & Sunderland, T. (1992). Increased cognitive sensitivity to scopolamine with age and a perspective on the scopolamine model. Brain Research Reviews, 17(3), 215–226. https://doi.org/10.1016/0165-0173(92)90017-g

Moore, L. D., Le, T., & Fan, G. (2012). DNA Methylation and Its Basic Function. Neuropsychopharmacology, 38(1), 23–38. https://doi.org/10.1038/npp.2012.112

Moore, M. (1995). Herbal Formulas For Clinic And Home (2nd ed.). Retrieved from http://www.swsbm.com/ManualsMM/Formulary2.pdf

Mordor Intelligence. (n.d.). Glyphosate Market | Growth, Trends, and Forecast (2019-2024). Retrieved from https://www.mordorintelligence.com/industry-reports/glyphosate-herbicide-market

Morones-Ramirez, J. R., Winkler, J. A., Spina, C. S., & Collins, J. J. (2013). Silver Enhances Antibiotic Activity Against Gram-Negative Bacteria. Science Translational Medicine, 5(190), 190ra81-190ra81. https://doi.org/10.1126/scitranslmed.3006276

Mountjoy, K. G., Caron, A., Hubbard, K., Shome, A., Grey, A. C., Sun, B., . . . Elmquist, J. K. (2018). Desacetyl-α-melanocyte stimulating hormone and α-melanocyte stimulating hormone are required to regulate energy balance. Molecular Metabolism, 9, 207–216. https://doi.org/10.1016/j.molmet.2017.11.008

Murthy, K. S., & Grider, J. R. (2013). VIP. Handbook of Biologically Active Peptides, 1354–1360. https://doi.org/10.1016/B978-0-12-385095-9.00184-6

Musto, J., Hrabec, G., & Moin, E. (2020). Report on the Effectiveness of the Antimicrobial Formula 1 NSB in Treating Multiple Antibiotic Resistant Coagulase Negative Staphylococcus (MARCoNS). Bedford, United States: MicrobiologyDX.

Nagel, T. (1974). What Is It Like to Be a Bat? The Philosophical Review, 83(4), 435. https://doi.org/10.2307/2183914

Nakatomi, Y., Mizuno, K., Ishii, A., Wada, Y., Tanaka, M., Tazawa, S., ... Watanabe, Y. (2014). Neuroinflammation in Patients with Chronic Fatigue Syndrome/Myalgic Encephalomyelitis: An 11C-(R)-PK11195 PET Study. Journal of Nuclear Medicine, 55(6), 945–950. Retrieved from http://jnm.snmjournals.org/content/55/6/945

National Center for Complementary and Integrative Health. (n.d.). Natural Products. Retrieved April 25, 2019, from https://nccih.nih.gov/taxonomy/term/8

National Center for Complementary and Integrative Health. (2017, September 24). Aromatherapy. Retrieved from https://nccih.nih.gov/health/aromatherapy

National Institutes of Health. (2002, December 20). NIH Guide: RESEARCH ON MICROBIAL BIOFILMS. Retrieved March 14, 2019, from https://grants.nih.gov/grants/guide/pa-files/pa-03-047.html

National Institutes of Health. (2018, November 28). Insights into MRSA Epidemic. Retrieved April 28, 2019, from https://www.nih.gov/news-events/nih-research-matters/insights-into-mrsa-epidemic

National Institutes of Health. (2019, April 10). National Center for Complementary and Integrative Health (NCCIH). Retrieved from https://www.nih.gov/about-nih/what-we-do/nih-almanac/national-center-complementary-integrative-health-nccih

National Organization of Rare Disorders. (2018, May 3). Mastocytosis. Retrieved from https://rarediseases.org/rare-diseases/mastocytosis/

National Women's Health Network. (2017, June 2). Are my breast implants causing my health problems? Retrieved from https://nwhn.org/breast-implants-causing-health-problems/

Nauser, T. D., & Stites, S. W. (2001, May 1). Diagnosis and Treatment of Pulmonary Hypertension. Retrieved from https://www.aafp.org/afp/2001/0501/p1789.html

New Directions Aromatics Inc. (2017, March 20). A Comprehensive Guide to Essential Oil Extraction Methods. Retrieved from https://www.newdirectionsaromatics.com/blog/articles/how-essential-oils-are-made.html

Newman, T. (2011, February 18). How do penicillins work? Retrieved from https://www.medicalnewstoday.com/articles/216798.php

Newman, T. (2017, November 17). How the immune system works. Retrieved from https://www.medicalnewstoday.com/articles/320101.php

Newsom, S. W. B. (2004). MRSA--past, present, future. JRSM, 97(11), 509–510. https://dx.doi.org/10.1258%2Fjrsm.97.11.509

Newton, W. (2001). Rationalism and Empiricism in Modern Medicine. Law and Contemporary Problems, 64(4), 299. https://doi.org/10.2307/1192299

NICHD - Eunice Kennedy Shriver National Institute of Child Health and Human Development. (2017, June 2). Early Intervention for Autism. Retrieved from https://www.nichd.nih.gov/health/topics/autism/conditioninfo/treatments/early-intervention

Nirmal, S. A., Pal, S. C., Otimenyin, S., Aye, T., Mostafa, E., Kundu, S., ... Mandal, S. (2013). Contribution of Herbal Products In Global Market. The Pharma Review, 95–104. Retrieved from https://www.researchgate.net/publication/320357308_Contribution_of_Herbal_Products_In_Global_Market

Norris, D. (2017). Short-term memory and long-term memory are still different. Psychological Bulletin, 143(9), 992–1009. Retrieved from https://www.ncbi.nlm.nih.gov/pmc/articles/PMC5578362/

Norton, J. D. (2017, February 14). Euclidean Geometry. Retrieved from https://www.pitt.edu/%7Ejdnorton/teaching/HPS_0410/chapters/non_Euclid_Euclid/index.html

O'Dwyer, L., Tanner, C., van Dongen, E. V., Greven, C. U., Bralten, J., Zwiers, M. P., ... Buitelaar, J. K. (2016). Decreased Left Caudate Volume Is Associated with Increased Severity of Autistic-Like Symptoms in a Cohort of ADHD Patients and Their Unaffected Siblings. PLOS ONE, 11(11). https://doi.org/10.1371/journal.pone.0165620

Occupational Safety and Health Administration. (2013, November 8). Safety and Health Information Bulletins | A Brief Guide to Mold in the Workplace | Occupational Safety and Health Administration. Retrieved from https://www.osha.gov/dts/shib/shib101003.html

Offit, P. A. (2008). Autism's False Prophets: Bad Science, Risky Medicine, and the Search for a Cure. New York, USA: Columbia University Press.

Oliva, A., Costantini, S., De Angelis, M., Garzoli, S., Božović, M., Mascellino, M., ... Ragno, R. (2018). High Potency of Melaleuca alternifolia Essential Oil against Multi-Drug Resistant Gram-Negative Bacteria and Methicillin-Resistant Staphylococcus aureus. Molecules, 23(10), 2584. https://doi.org/10.3390/molecules23102584

Oncul, S., Cuce, E. M., Aksu, B., & Inhan Garip, A. (2015). Effect of extremely low frequency electromagnetic fields on bacterial membrane. International Journal of Radiation Biology, 92(1), 42–49. https://doi.org/10.3109/09553002.2015.1101500

Osafo, N., Mensah, K. B., & Yeboah, O. K. (2017). Phytochemical and Pharmacological Review of Cryptolepis sanguinolenta (Lindl.) Schlechter. Advances in Pharmacological Sciences, 2017, 1–13. https://doi.org/10.1155/2017/3026370

Page AV, Liles WC. Posaconazole: a new agent for the prevention and management of severe, refractory or invasive fungal infections. Can J Infect Dis Med Microbiol. 2008:297–305.

Pal, S. (2016, December 1). J C Bose: The Little Known Story of How India's First Biophysicist Proved Plants Have Life. Retrieved from https://www.thebetterindia.com/76587/jagdish-chandra-bose-indian-biophysicist-radio-plant-physiology/

Panda, S., & Ding, J. L. (2014). Natural Antibodies Bridge Innate and Adaptive Immunity. The Journal of Immunology, 194(1), 13–20. https://doi.org/10.4049/jimmunol.1400844

Paulo, A., Duarte, A., & Gomes, E. T. (1994). In vitro antibacterial screening of Cryptolepis sanguinolenta alkaloids. Journal of Ethnopharmacology, 44(2), 127–130. https://doi.org/10.1016/0378-8741(94)90079-5

Pei, L., & Flock, J. (2001). Lack of fbe, the gene for a fibrinogen-binding protein from Staphylococcus epidermidis, reduces its adherence to fibrinogen coated surfaces. Microbial Pathogenesis, 31(4), 185–193. https://doi.org/10.1006/mpat.2001.0462

Penetar, D. M., Toto, L. H., Lee, D. Y. W., & Lukas, S. E. (2015). A single dose of kudzu extract reduces alcohol consumption in a binge drinking paradigm. Drug and Alcohol Dependence, 153, 194–200. https://doi.org/10.1016/j.drugalcdep.2015.05.025

Peng, Q., Li, K., Sacks, S., & Zhou, W. (2009). The Role of Anaphylatoxins C3a and C5a in Regulating Innate and Adaptive Immune Responses. Inflammation & Allergy - Drug Targets, 8(3), 236–246. https://doi.org/10.2174/187152809788681038

Peralta, V., & Cuesta, M. J. (2011). Eugen Bleuler and the Schizophrenias: 100 Years After. Schizophrenia Bulletin, 37(6), 1118–1120. https://doi.org/10.1093/schbul/sbr126

Pharmacy Solution. (n.d.). Drug Induced Nutrient Depletion. Retrieved from https://pharmacysolutionsonline.com/drug-induced-nutrient-depletion.php

Pope, C. (2003). Resisting Evidence: The Study of Evidence-Based Medicine as a Contemporary Social Movement. Health: An Interdisciplinary Journal for the Social Study of Health, Illness and Medicine, 7(3), 267–282. https://doi.org/10.1177/1363459303007003002

Popkin, B. M. (2002). Part II. What is unique about the experience in lower-and middle-income less-industrialised countries compared with the very-high income industrialised countries? Public Health Nutrition, 5(1a), 205–214. https://doi.org/10.1079/phn2001295

Popp, F. A., Nagl, W., Li, K. H., Scholz, W., Weingärtner, O., & Wolf, R. (1984). Biophoton emission. Cell Biophysics, 6(1), 33–52. https://doi.org/10.1007/BF02788579

Popp F.A., (1999) About the coherence of biophotons. In: Sassaroli E, Srivastava Y, Swain J, Widom A., eds. Macroscopic Quantum Coherence. River Edge, NJ: World Scientific.

Powell, A. (2008, January 9). Chromosomal abnormality linked to autism disorders. The Harvard Gazette. Retrieved from https://news.harvard.edu/gazette/story/2008/01/chromosomal-abnormality-linked-to-autism-disorders/

Prousky, J. (2008). The Treatment of Pulmonary Diseases and Respiratory-Related Conditions with Inhaled (Nebulized or Aerosolized) Glutathione. Evidence-Based Complementary and Alternative Medicine, 5(1), 27–35. https://doi.org/10.1093/ecam/nem040

Qin, Z., Ou, Y., Yang, L., Zhu, Y., Tolker-Nielsen, T., Molin, S., & Qu, D. (2007). Role of autolysin-mediated DNA release in biofilm formation of Staphylococcus epidermidis. Microbiology, 153(7), 2083–2092. https://doi.org/10.1099/mic.0.2007/006031-0

Qin, Z., Yang, X., Yang, L., Jiang, J., Ou, Y., Molin, S., & Qu, D. (2007). Formation and properties of in vitro biofilms of ica-negative Staphylococcus epidermidis clinical isolates. Journal of Medical Microbiology, 56(1), 83–93. https://doi.org/10.1099/jmm.0.46799-0

Radtke, K. M., Ruf, M., Gunter, H. M., Dohrmann, K., Schauer, M., Meyer, A., & Elbert, T. (2011). Transgenerational impact of intimate partner violence on methylation in the promoter of the glucocorticoid receptor. Translational Psychiatry, 1(7), e21–e21. https://doi.org/10.1038/tp.2011.21

Rago, J., Vath, G., Tripp, T., Bohach, G., Ohlendorf, D., & Schlievert, P. (2000, April). Staphylococcal Exfoliative Toxins Cleave α- and β-Melanocyte-Stimulating Hormones. Retrieved from https://www.ncbi.nlm.nih.gov/pmc/articles/PMC97430/

Raman, A., Weir, U., & Bloomfield, S. F. (1995). Antimicrobial effects of tea-tree oil and its major components on Staphylococcus aureus, Staph. epidermidis and Propionibacterium acnes. Letters in Applied Microbiology, 21(4), 242–245. https://doi.org/10.1111/j.1472-765X.1995.tb01051.x

Ravizza, S. M., Solomon, M., Ivry, R. B., & Carter, C. S. (2013). Restricted and repetitive behaviors in autism spectrum disorders: The relationship of attention and motor deficits. Development and Psychopathology, 25(3), 773–784. https://doi.org/10.1017/S0954579413000163

Ray, P., & Gupta, H. (1965). Caraka Samhita: A Scientific Synopsis. Retrieved from https://archive.org/details/CarakaSamhitaAScientificSynopsis

Raymond, C. A., Davies, N. W., & Larkman, T. (2017). GC-MS method validation and levels of methyl eugenol in a diverse range of tea tree (Melaleuca alternifolia) oils. Analytical and Bioanalytical Chemistry, 409(7), 1779–1787. https://doi.org/10.1007/s00216-016-0134-4

Reed, J. C. (1990). Magnesium therapy in musculoskeletal pain syndromes retrospective review of clinical results. Magnesium Trace Elem, 9, 330.

Reiersen, A. M., & Todd, R. D. (2008). Co-occurrence of ADHD and autism spectrum disorders: phenomenology and treatment. Expert Review of Neurotherapeutics, 8(4), 657–669. https://doi.org/10.1586/14737175.8.4.657

Reifschneider, K., Auble, B., & Rose, S. (2015). Update of Endocrine Dysfunction following Pediatric Traumatic Brain Injury. Journal of Clinical Medicine, 4(8), 1536–1560. Retrieved from https://pdfs.semanticscholar.org/8c82/6ccc382241803ece150cc194fc8e940b20ee.pdf

Resch, A., Rosenstein, R., Nerz, C., & Gotz, F. (2005). Differential Gene Expression Profiling of Staphylococcus aureus Cultivated under Biofilm and Planktonic Conditions. Applied and Environmental Microbiology, 71(5), 2663–2676. https://doi.org/10.1128/aem.71.5.2663-2676.2005

Revathi, M., Senthilkumar, G., Panneerselvam, A., Karthy, E. S., & Gopika, R. (2016). In Vitro Assessment of Terminalia chebula Retz. Fruits Against Methicillin Resistant Staphylococcus aureus. International Journal of Pharma Sciences and Research, 7(11). Retrieved from http://www.ijpsr.info/docs/IJPSR16-07-11-007.pdf

Reynolds, L. A., & Tansey, E. M. (2008). Superbugs and Superdrugs: A history of MRSA. Wellcome Witnesses to Twentieth Century Medicine, vol. 32. London: Wellcome Trust Centre for the History of Medicine at UCL (Rev. ed.). Retrieved from http://www.histmodbiomed.org/sites/default/files/44862.pdf

Rice, K. C., Mann, E. E., Endres, J. L., Weiss, E. C., Cassat, J. E., Smeltzer, M. S., & Bayles, K. W. (2007). The cidA murein hydrolase regulator contributes to DNA release and biofilm development in Staphylococcus aureus. Proceedings of the National Academy of Sciences, 104(19), 8113–8118. https://doi.org/10.1073/pnas.0610226104

Richards, E. J. (2006). Inherited epigenetic variation — revisiting soft inheritance. Nature Reviews Genetics, 7(5), 395–401. https://doi.org/10.1038/nrg1834

Roberts, J. A., Kruger, P., Paterson, D. L., & Lipman, J. (2008). Antibiotic resistance—What's dosing got to do with it? Critical Care Medicine, 36(8), 2433–2440. https://doi.org/10.1097/ccm.0b013e318180fe62

Rohde, H., Burandt, E. C., Siemssen, N., Frommelt, L., Burdelski, C., Wurster, S., . . . Mack, D. (2007). Polysaccharide intercellular adhesin or protein factors in biofilm accumulation of Staphylococcus epidermidis and Staphylococcus aureus isolated from prosthetic hip and knee joint infections. Biomaterials, 28(9), 1711–1720. https://doi.org/10.1016/j.biomaterials.2006.11.046

Ronaldson, P. T., DeMarco, K. M., Sanchez-Covarrubias, L., Solinsky, C. M., & Davis, T. P. (2009). Transforming Growth Factor-β Signaling Alters Substrate Permeability and Tight Junction Protein Expression at the Blood-Brain Barrier during Inflammatory Pain. Journal of Cerebral Blood Flow & Metabolism, 29(6), 1084–1098. https://doi.org/10.1038/jcbfm.2009.32

Rosenberg, W., & Donald, A. (1995). Evidence based medicine: an approach to clinical problem-solving. BMJ, 310(6987), 1122–1126. https://doi.org/10.1136/bmj.310.6987.1122

Rosenstein, R., Nerz, C., Biswas, L., Resch, A., Raddatz, G., Schuster, S., & Götz, F. (2009, February). Genome Analysis of the Meat Starter Culture Bacterium Staphylococcus carnosus TM300. Retrieved from https://www.ncbi.nlm.nih.gov/pmc/articles/PMC2632126/

Rubbia, C. Nobel Lecture. The Nobel Prize in Physics 1984. Retrieved from https://www.nobelprize.org/uploads/2018/06/rubbia-lecture.pdf

Rupp, M., & Archer, G. (1994). Coagulase-Negative Staphylococci: Pathogens Associated with Medical Progress. Clinical Infectious Diseases, 19(2), 231–245. https://doi.org/10.1093/clinids/19.2.231

Russell, Deb. (2019, January 21). Bell Curve and Normal Distribution Definition. Retrieved from https://www.thoughtco.com/bell-curve-normal-distribution-defined-2312350

Rustenhoven, J., Aalderink, M., Scotter, E. L., Oldfield, R. L., Bergin, P. S., Mee, E. W., … Dragunow, M. (2016). TGF-beta1 regulates human brain pericyte inflammatory processes involved in neurovasculature function. Journal of Neuroinflammation, 13(1). https://doi.org/10.1186/s12974-016-0503-0

Rutter, Michael, Shaffer, David, Shepherd, Michael & World Health Organization. (1975). A multi-axial classification of child psychiatric disorders : an evaluation of a proposal. World Health Organization. https://apps.who.int/iris/handle/10665/40147

Sackett, D. L., & Rosenberg, W. M. (1995). The need for evidence-based medicine. Journal of the Royal Society of Medicine, 88(11), 620–624.

Sackett, D. L., Rosenberg, W. M. C., Gray, J. A. M., Haynes, R. B., & Richardson, W. S. (1996). Evidence based medicine: what it is and what it isn't. BMJ, 312(7023), 71–72. https://doi.org/10.1136/bmj.312.7023.71

Said, S. I., Chappe, V., & Hamidi, S. A. (2013). VIP. Handbook of Biologically Active Peptides, 1535–1542. https://doi.org/10.1016/B978-0-12-385095-9.00209-8

Sajid, M., & Ilyas, M. (2017). PTFE-coated non-stick cookware and toxicity concerns: a perspective. Environmental Science and Pollution Research, 24(30), 23436–23440. https://doi.org/10.1007/s11356-017-0095-y

Salari, M. H., Amine, G., Shirazi, M. H., Hafezi, R., & Mohammadypour, M. (2006). Antibacterial effects of Eucalyptus globulus leaf extract on pathogenic bacteria isolated from specimens of patients with respiratory tract disorders. Clinical Microbiology and Infection, 12(2), 194–196. https://doi.org/10.1111/j.1469-0691.2005.01284.x

Salin, M. L., & Bridges, S. M. (1981). Chemiluminescence in Wounded Root Tissue : Evidence For Peroxidase Involvement. Plant Physiology, 67(1), 43–46. https://doi.org/10.1104/pp.67.1.43

Sallows, G. O., & Graupner, T. D. (2005). Intensive Behavioral Treatment for Children With Autism: Four-Year Outcome and Predictors. American Journal on Mental Retardation, 110(6), 417. https://doi.org/https://doi.org/10.1352/0895-8017(2005)110[417:IBTFCW]2.0.CO;2

Samsel, A., & Seneff, S. (2013). Glyphosate's Suppression of Cytochrome P450 Enzymes and Amino Acid Biosynthesis by the Gut Microbiome: Pathways to Modern Diseases. Entropy, 15(12), 1416–1463. https://doi.org/10.3390/e15041416

Sanctuary, M. R., Kain, J. N., Angkustsiri, K., & German, J. B. (2018). Dietary Considerations in Autism Spectrum Disorders: The Potential Role of Protein Digestion and Microbial Putrefaction in the Gut-Brain Axis. Frontiers in Nutrition, 5. https://doi.org/10.3389/fnut.2018.00040

Sandra, F. (2018). Role of Herbal Extract in Stem Cell Development. Molecular and Cellular Biomedical Sciences, 2(1). https://doi.org/10.21705/mcbs.v2i1.19

Schaberg, D., Culver, D., & Gaynes, R. (1991). Major Trends in the Microbial Etiology of Nosocomial Infection. The American Journal of Medicine, 91(Supp 3B), 72–75. Retrieved from https://pdfs.semanticscholar.org/497d/fb0dac058bd84ecd30a91dda65c7da06378b.pdf

Schlummer, M., Sölch, C., Meisel, T., Still, M., Gruber, L., & Wolz, G. (2015). Emission of perfluoroalkyl carboxylic acids (PFCA) from heated surfaces made of polytetrafluoroethylene (PTFE) applied in food contact materials and consumer products. Chemosphere, 129, 46–53. https://doi.org/10.1016/j.chemosphere.2014.11.036

Schmid, D., Schurch, P., Belser, E., & Zulli, F. (2008). Plant Stem Cell Extract for Longevity of Skin and Hair. International Journal for Applied Science, 30–35. Retrieved from https://pdfs.semanticscholar.org/117a/4f1c63ec31bb283f3eef9c1bbb9ed5ccf408.pdf

Schnaper, H. W., Hayashida, T., Hubchak, S. C., & Poncelet, A. (2003). TGF-β signal transduction and mesangial cell fibrogenesis. American Journal of Physiology-Renal Physiology, 284(2), F243–F252. https://doi.org/10.1152/ajprenal.00300.2002

Scholey, A. B., & Kennedy, D. O. (2002). Acute, dose-dependent cognitive effects ofGinkgo biloba, Panax ginseng and their combination in healthy young volunteers: differential interactions with cognitive demand. Human Psychopharmacology: Clinical and Experimental, 17(1), 35–44. https://doi.org/10.1002/hup.352

Schombert, J. (2018). Newtonian Physics. Retrieved from http://abyss.uoregon.edu/%7Ejs/21st_century_science/lectures/lec03.html

Schreiber, J. S., Hudnell, H. K., Geller, A. M., House, D. E., Aldous, K. M., Force, M. S., … Parker, J. C. (2002). Apartment residents' and day care workers' exposures to tetrachloroethylene and deficits in visual contrast sensitivity. Environmental Health Perspectives, 110(7), 655–664. https://doi.org/10.1289/ehp.02110655

Schultz, J. C. (2002). Shared Signals and the Potential for Phylogenetic Espionage Between Plants and Animals. Integrative and Comparative Biology, 42(3), 454–462. https://doi.org/10.1093/icb/42.3.454

ScienceDirect. (2020). REM Rebound - an overview | ScienceDirect Topics. Retrieved from https://www.sciencedirect.com/topics/medicine-and-dentistry/rem-rebound

Science History Institute. (2017, December 1). Elizabeth Lee Hazen and Rachel Fuller Brown. Retrieved from https://www.sciencehistory.org/historical-profile/elizabeth-lee-hazen-and-rachel-fuller-brown

Science History Institute. (2017, December 5). Alexander Fleming. Retrieved from https://www.sciencehistory.org/historical-profile/alexander-fleming

Scoffone, H. M., Krajewski, M., Zorca, S., Bereal-Williams, C., Littel, P., Seamon, C., … Kato, G. J. (2013). Effect of Extended-Release Niacin on Serum Lipids and on Endothelial Function in Adults With Sickle Cell Anemia and Low High-Density Lipoprotein Cholesterol Levels. The American Journal of Cardiology, 112(9), 1499–1504. https://doi.org/10.1016/j.amjcard.2013.06.035

Scotti, L., Genovese, S., Bucciarelli, T., Martini, F., Epifano, F., Fiorito, S., …
Taddeo, V. A. (2018). Analysis of biologically active oxyprenylated phenylpropanoids in Tea tree oil using selective solid-phase extraction with UHPLC-PDA detection. Journal of Pharmaceutical and Biomedical Analysis, 154, 174–179. https://doi.org/10.1016/j.jpba.2018.03.004

Selander, J., & Buys, N. (2010). Sickness Absence as an Indicator of Health in Sweden. International Journal of Disability Management, 5(2), 40–47. https://doi.org/10.1375/jdmr.5.2.40

Selin, H. (2008). Encyclopaedia of the History of Science, Technology, and Medicine in Non-Western Cultures. Netherlands: Springer.

Sener, E. F., Oztop, D. B., & Ozkul, Y. (2014). MTHFRGene C677T Polymorphism in Autism Spectrum Disorders. Genetics Research International, 2014, 1–5. https://doi.org/10.1155/2014/698574

Shabo, Y., & Yagil, R. (2005). Etiology of autism and camel milk as therapy. International Journal on Disability and Human Development, 4(2). https://doi.org/10.1515/IJDHD.2005.4.2.67

Shabo, Y., Barzel, R., Margoulis, M., & Yagil, R. (2005). Camel Milk for Food Allergies in Children. Immunology and Allergies, 7, 796–798. Retrieved from https://www.researchgate.net/profile/Reuven_Yagil/publication/7388076_Camel_Milk_for_Food_Allergies_in_Children/links/572a08de08ae2efbfdbc14da/Camel-Milk-for-Food-Allergies-in-Children.pdf

Shah, S. A., Yoon, G. H., Kim, H.-O., & Kim, M. O. (2015). Vitamin C Neuroprotection Against Dose-Dependent Glutamate-Induced Neurodegeneration in the Postnatal Brain. Neurochemical Research, 40(5), 875–884. https://doi.org/10.1007/s11064-015-1540-2

Shapiro, J. (2007). Bacteria are small but not stupid: cognition, natural genetic engineering and socio-bacteriology. Studies in History and Philosophy of Science Part C: Studies in History and Philosophy of Biological and Biomedical Sciences, 38(4), 807–819. Retrieved from https://pdfs.semanticscholar.org/41bd/97eb735eff64874b5bcdf0a4f72ce0b514c9.pdf?_ga=2.21987323.191435096.1547128852-1314994624.1544805058

Sharifi-Rad, J., Salehi, B., Varoni, E. M., Sharopov, F., Yousaf, Z., Ayatollahi, S. A., … Iriti, M. (2017). Plants of the Melaleuca Genus as Antimicrobial Agents: From Farm to Pharmacy. Phytotherapy Research, 31(10), 1475–1494. https://doi.org/10.1002/ptr.5880

Shaul, P. W., Towbin, R. B., & Chernausek, S. D. (1985, May). Precocious puberty following severe head trauma. - PubMed - NCBI. Retrieved March 15, 2019, from https://www.ncbi.nlm.nih.gov/pubmed/3157313

Sheehan D.J., Hitchcock C.A. and Sibley C.M. (1999) Current and emerging azole antifungal agents. Clin. Microbiol. Rev. 12, 40–79.

Shen, W., Li, S., Chung, S. H., Zhu, L., Stayt, J., Su, T., … Gillies, M. C. (2011). Tyrosine phosphorylation of VE-cadherin and claudin-5 is associated with TGF-β1-induced permeability of centrally derived vascular endothelium. European Journal of Cell Biology, 90(4), 323–332. https://doi.org/10.1016/j.ejcb.2010.10.013

Shephard G, Burger H, Gambacorta L, Gong Y, Krska R, Rheeder J, Solfrizzo M, Srey C, Sulyok M, Visconti A, Waarth V, van der Westhuizen L. (2013) Multiple mycotoxin exposure determined by urinary biomarkers in rural subsistence farmers in the former Transkei, South Africa. Food Chem Toxicol, 62: 217-25.

Shoemaker, R. C. (1998). Pfiesteria: Crossing Dark Waters. Baltimore, United States of America: Gateway Press.

Shoemaker, R. C. (2001a). Residential and recreational acquisition of possible estuary-associated syndrome: a new approach to successful diagnosis and treatment. Environmental Health Perspectives, 109(suppl 5), 791–796. https://doi.org/10.1289/ehp.01109s5791

Shoemaker, R. C. (2001b). Desperation Medicine. Baltimore, United States of America: Gateway Press.

Shoemaker, R. (2010). Surviving Mold: Life in the Era of Dangerous Buildings. Baltimore, United States of America: Otter Bay Books.

Shoemaker, R. C. (2011). ACOEM 2011 Report Review . Retrieved from https://irp-cdn.multiscreensite.com/562d25c6/files/uploaded/GywTPxuSTmqI1M6g8s4l_Shoemaker_A%20review%20of%20ACOEM%202011%20paper.pdf

Shoemaker, R. C. (2014). Repetitive Exposure Protocol: CIRS-WDB Conference 2014 [Document provided as part of physician information packet].

Shoemaker, R. C. (2019). Use of GENIE in clinical management of CIRS patients. Retrieved from https://www.survivingmold.com/shoemaker-protocol/community/use-of-genie-in-clinical-management-of-cirs-patients

Shoemaker, R. C., Domenico, P., & Shirtliff, M. (2004). MSH Deficiency in Chronic Fatigue Syndrome Associated with Nasal Carriage of MARCoNS [Presentation slides]. Retrieved from https://www.survivingmold.com/store1/presentations/msh-deficiency-in-chronic-fatigue-syndrome-associated-with-nasal-carriage-of-marcons

Shoemaker, R. C., Giclas, P. C., Crowder, C., House, D., & Glovsky, M. M. (2008). Complement Split Products C3a and C4a Are Early Markers of Acute Lyme Disease in Tick Bite Patients in the United States. International Archives of Allergy and Immunology, 146(3), 255–261. https://doi.org/10.1159/000116362

Shoemaker, R. C., House, D., & Ryan, J. C. (2013). Vasoactive intestinal polypeptide (VIP) corrects chronic inflammatory response syndrome (CIRS) acquired following exposure to water-damaged buildings. Health, 05(03), 396–401. Retrieved from https://www.survivingmold.com/docs/VIP_published_3_2013.pdf

Shoemaker, R. C., & House, D. E. (2006). Sick building syndrome (SBS) and exposure to water-damaged buildings: Time series study, clinical trial and mechanisms. Neurotoxicology and Teratology, 28(5), 573–588. Retrieved from https://www.survivingmold.com/docs/Resources/Shoemaker%20Papers/Johanning_book_5_06.pdf

Shoemaker, R. C., House, D., & Ryan, J. C. (2014). Structural brain abnormalities in patients with inflammatory illness acquired following exposure to water-damaged buildings: A volumetric MRI study using NeuroQuant®. Neurotoxicology and Teratology, 45, 18–26. Retrieved from https://www.sciencedirect.com/science/article/pii/S0892036214001329?via%3Dihub

Shoemaker, R. C., Heyman, A., Mancia, A., & Ryan, J. (2017). Inflammation Induced Chronic Fatiguing Illnesses: A steady march towards understanding mechanisms and identifying new biomarkers and therapies.. Internal Medicine Review, 3(10). Retrieved from https://www.internalmedicinereview.org/index.php/imr/article/view/585/pdf

Shoemaker, R.C., & Hudnell, H. K. (2001). Possible estuary-associated syndrome: symptoms, vision, and treatment. Environmental Health Perspectives, 109(5), 539–545. https://doi.org/10.1289/ehp.01109539

Shoemaker, R.C., & Katz, D. (2013). BEG, CSM, VIP [DVD Training Modules]. Retrieved July 14, 2018, from https://www.survivingmold.com/

Shoemaker, R.C., Katz, D., Ackerley, M., Rapaport, S., McMahon, S., Berndtson, K., & Ryan, J. (2017). Intranasal VIP safely restores volume to multiple grey matter nuclei in patients with CIRS. Internal Medicine Review, 3(4). https://doi.org/10.18103/imr.v3i4.412

Shoemaker, R. C., & Lark, D. (2019). Urinary Mycotoxins: A Review of Contaminated Buildings and Food in Search of a Biomarker Separating Sick Patients from Controls. Internal Medicine Review, 5(6). Retrieved from https://www.survivingmold.com/Publications/Urinary_mycotoxins_10_8_19_RS_published.pdf

Shoemaker, R. C., Lark, D., & Ryan, J. (2019, October 26). Moldy Buildings, CIRS, Sick People and Damaged Brains, Part 3: 25 Years of Research Brought Us to the Cure Word. Retrieved from https://www.townsendletter.com/article/435-moldy-buildings-water-damage-cirs-antifungals/

Shoemaker, R.C., & Maizel, M.S. (2009). Innate immunity, MR spectroscopy, HLA DR, TGF-beta1, VIP and capillary hypoperfusion define acute and chronic human illness acquired following exposure to water-damaged buildings.

Shoemaker, R.C., Mark, L.V., McMahon, S., Thrasher, J.D., & Hhs, C.G. (2010). Research Committee Report on Diagnosis and Treatment of Chronic Inflammatory Response Syndrome Caused by Exposure to the Interior Environment of Water-Damaged Buildings.

Shoemaker, R.C., Rash, J., & Simon, E. (2006). Sick Building Syndrome In water-damaged Buildings: Generalization Of The Chronic Biotoxin-associated Illness Paradigm To Indoor Toxigenic Fungi. Retrieved from https://survivingmold.fivetechdev.com/docs/Resources/Shoemaker%20Papers/Johanning_book_5_06.pdf

Shoemaker, R. C., Schaller, J. L., & Schmidt, P. (2005). Mold warriors: fighting America's hidden health threat (3rd ed.). Baltimore, United States of America: Otter Bay Books.

Shoemaker, R. C., & Schmidt, P. (2010). Mold Warriors: Fighting America's hidden health threat. Baltimore, United States of America: Otter Bay Books.

Shoemaker, R. C., & Surviving Mold. (n.d.). The Biotoxin Pathway. Retrieved from https://www.survivingmold.com/diagnosis/the-biotoxin-pathway

Siasos, G., Tsigkou, V., Kosmopoulos, M., Theodosiadis, D., Simantiris, S., Tagkou, N. M., ... Papavassiliou, A. G. (2018). Mitochondria and cardiovascular diseases—from pathophysiology to treatment. Annals of Translational Medicine, 6(12), 256–256. https://doi.org/10.21037/atm.2018.06.21

Singh, V., Singh, N., & Mohammad, S. (2012). Herbs and surgery. National Journal of Maxillofacial Surgery, 3(1), 101. https://dx.doi.org/10.4103%2F0975-5950.102180

Sinha, A., & Bagga, A. (2008). Pulse Steroid Therapy. Indian Journal of Pediatrics, 75, 1057–1066. Retrieved from http://medind.nic.in/icb/t08/i10/icbt08i10p1057.pdf

Siu, M. T., & Weksberg, R. (2017). Epigenetics of Autism Spectrum Disorder. Advances in Experimental Medicine and Biology, 63–90. https://doi.org/10.1007/978-3-319-53889-1_4

Skobeloff, E. M. (1989). Intravenous Magnesium Sulfate for the Treatment of Acute Asthma in the Emergency Department. JAMA: The Journal of the American Medical Association, 262(9), 1210. https://doi.org/10.1001/jama.1989.03430090072036

Song, Y., Manson, J. E., Cook, N. R., Albert, C. M., Buring, J. E., & Liu, S. (2005). Dietary Magnesium Intake and Risk of Cardiovascular Disease Among Women. The American Journal of Cardiology, 96(8), 1135–1141. https://doi.org/10.1016/j.amjcard.2005.06.045

Soto, S. M. (2013). Role of efflux pumps in the antibiotic resistance of bacteria embedded in a biofilm. Virulence, 4(3), 223–229. https://doi.org/10.4161/viru.23724

Souza, M. E., Lopes, L. Q. S., Bonez, P. C., Gündel, A., Martinez, D. S. T., Sagrillo, M. R., Santos, R. C. V. (2017). Melaleuca alternifolia nanoparticles against Candida species biofilms. Microbial Pathogenesis, 104, 125–132. https://doi.org/10.1016/j.micpath.2017.01.023

Spellberg, B., & Gilbert, D. N. (2014). The Future of Antibiotics and Resistance: A Tribute to a Career of Leadership by John Bartlett. Clinical Infectious Diseases, 59(suppl 2), S71–S75. https://doi.org/10.1093/cid/ciu392

Stauffer, K. (1950). Homöotherapie (4th ed.). Stuttgart, Germany: Hippokrates Verlag Marquardt & Cie.

Steere, A., Klitz, W., Drouin, E., Falk, B., Kwok, W., Nepom, G., & Baxter-Lowe, L. (2006, April 17). Antibiotic-refractory Lyme arthritis is associated with HLA-DR molecules that bind a Borrelia burgdorferi peptide. Retrieved from https://www.ncbi.nlm.nih.gov/pmc/articles/PMC3212725/

Stewart, P. S., & Franklin, M. J. (2008). Physiological heterogeneity in biofilms. Nature Reviews Microbiology, 6(3), 199–210. https://doi.org/10.1038/nrmicro1838

Stiegel, M. A., Pleil, J. D., Sobus, J. R., & Madden, M. C. (2016). Inflammatory Cytokines and White Blood Cell Counts Response to Environmental Levels of Diesel Exhaust and Ozone Inhalation Exposures. PLoS ONE, 11(4), e0152458. https://doi.org/10.1371/journal.pone.0152458

Stocco, A., Lebiere, C., & Anderson, J. R. (2010). Conditional routing of information to the cortex: A model of the basal ganglia's role in cognitive coordination. Psychological Review, 117(2), 541–574. https://doi.org/10.1037/a0019077

Strawson, G. (2016, May 16). Consciousness Isn't a Mystery. It's Matter. The New York Times. Retrieved from https://www.nytimes.com/2016/05/16/opinion/consciousness-isnt-a-mystery-its-matter.html

Stricker, R. B., Savely, V. R., Motanya, N. C., & Giclas, P. C. (2009). Complement Split Products C3a and C4a in Chronic Lyme Disease. Scandinavian Journal of Immunology, 69(1), 64–69. https://doi.org/10.1111/j.1365-3083.2008.02191.x

Stubbs, E. G., Ritvo, E. R., & Mason-Brothers, A. (1985). Autism and Shared Parental HLA Antigens. Journal of the American Academy of Child Psychiatry, 24(2), 182–185. https://doi.org/10.1016/S0002-7138(09)60445-3

Surviving Mold. (2011). The Biotoxin Pathway. Retrieved from https://www.survivingmold.com/diagnosis/the-biotoxin-pathway

Swinker, M. (2003). Neuropsychologic testing versus visual contrast sensitivity in diagnosing PEAS. Environmental Health Perspectives, 111(1). https://doi.org/10.1289/ehp.111-a17

Szatmari, P. (1992). A review of the DSM-III-R criteria for autistic disorder. Journal of Autism and Developmental Disorders, 22(4), 507–523. Retrieved from https://link.springer.com/article/10.1007/BF01046325

Tang, X., & Chen, S. (2015). Epigenetic Regulation of Cytochrome P450 Enzymes and Clinical Implication. Current Drug Metabolism, 16(2), 86–96. https://doi.org/ 10.2174/1389200021602150713114159

Taylor, A. W. (2007). Ocular Immunosuppressive Microenvironment. Immune Response and the Eye, , 71–85. https://doi.org/10.1159/000099255

Taylor, A. W. (2013). Alpha-Melanocyte Stimulating Hormone (α-MSH) Is a Post-Caspase Suppressor of Apoptosis in RAW 264.7 Macrophages. PLoS ONE, 8(8). https://doi.org/10.1371/ journal.pone.0074488

Thakur, M., Rana, R.C., & Thakur, S. (2008). Physiochemical evaluation of Terminalia chebula fruits. J Non Timber Forest Prod. 15. 37-42.

U.S. Department of Energy, & U.S. Department of Energy Office of Science, Office of Biological and Environmental Research. (n.d.). History of the Human Genome Project. Retrieved from https://web.ornl.gov/sci/techresources/Human_Genome/project/hgp.shtml

U.S. Environmental Protection Agency. (2011, September 7). Mold - Glossary of Terms. Retrieved from https://ofmpub.epa.gov/sor_internet/registry/termreg/searchandretrieve/ glossariesandkeywordlists/search.do?details=

U.S. Environmental Protection Agency. (2018, September 4). Building Assessment Survey and Evaluation Study | US EPA. Retrieved from https://www.epa.gov/indoor-air-quality-iaq/building-assessment-survey-and-evaluation-study

U.S. Environmental Protection Agency. (2018, July 16). Indoor Air Quality. Retrieved from https:// www.epa.gov/report-environment/indoor-air-quality

U.S. Environmental Protection Agency. (2019, January 27). Mold Course Chapter 2: | US EPA. Retrieved March 23, 2019, from https://www.epa.gov/mold/mold-course-chapter-2

U.S. Environmental Protection Agency. (2019, December 18). Proposed Revisions to the Lead and Copper Rule. Retrieved from https://www.epa.gov/ground-water-and-drinking-water/proposed-revisions-lead-and-copper-rule

U.S. Environmental Protection Agency. (2020, January 28). What is Endocrine Disruption? Retrieved from https://www.epa.gov/endocrine-disruption/what-endocrine-disruption

U.S. Food and Drug Administration. (2019, October 23). Risks of Breast Implants. Retrieved from https://www.fda.gov/medical-devices/breast-implants/risks-and-complications-breast-implants

U.S. Government Accountability Office. (2008). Indoor Mold: Better Coordination of Research on Health Effects and More Consistent Guidance Would Improve Federal Efforts (GAO-08-980). Retrieved from https://www.gao.gov/new.items/d08980.pdf

U.S. National Library of Medicine. (2018, August 11). List of Herbs in the NLM Herb Garden. Retrieved from https://www.nlm.nih.gov/about/herbgarden/list.html

University of Illinois at Chicago. (2011, July 18). Subject & Course Guides: Evidence Based Medicine: Home. Retrieved from https://researchguides.uic.edu/c.php?g=252338

Vadhana, P., Singh, B. R., & Bharadwaj, M. (2015). Emergence of Herbal Antimicrobial Drug Resistance in Clinical Bacterial Isolates. Pharmaceutica Analytica Acta, 6(10). https://doi.org/ 10.4172/2153-2435.1000434

Valdearcos, M., Xu, A. W., & Koliwad, S. K. (2015). Hypothalamic Inflammation in the Control of Metabolic Function. Annual Review of Physiology, 77(1), 131–160. Retrieved from https://www.ncbi.nlm.nih.gov/pubmed/25668019

Valiathan, M.S. (2009), An Ayurvedic view of life, Current Science, Volume 96, Issue 9, pages 1186-1192

van der Meer, J. (2013). The infectious disease challenges of our time. Frontiers in Public Health, 1. https://doi.org/10.3389/fpubh.2013.00007

van der Toorn, M., Smit-de Vries, M. P., Slebos, D.-J., de Bruin, H. G., Abello, N., van Oosterhout, A. J. M., ... Kauffman, H. F. (2007). Cigarette smoke irreversibly modifies glutathione in airway epithelial cells. American Journal of Physiology-Lung Cellular and Molecular Physiology, 293(5), L1156–L1162. https://doi.org/10.1152/ajplung.00081.2007

Vargas, D. L., Nascimbene, C., Krishnan, C., Zimmerman, A. W., & Pardo, C. A. (2004). Neuroglial activation and neuroinflammation in the brain of patients with autism. Annals of Neurology, 57(1), 67–81. https://doi.org/10.1002/ana.20315

Vasic, V., & Schmidt, M. (2017). Resilience and Vulnerability to Pain and Inflammation in the Hippocampus. International Journal of Molecular Sciences, 18(4), 739. Retrieved from https://www.ncbi.nlm.nih.gov/pmc/articles/PMC5412324/

Ventola, C. (2015, April 1). The Antibiotic Resistance Crisis: Part 1: Causes and Threats. Retrieved March 13, 2019, from https://www.ncbi.nlm.nih.gov/pmc/articles/PMC4378521/

Voelbel, G. T., Bates, M. E., Buckman, J. F., Pandina, G., & Hendren, R. L. (2006). Caudate Nucleus Volume and Cognitive Performance: Are They Related in Childhood Psychopathology? Biological Psychiatry, 60(9), 942–950. Retrieved from https://www.biologicalpsychiatryjournal.com/article/S0006-3223(06)00555-5/fulltext

Volkmar, F. R., Cohen, D. J., & Paul, R. (1986). An Evaluation of DSM-III Criteria for Infantile Autism. Journal of the American Academy of Child Psychiatry, 25(2), 190–197. Retrieved from https://www.jaacap.org/article/S0002-7138(09)60226-0/pdf

Von Eiff, C., Peters, G., & Heilmann, C. (2002). Pathogenesis of infections due to coagulasenegative staphylococci. The Lancet Infectious Diseases, 2(11), 677–685. https://doi.org/10.1016/s1473-3099(02)00438-3

Vuong, C., Kocianova, S., Yao, Y., Carmody, A., & Otto, M. (2004). Increased Colonization of Indwelling Medical Devices by Quorum-Sensing Mutants of Staphylococcus epidermidis In Vivo. The Journal of Infectious Diseases, 190(8), 1498–1505. https://doi.org/10.1086/424487

Wahl, S. M. (2007). Transforming growth factor-β: innately bipolar. Current Opinion in Immunology, 19(1), 55–62. https://doi.org/10.1016/j.coi.2006.11.008

Wan, X., Takano, D., Asamizuya, T., Suzuki, C., Ueno, K., Cheng, K., ... Tanaka, K. (2012). Developing Intuition: Neural Correlates of Cognitive-Skill Learning in Caudate Nucleus. Journal of Neuroscience, 32(48), 17492–17501. https://doi.org/10.1523/jneurosci.2312-12.2012

Wan, Y., & Flavell, R. (2007, December). 'Yin-Yang' functions of TGF-β and Tregs in immune regulation. Retrieved from https://www.ncbi.nlm.nih.gov/pmc/articles/PMC2614905/

Warth B, Sulyok M, Krska R. (2013). LC-MS/MS-based multi-biomarker approaches for the assessment of human exposure to mycotoxins. Anal Bioanal Chem, 405: 5687-95.

Watson, J. B. (1919). Psychology from the standpoint of a behaviorist. https://doi.org/10.1037/10016-000

Weber, C., & Noels, H. (2011). Atherosclerosis: current pathogenesis and therapeutic options. Nature Medicine, 17(11), 1410–1422. https://doi.org/10.1038/nm.2538

Webb, W. (2018). Rationalism, Empiricism, and Evidence-Based Medicine: A Call for a New Galenic Synthesis. Medicines, 5(2), 40. https://doi.org/10.3390/medicines5020040

Webber, M. A. (2002). The importance of efflux pumps in bacterial antibiotic resistance. Journal of Antimicrobial Chemotherapy, 51(1), 9–11. https://doi.org/10.1093/jac/dkg050

Wei, Y., Schatten, H., & Sun, Q. (2014). Environmental epigenetic inheritance through gametes and implications for human reproduction. Human Reproduction Update, 21(2), 194–208. https://doi.org/10.1093/humupd/dmu061

Weiss, L. A., Shen, Y., Korn, J. M., Arking, D. E., Miller, D. T., Fossdal, R., Weyhenmeyer, J. A., & Gallman, E. A. (2007). Rapid Review of Neuroscience. Maryland Heights: Mosby Elsevier.

White, S. W., Oswald, D., Ollendick, T., & Scahill, L. (2009). Anxiety in children and adolescents with autism spectrum disorders. Clinical Psychology Review, 29(3), 216–229. https://doi.org/10.1016/j.cpr.2009.01.003

Wiederhold, N. (2017). Antifungal resistance: current trends and future strategies to combat. Infection and Drug Resistance, Volume 10, 249–259. https://doi.org/10.2147/IDR.S124918

Wilmott, R. W., Bush, A., Deterding, R. R., Sly, P., Ratjen, F., Zar, H., & Li, A. P. (2018). Kendig's Disorders of the Respiratory Tract in Children. Philadelphia, USA: Elsevier Gezondheidszorg.

Wing, L. (1981). Asperger's syndrome: a clinical account. Psychological Medicine, 11(1), 115–129. https://doi.org/10.1017/S0033291700053332

Wing. L., & Attwood, A. (1987). Syndromes of autism and atypical development. In D. Cohen, A. Donellan, & R. Paul (Eds.), Handbook of autism and pervasive developmental disorders (pp. 3-19). New York: Wiley.

Wiseman, G. (1975, December). The hemolysins of Staphylococcus aureus.. Retrieved from https://www.ncbi.nlm.nih.gov/pmc/articles/PMC408339/

World Health Organization. (1998). The world health report 1998 - Life in the 21st century: A vision for all. Retrieved from https://www.who.int/whr/1998/en/

World Health Organization. (2000). Nutrition for health and development : a global agenda for combating malnutrition. World Health Organization. https://apps.who.int/iris/handle/10665/66509

World Health Organization. (2001). Legal Status of Traditional Medicine and Complementary/Alternative Medicine: A Worldwide Review: South-East Asia: India. Retrieved from http://apps.who.int/medicinedocs/en/d/Jh2943e/8.4.html

World Health Organization. (2002). Aetheroleum Melaleucae Alternifoliae. In WHO Monographs on Selected Medicinal Plants, Volume 2 (pp. 172–179). Geneva, Switzerland: World Health Organization.

World Health Organization. (2006, October). Constitution of the World Health Organization. Retrieved from https://www.who.int/governance/eb/who_constitution_en.pdf

World Health Organization. (2010, December 8). WHO | New WHO guidelines to promote proper use of alternative medicines. Retrieved from https://www.who.int/mediacentre/news/releases/2004/pr44/en/

World Health Organization. (2017, November 7). WHO guidelines for indoor air quality: dampness and mould. Retrieved from https://www.who.int/airpollution/guidelines/dampness-mould/en/

World Health Organization. (2018). How air pollution is destroying our health. Retrieved from https://www.who.int/air-pollution/news-and-events/how-air-pollution-is-destroying-our-health

World Health Organization - Interagency Coordination Group on Antimicrobial Resistance. (2019). No Time To Wait: Securing The Future From Drug-Resistant Infections. Retrieved from https://www.who.int/antimicrobial-resistance/interagency-coordination-group/IACG_final_report_EN.pdf

World Health Organization . (2019). World Health Organization Model List of Essential Medicines (21). Retrieved from https://apps.who.int/iris/bitstream/handle/10665/325771/WHO-MVP-EMP-IAU-2019.06-eng.pdf

Wujastyk, D. (2012). Well-Mannered Medicine: Medical Ethics and Etiquette in Classical Ayurveda. England: Oxford University Press.

Xutian, S., Zhang, J., & Louise, W. (2009). New Exploration and Understanding of Traditional Chinese Medicine. The American Journal of Chinese Medicine, 37(03), 411–426. https://doi.org/10.1142/S0192415X09006941

Yang, X. W., & Guo, Q. M. (2007). Studies on chemical constituents in fruits of Eucalyptus globulus. Zhongguo Zhong Yao Za Zhi, 32(6). Retrieved from https://www.ncbi.nlm.nih.gov/pubmed/17552153

Yarwood, J. M., Bartels, D. J., Volper, E. M., & Greenberg, E. P. (2004). Quorum Sensing in Staphylococcus aureus Biofilms. Journal of Bacteriology, 186(6), 1838–1850. Retrieved from https://jb.asm.org/content/186/6/1838

Zafeiriou, D. I., Ververi, A., & Vargiami, E. (2007). Childhood autism and associated comorbidities. Brain and Development, 29(5), 257–272. https://doi.org/10.1016/j.braindev.2006.09.003

Zambrano-Zaragoza, J. F., Romo-Martínez, E. J., Durán-Avelar, M. J., García-Magallanes, N., & Vibanco-Pérez, N. (2014). Th17 Cells in Autoimmune and Infectious Diseases. International Journal of Inflammation, 2014, 1–12. https://doi.org/10.1155/2014/651503

Zeddou, M., Briquet, A., Relic, B., Josse, C., Malaise, M. G., Gothot, A., … Beguin, Y. (2010). The umbilical cord matrix is a better source of mesenchymal stem cells (MSC) than the umbilical cord blood. Cell Biology International, 34(7), 693–701. https://doi.org/10.1042/CBI20090414

Zhang, A., Sun, H., & Wang, X. (2013). Potentiating Therapeutic Effects by Enhancing Synergism Based on Active Constituents from Traditional Medicine. Phytotherapy Research, 28(4), 526–533. https://doi.org/10.1002/ptr.5032

Zhang, X, Chen, C., He, S., & Ge, F. (1997). Supercritical-CO2 fluid extraction of the fatty oil in Terminalia chebula and GC-MS analysis. Journal of Chinese Medicine Materials, 20(9), 463–464. Retrieved from https://www.ncbi.nlm.nih.gov/pubmed/12572426

Zhou, X., Seto, S. W., Chang, D., Kiat, H., Razmovski-Naumovski, V., Chan, K., & Bensoussan, A. (2016). Synergistic Effects of Chinese Herbal Medicine: A Comprehensive Review of Methodology and Current Research. Frontiers in Pharmacology, 7. https://doi.org/10.3389/fphar.2016.00201

Zibaee, S., Hosseini, S. M. al-reza, Yousefi, M., Taghipour, A., Kiani, M. A., & Noras, M. R. (2015). Nutritional and Therapeutic Characteristics of Camel Milk in Children: A Systematic Review. Electronic Physician, 7(7), 1523–1528. https://doi.org/10.19082/1523

www.ingramcontent.com/pod-product-compliance
Lightning Source LLC
Chambersburg PA
CBHW060127280326
41932CB00012B/1449